Cancer Chemotherapy

FRONTIERS IN PHARMACOLOGY & THERAPEUTICS

FRONTIERS IN PHARMACOLOGY & THERAPEUTICS

Cancer Chemotherapy

edited by

John A. Hickman MSc, PhD, DSc

CRC Molecular and Cellular Pharmacology Group,
School of Biological Sciences, University of Manchester M13 9PT, UK

Thomas R. Tritton PhD

Department of Pharmacology and Vermont Cancer Center,
University of Vermont College of Medicine,
Berlington, Vermont 05405, USA

OXFORD

BLACKWELL SCIENTIFIC PUBLICATIONS

LONDON EDINBURGH BOSTON

MELBOURNE PARIS BERLIN VIENNA

© 1993 by Blackwell Scientific Publications
Editorial Offices:
Osney Mead, Oxford OX2 0EL
25 John Street, London WC1N 2BL
23 Ainslie Place, Edinburgh EH3 6AJ
238 Main Street, Cambridge
    Massachusetts 02142, USA
54 University Street, Carlton
    Victoria 3053, Australia

Other Editorial Offices:
Librairie Arnette SA
2 rue Casimir-Delavigne
75006 Paris
France

Blackwell Wissenschafts-Verlag
Meinekestrasse 4
D-1000 Berlin 15
Germany

Blackwell MZV
Feldgasse 13
A-1238 Wien
Austria

First published 1993

Set by Alden Multimedia Ltd, Northampton
Printed and bound in Great Britain by
Hartnolls Ltd, Bodmin, Cornwall

DISTRIBUTORS

  Marston Book Services Ltd
  PO Box 87
  Oxford OX2 0DT
  (*Orders*: Tel: 0865 791155
        Fax: 0865 791927
        Telex: 837515)

USA
  Blackwell Scientific Publications, Inc.
  238 Main Street
  Cambridge, MA 02142
  (*Orders*: Tel: 800 759-6102)
         617 876-7000)

Canada
  Times Mirror Professional Publishing Ltd
  130 Flaska Drive
  Markham, Ontario L6G 1B8
  (*Orders*: Tel: 800 268-4178
         416 470-6739)

Australia
  Blackwell Scientific Publications Pty Ltd
  54 University Street
  Carlton, Victoria 3053
  (*Orders*: Tel: 03 347-5552)

A catalogue record for this title is available
from the British Library.

ISBN 0-632-03441-6

Library of Congress
Cataloging-in-Publication Data

Cancer chemotherapy/edited by John A.
Hickman, Thomas R. Tritton.
        p.   cm.—(Frontiers in
        pharmacology & therapeutics)
        Includes bibliographical references and
        index.
        ISBN 0-632-03441-6
        1. Cancer—Chemotherapy. 2. Antineo-
plastic agents—Mechanism of action.
I. Hickman, John A. II. Tritton, Thomas R.
III. Series.
        [DNLM: 1. Antineoplastic Agents—
therapeutic use. 2. Neoplasms—
drug.   QZ267 C2146]
RC271.C5C29   1992
616.99′4061—dc20

Contents

Contributors

Shakeel Ahmad *Department of Pharmacology, Georgetown University Medical Center, Washington, Washington DC 20007, USA*

Flavia Borellini *Department of Pharmacology, Georgetown University Medical Center, Washington, Washington DC 20007, USA*

Robert H. Connamacher *Department of Pharmacology, School of Medicine, University of Pittsburgh, Pittsburgh, Pennsylvania 15261, USA*

Larry W. Daniel *Department of Biochemistry, Wake Forest University Medical Center, Winston-Salem, North Carolina 27157-1016, USA*

T. Michael Dexter *CRC Department of Experimental Haematology, Paterson Institute for Cancer Research, Christie Hospital, Manchester M20 9BX, UK*

Caroline Dive *CRC Molecular and Cellular Pharmacology Group, Department of Physiological Sciences, Manchester University School of Biological Sciences, Stopford Building, Manchester M13 9PT, UK*

Amy L. Ellis *Department of Medical Oncology, Division of Medicine, MD Anderson Cancer Center, Houston, Texas 77030, USA*

Paul H. Fischer *Cancer Department, Pfizer Central Research, Groton, Connecticut 06340, USA*

Chaim Gilon *Department of Organic Chemistry, The Hebrew University of Jerusalem, Jerusalem 91904, Israel*

Robert I. Glazer *Department of Pharmacology and Lombardi Cancer Research Center, Georgetown University Medical Center, Washington DC 20007, USA*

Irving H. Goldberg *Department of Biological Chemistry and Molecular Pharmacology, Harvard Medical School, Boston, Massachusetts 02115, USA*

John A. Hartley *Department of Oncology, University College and Middlesex School of Medicine, London W1P 8BT, UK*

John T. Isaacs *Department of Urology and Oncology, The Brady Urological Institute, The Johns Hopkins University School of Medicine, Baltimore, Maryland 21205, USA*

John S. Lazo *Department of Pharmacology, School of Medicine and the Experimental Therapeutics Program, Pittsburgh Cancer Institute, University of Pittsburgh, Pittsburgh, Pennsylvania 15261, USA*

Alexander Levitzki *Department of Biological Chemistry, The Hebrew University of Jerusalem, Jerusalem 91904, Israel*

James D. Moyer *Cancer Department, Pfizer Central Research, Groton, Connecticut 06340, USA*

Yves Pommier *Laboratory of Molecular Pharmacology, Developmental Therapeutics Program, Division of Cancer Treatment, National Cancer Institute, Bethesda, Maryland 20892, USA*

Enrique Rozengurt *Growth Regulation Laboratory, Imperial Cancer Research Fund, London WC2A 3PX, UK*

Tariq Sethi *Growth Regulation Laboratory, Imperial Cancer Research Fund, London WC2A 3PX, UK*

Robert L. Souhami *Department of Oncology, University College and Middlesex School of Medicine, London W1P 8BT, UK*

Lisa A. Speicher *Department of Pharmacology, Fox Chase Cancer Center, Philadelphia, Pennsylvania 19111, USA*

Gary D. Steinberg *Department of Urology and Oncology, The Brady Urological Institute, The Johns Hopkins University School of Medicine, Baltimore, Maryland 21205, USA*

Akihiko Tanizawa *Laboratory of Molecular Pharmacology, Developmental Therapeutics Program, Division of Cancer Treatment, National Cancer Institute, Bethesda, Maryland 20892, USA*

Claire M. Tenny *Department of Medicine, School of Medicine, Pittsburgh Cancer Institute, University of Pittsburgh, Pittsburgh, Pennsylvania 15261, USA*

Nydia G. Testa *CRC Department of Experimental Haematology, Paterson Institute for Cancer Research, Christie Hospital, Manchester M20 9BX, UK*

Kenneth D. Tew *Department of Pharmacology, Fox Chase Cancer Center, Philadelphia, Pennsylvania 19111, USA*

Penella J. Woll *CRC Department of Medical Oncology, Christie Hospital, Manchester M20 9BX, UK*

Andrew H. Wyllie *Department of Pathology, Edinburgh University Medical School, Edinburgh EH4 9AG, UK*

Gang Yu *Laboratory of Biological Chemistry, National Cancer Institute, National Institutes of Health, Bethesda, Maryland 20892, USA*

Leonard A. Zwelling *Department of Medical Oncology, Division of Medicine, MD Anderson Cancer Center, Houston, Texas 77030, USA*

Preface

Experimental cancer chemotherapy is a constant struggle between the desire for immediate results that will help the sick patient, and the striving to develop concepts that may have no immediate practicality, but which lay the foundation for more refined and rational treatments. Efforts in the former category include: synthesizing new congeners based on existing successful drugs, optimizing delivery schedules that provide the best medicinal action, defining the pharmacokinetics and pharmacodynamics necessary for optimal drug use, and trying combinations of agents to minimize both toxic repercussions and the emergence of drug resistance. These are admirable efforts without which progress in disease treatment would be slow and fitful. In this volume, however, we have chosen to de-emphasize studies of this type, focusing instead on some new mechanistic possibilities from which we expect the next generation of drugs to emerge. This is not without risk, of course, because one cannot afford to be dissociated from the main stream of efforts in a discipline, but the standard approaches have been amply treated in a continuing variety of books and review articles. Consequently, we have asked each author to take a prospective view of his or her subject. Of necessity there is a significant content of review material, but this is intended to set the stage for thoughtful speculations, by both the writer and the reader, on where we might go from here.

A number of important subjects are *not* covered. This was dictated by three forces: (i) the necessity to keep the volume to a reasonable length, (ii) our inability to convince outstanding scientists in some areas to take the time away from their busy schedules to write yet another chapter, and (iii) personal biases about what areas offer the best promise for real development. Some of the important subjects not covered, but which could easily fill a successor volume, include antisense oligonucleotides, triple helix-forming sequences, immunomodulation, angiogenesis as a drug target, reversal of drug resistance, tumour cell differentiation and the cell division control apparatus as a locus for drug action.

Cancer chemotherapy has been a successful science for about four decades. There can be little doubt that the development of the 50 or so truly effective agents has improved both the quality and quantity of human life, and that there are many people walking the earth today who would not be were it not for alkylating agents, antimetabolites and the natural product 'mycins'. On the negative side of the ledger, however, are the propensity of these agents to cause obnoxious side effects, to select for resistant subpopulations and to fail to act as effectively in one person as in the next. We make the presupposition that these are not insoluble problems, and each chapter in the volume operates with the optimistic, even if unstated, assumption that new ideas can lead the way past current obstacles. This does not mean that our enthusiasm for future prospects is unbounded by any realization of the difficulty of the task. Each of the working scientists whose thoughts are set to paper here have, however, in the quiet of their offices come up with a surprisingly large number of original and hopeful ideas that may light the roadway that has to be travelled in the quest to eradicate cancer.

John A. Hickman

Thomas R. Tritton

Abbreviations

ACTH	adrenocorticotropic hormone
ADP	adenosine diphosphate
ADR	Adriamycin
aFGF	acidic fibroblast growth hormone
ALP	alkyl-lysophospholipid
AML	acute myeloblastic leukaemia
ara-C	arabinofuranosylcytosine
ATP	adenosine triphosphate
ATPase	adenosine triphosphatase
BCNU	1,3-*bis*-(2-chloroethyl)-1-nitrosurea
bFGF	basic fibroblast growth factor
BL	Burkitt's lymphoma
bp	base pair
cAMP	cyclic adenosine monophosphate
CAT	chloramphenicol acetyltransferase
CCK	cholecystokinin
CDDP	*cis*-dichlorodiamine-platinum
CFC	colony-forming cell
cGMP	cyclic guanosine monophosphate
CHO	Chinese hamster ovary
CNS	central nervous system
CPZ	chlorpromazine
CRE	cAMP responsive element
CRF	corticotropin-releasing factor
CSF	colony-stimulating factor
DAG	1,2-diacylglycerol
DCBT	2,4-dichlorobenzyl thiocyanate
DDP	5,6-diphenylpyriadazin-3-one
DES	diethylstilboestrol
DHAP	dihydroxyacetone phosphate
DHT	5α-dihydrotestosterone
DS	double strand
DZQ	3,6-diaziridinyl-1,4-benzoquinone

EBV	Epstein–Barr virus
EGF	epidermal growth factor
EGFRK	EGF-receptor kinase
EMS	ethylmethane sulphonate
Epo	erythropoietin
ET-18-OCH$_3$	1-O-octadecyl-2-O-methyl-rac-glycero-3-phosphocholine
FAA	flavone acetic acid
Fn	fibronectin
FSH	follicle-stimulating hormone
5FU	5-fluorouracil
GAP	GTPase-activating protein
GDP	guanosine diphosphate
GM-CSF	granulocyte-macrophage colony-stimulating factor
GRP	gastrin-releasing peptide
GTP	guanosine triphosphate
GTPase	guanosine triphosphatase
HDL	high-density lipoprotein
HePC	hexadecylphosphocholine
HIV	human immunodeficiency virus
HMG	high mobility group
Hsp70	heat shock protein 70
IF	intermediate filament
IFN	interferon
IGF-I	insulin-like growth factor-I
IL-1	interleukin-1
Ins(1,4,5)P$_3$	inositol 1,4,5-trisphosphate
KGF	keratinocyte growth factor
KGFRK	keratinocyte growth factor receptor kinase
LDL	low-density lipoprotein
LH	luteinizing hormone
LHRH	luteinizing hormone-releasing hormone
MAP	MT-associated protein
MDCK	Madin Darby canine kidney
MDR	multidrug resistance
MF	microfilament
MIP-1α	macrophage inflammatory protein-1α
MP	methylprednisolone
MPTP	2-methoxy-5-(2′,3′,4′-trimethoxy-phenyl)tropone
MS	mass spectrometry
MT	microtubule
MTT	methylthiazotetrazolium
MTX	methotrexate
NADP	nicotinamide–adenine dinucleotide phosphate
NCME	4-N-acetylcolchinol O-methyl ether

NCS	neocarzinostatin
NEM	N-ethylmaleimide
NGF	nerve growth factor
NK	natural killer
NMR	nuclear magnetic resonance
NSCLC	non-small cell lung cancer
PAF	platelet-activating factor
PCD	programmed cell death
PCMBS	p-chloromercuribenzene sulphonic acid
PDGF	platelet-derived growth factor
PGE_2	prostaglandin E_2
PIP_2	phosphatidylinositol 4,5-bisphosphate
PI-PLC	phosphatidylinositol-specific phospolipase C
PKA	protein kinase A
PKC	protein kinase C
PLC	phospholipase C
PMA	phorbol 2-myristate 13-acetate
PMN	polymorphonuclear neutrophils
$PtdIns(4,5)P_2$	phosphatidylinositol 4,5-bisphosphate
PTK	protein tyrosine kinase
RA	retinoic acid
RB	retinoblastoma gene
RSV	Rous sarcoma virus
SAR	structure–activity relationship
SCF	stem cell factor
SCLC	small cell lung cancer
SDS	sodium dodecylsulphate
SGP-2	sulphated glycoprotein-2
SS	single strand
STOP	stable tubule only peptide
SV40	simian virus 40
T	testosterone
TAF	tumour angiogenesis factor
TGF	transforming growth factor
TNF	tumour necrosis factor
topo II	topoisomerase II
TPA	12-O-tetradecanoylphorbol 13-acetate
TRPM-2	testosterone-repressed prostate message-2
u.v.	ultraviolet
Vn	vibronectin

Chapter 1
The promise of oncogene inhibitors as novel antitumour agents

James D. Moyer and Paul H. Fischer

Introduction
Would inhibition of oncogene function
    slow tumour growth?
What are the bases for selectivity of
    oncogene inhibitors?
    The oncogenic protein or gene may
        not be expressed in any normal
        tissue
    The cells of the normal tissues may
        have adequate alternative pathways
        that bypass the oncogenic protein
    The oncogenic protein is dispensible
        for cell replication in the adult
    The oncogenic protein may be essen-
        tial for replication of some normal
        tissue, but the cessation of cell rep-
        lication in this tissue is an accept-
        able toxicity in the cancer patient
    Altered regulation of oncogene trans-
        cription may provide opportunities

        for preferential inhibition of
        selected oncogenes
What would be the consequences of
    inhibition of an oncogene?
Ras as an example of an oncogene to
    target for chemotherapy
    Approaches based on inhibition of
        nucleotide binding or activation of
        guanosine triphosphatase (GTPase)
        activity
    Approaches based on disruption of
        the effector/p21^{ras} interaction
    Approaches based on blocking p21^{ras}
        post-translational processing
    Inhibition of *ras* transcription
    Ras-induced vulnerability
    Antisense oligonucleotides
Conclusion
Acknowledgements
References

Introduction

Our primary aim is to discuss the suitability of oncogenes and oncoproteins as new targets for the treatment of cancer. The frequency of
oncogene activation in human cancer and the contribution of oncogenes
to the malignant progression of human cancer have been intensely investigated over the past decade. Amplification or mutation of growth-
promoting genes (oncogenes), overexpression of the protein products of
the oncogenes, and the loss of tumour-suppressor genes clearly are
frequent events in most human cancers (Bishop, 1987, 1989, 1991;
Weinberg, 1989a; Fearon & Vogelstein, 1990). Activation of more than
one oncogene is necessary to transform normal cells, and distinct signalling pathways mediated by different oncogenes may often be involved
(Weinberg, 1989b; Cantley *et al.*, 1991; Hunter, 1991).

The identification of specific genetic changes in these key regulatory

1

genes of human tumours provides, for the first time, tumour-specific molecules (either protein or nucleic acid) as targets for drug discovery. However, the genetic changes identified are often subtle: changes in regulatory sequences or point mutations producing single amino acid changes. In the case of tumour-suppressor genes such as retinoblastoma gene (RB) the defect is a deletion—replacement of function rather than inhibition may be required as a treatment strategy. Does this recent information about the genetic basis of transformation permit the design or discovery of more selective and effective chemotherapy? Anticipated improvements in efficacy, toleration or both would warrant a major investment in the search for such compounds.

Although the crucial role of oncogenes in human carcinogenesis provokes consideration of these genes and their oncoproteins as new therapeutic targets, several issues which will greatly influence the ultimate medical utility of oncogene inhibitors as antitumour agents are still unresolved. What is the evidence that inhibition of a single oncogene will suppress the replication of tumour cells likely to have multiple genetic alterations? What will be the key toleration issues with such inhibitors? If growth inhibition is achieved by these agents, will this lead to cell death, differentiation or only transient stasis? How might tumour-selective effects be achieved by inhibition of oncogenic proteins? We will provide a general framework for addressing these questions and then review, as an example, the advantages and disadvantages of different approaches to the discovery of *ras* inhibitors.

Would inhibition of oncogene function slow tumour growth?

Several lines of evidence suggest that interference with a specific oncogene can inhibit tumour cell replication both in cell cultures and *in vivo*. Studies of transfection of oncogenes into fibroblasts provide presumptive evidence for an ongoing role for oncogenes in transformation, and this has been substantiated by studies of inducible or temperature sensitive forms of several oncogenes. Inducible v-*ras* and v-*src* genes have been used to define a threshold level of oncogene expression required for transformation of fibroblasts; a two- to 30-fold induction of the oncogene was sufficient to convert a cell from a 'normal' to a transformed phenotype in some instances (Huang *et al.*, 1981; Jakobovits *et al.*, 1984). By analogy, a 50–97% inhibition of the oncogenic protein function by a drug might restore the normal phenotype. Evidence for an antiproliferative consequence of oncogene inhibition in human tumour cells has been obtained by use of antibodies to the oncogenic protein or antisense oligonucleotides. As examples, inhibition of the expression or function of *myc*, *erb*B-2, or *ras* have been shown to slow the replication of cells transformed by these oncogenes.

HL-60 promyelocytic leukaemia cells express high levels of c-*myc* as a result of gene amplification, and also express mutant *ras*; treatment with c-*myc* antisense oligomers inhibits the replication of these cells and induces their differentiation (Holt *et al.*, 1988). Similarly, the down-regulation of *myc* by antisense sequences inhibits the replication of Friend erythroleukaemia cells (Prochovnik *et al.*, 1988). Reduction of *myc* in *ras*-transformed 3T3 fibroblasts by antisense sequences greatly decreases the soft-agar colony formation and tumorigenicity of the cells, even though the transforming *ras* protein continues to be expressed (Sklar *et al.*, 1991)—this is a clear example of an inhibition of replication by blocking a proto-oncogene (c-*myc*) in cells that are transformed by a different oncogene.

Antibodies to the *erb*B-2 receptor selectively inhibit the growth of cells transformed by mutant *erb*B-2 *in vitro* and *in vivo* (Drebin *et al.*, 1986, 1988a,b; Hudziak *et al.*, 1989) and prevented the growth in soft agar of fibroblasts transformed by activated *erb*B-2 or of human breast cells overexpressing c-*erb*B-2 (Drebin *et al.*, 1985; Hudziak *et al.*, 1989; Lupu *et al.*, 1990). An independent line of evidence is provided by studies with antisense oligonucleotides complementary to the *erb*B-2 gene; these oligonucleotides greatly reduce tyrosine kinase activity of SKBR3 cells and inhibit DNA synthesis (Brysch *et al.*, 1991). A pharmacological inhibitor of p185 kinase might also inhibit the replication of cells overexpressing p185 (*erb*B-2).

There is convincing evidence for a role of mutant *ras* in driving tumour cell replication. Microinjection of antibodies to $p21^{ras}$ inhibits the replication of various human tumour cell lines expressing mutant *ras* (Stacey *et al.*, 1987) as well as fibroblasts transformed by transfection with v-*ras* (Smith *et al.*, 1986)—in the latter case the antibody also produces morphological reversion of the cells to a normal phenotype. Complementary evidence for a role of mutant *ras* in driving neoplastic cell replication comes from studies with antisense DNA; reduction of the expression of mutant *ras* in a human lung tumour cell line by antisense DNA leads to reduced proliferation in cultures and reduced tumorigenicity in nude mice (Mukhopadhyay *et al.*, 1991). Similarly, antisense to mutant *ras* reduces anchorage-independent cell growth in a *ras*-transformed 3T3 line (Daaka & Wickstrom, 1990).

The evidence reviewed above suggests strongly that an effective inhibition of oncogene function will inhibit the growth of some tumours, although subsequent activation of other oncogenes may override this inhibition; for example, fibroblasts transformed by *raf* or *mos* are not inhibited by antibodies to $p21^{ras}$ (Smith *et al.*, 1986). Inhibition may be obtained not only in instances wherein the target oncogene has been mutated or overexpressed and therefore is responsible for the transformed properties, but also where the proto-oncogene is required for replication but is properly regulated and not mutated. In the examples above some selectivity in inhibition of replication of transformed cells has often been achieved, but effective pharmacological agents are not available to determine the consequences of systemic inhibition of an oncogene to normal tissues *in vivo*. The possibility that oncogene inhibitors might combine efficacy with reduced toxicity to normal replicating cells is the major promise of this approach.

What are the bases for selectivity of oncogene inhibitors?

Several bases for a selective effect of oncogene inhibitors on tumour cell replication can be proposed: (i) the oncogenic protein (or gene) may not be expressed in any normal tissue; (ii) key normal tissues may have alternative pathways for the stimulation of prolifcration that bypass the oncogene protein; (iii) the oncogene product may be a component of a pathway that is not critical for any tissue in the adult; (iv) the oncogenic protein may be essential for replication of some normal tissue, but the cessation of cell replication in this tissue is an acceptable toxicity in the cancer patient; or (v) altered regulation of oncogene transcription may provide opportunities for preferential inhibition of selected oncogenes. Some of the evidence for each of these is described below.

The oncogenic protein or gene may not be expressed in any normal tissue

If the oncogene target is unique to cancer cells, then an extremely high level of therapeutic selectivity is theoretically possible for a drug that inhibits that target. In these circumstances cancer therapy could attain the selectivity achieved in the chemotherapy of bacterial infections. It is now clear that mutations in the *ras* gene family are frequent events in human cancer (Bos, 1989). These mutations result in activated *ras* proteins with slightly altered structure and their activation is implicated in the development of important tumours. Thus, the development of *ras* inhibitors that selectively inhibit function of the mutant protein and not that of normal *ras* proteins would have enormous selectivity for the cancer cells. Similarly, *bcr-abl* is a chimeric protein uniquely expressed in chronic myelogenous leukaemia cells and not in any normal host tissues (Ramakrishnan & Rosenberg, 1989). Preferential inhibition of this activated tyrosine kinase should result in considerable therapeutic selectivity.

Oncogenic mutations present tumour-specific targets at the level of the genes and mRNA as well as at the level of the encoded proteins. A particularly striking example of selectivity resulting from expression of a unique gene in the tumour cells is provided by studies with chronic myelogenous leukaemia cells. In these cells translocation of the proto-oncogene *abl* produces a hybrid *bcr-abl* gene present only in the tumour cells. This *bcr-abl* gene encodes an oncogenic tyrosine kinase. Antisense oligonucleotides complementary to the splice-junction formed by this translocation markedly inhibit the formation of colonies by leukaemia cells from patients with chronic myelogenous leukaemia without inhibiting the formation of colonies from normal marrow progenitor cells (Syczylik *et al.*, 1991). Because this approach targets the tumour-specific gene, it should (theoretically) be without effect even on cells dependent on the expression of the normal c-*abl* gene.

Mutated cell surface oncoproteins could provide attractive targets for immunologically based therapeutic approaches. Many efforts to exploit overexpression of normal oncoproteins with antireceptor monoclonal antibodies are ongoing, as in the case of the epidermal growth factor (EGF) receptor (Mendelsohn, 1990). Occasionally, however, the EGF receptor gene is rearranged and a modified protein is produced (Libermann *et al.*, 1985; Merlino, 1990). It may be possible, therefore, to use immunotoxins directed toward the mutant EGF receptors and achieve enhanced selectivity in the therapy of certain brain tumours.

The cells of the normal tissues may have adequate alternative pathways that bypass the oncogenic protein

Alternative pathways that functionally replace an oncogenic target could provide a basis for therapeutic selectivity, i.e. in normal cells redundant pathways may replace key functions lost as a consequence of inhibition of a proto-oncogene. In cancer cells the alternative pathways would still be under normal regulation and, therefore, they would not replace the oncogene's transforming function. At least two types of redundancy can be envisioned, distinct mitogenic signalling pathways and replacement of function by related members of the oncogene gene family.

As an example of distinct mitogenic signalling pathways, a single oncogene expressed in 3T3 cells can convert the cell from an immortalized cell to a fully transformed cell. Thus, either expression of v-*erb*B or overexpression of c-*erb*B in the presence of its ligand, EGF, transforms 3T3 cells. 3T3 cells are not, however, dependent on EGF (or its receptor c-*erb*B) under all circumstances and can be driven to proliferate by other mitogens, such as platelet-derived growth factor (PDGF) or bombesin, that act through distinct receptors (Rozengurt, 1986; and see Chapter 5). A pharmacological block of the *erb*B-receptor kinase should block transformation in these cells but permit regulated proliferation of fibroblasts under the control of other stimuli. This selectivity has been achieved to an extent with the tyrphostins, inhibitors of the EGF-receptor tyrosine kinase: these compounds are more potent inhibitors of EGF-stimulated DNA synthesis than of serum simulated DNA synthesis, presumably because serum stimulates alternative pathways (Gazit *et al.*, 1991; and see Chapter 4). The key question is to what extent redundant mitogenic pathways are operative in normal cells in intact animals. Selective inhibitors should provide an answer to this question.

If the activated oncogene is a member of a gene family then it is possible that one or another member of the family may replace some of the target protein's functions. Such redundancy could sustain normal cell function, but it is unlikely that the transforming actions of the activated oncogene would be replaced in the cancer cells since the other gene family members are not activated. This can be readily imagined if the pharmacological agent selectively inhibited the biochemical function of the activated oncogene. Similarly, preferential interference with transcription, RNA processing, translation or post-translational protein modifications of the target oncogene could have therapeutic selectivity. For example, in the *myc* family, N-*myc*, L-*myc* and c-*myc* have been amplified or overexpressed in different tumour cell types (Ingvarsson, 1990). The proteins coded for by these genes show some structural and functional similarity, but regulation of their expression appears quite divergent (Cesarman *et al.*, 1987; DePinho *et al.*, 1987; Krystal *et al.*, 1988). An agent that selectively inhibited N-*myc* expression may control the growth of tumours by inhibiting the overexpression of N-*myc* needed for malignant transformation. The deleted N-*myc* functions may be replaced by c-*myc*, which is expressed in most tissues, and thereby normal cell replication may be possible.

The toxicities of existing cancer therapeutic agents are often manifest on the bone marrow stem cells and on gastrointestinal mucosal cells. The identification of the key regulators of replication of these important cells could allow us to select targets that would avoid these toxicities.

The oncogenic protein is dispensible for cell replication in the adult

An interesting illustration of the potential for selectivity with oncogene inhibitors is the case of the *src* oncogene. Transfection of v-*src* oncogene transforms fibroblasts, and activation of *src* has been implicated in human colon cancer (Bolen *et al.*, 1987). Until very recently it seemed possible that c-*src* played an essential role in the replication or function of various cell types, and therefore that inhibition of the c-*src* kinase would be toxic to replicating tissues. Studies with *src*⁻ transgenic mice have now shown that c-*src* is not necessary for replication of any essential cell type even during embryonic development (Soriano *et al.*, 1991). Based on these findings, one could reasonably expect that a pharmacological agent that effectively and specifically blocked c-*src in vivo* could inhibit the growth of a c-*src*-driven tumour without grossly inhibiting rapidly dividing tissues such as bone marrow, gut or skin. Other oncogenic kinases shown to be important for tumour growth would also be attractive targets if they were dispensible in normal tissues.

In many instances the oncogenes implicated in human cancer have been found to be highly conserved. How likely then is it that inhibitors would be without toxicity if they target essential proteins? One possibility is that some oncogenes will prove to be essential only during embryogenesis and not in the adult. The *sevenless* gene of *Drosophila* encodes a protein tyrosine kinase with homology to the *ros* oncogene (Basler & Hafen, 1988). *Drosophila* with *sevenless* mutations fail to develop the seventh cell of the eye unit, but are otherwise viable. By analogy, some oncogenic tyrosine kinases may eventually be found to be dispensable in the adult, but essential in embryonic development, although no clear examples are currently known.

The oncogenic protein may be essential for replication of some normal tissue, but the cessation of cell replication in this tissue is an acceptable toxicity in the cancer patient

Endocrine-dependent tumours including breast (Lerner & Jordan, 1990) and prostate cancer (see Chapter 13) have been successfully treated using a variety of hormonal manipulations. Although these approaches are not cancer-specific, their side effects are not as problematic as those associated with most cytotoxic therapy since the adverse effects are generally confined to other tissues responsive to the particular hormone. Tamoxifen, an anti-oestrogen used in the treatment of breast cancer, is a well-tolerated endocrine therapy (Patterson *et al.*, 1981) in which the side effects are primarily related to actions on oestrogen-sensitive tissues. In an analogous fashion, therapeutic selectivity could be achieved with oncogene inhibitors if expression of the oncogene was limited to tissues in which inhibition of cell replication is acceptable. The *lck* oncogene may be a case in point. It appears that *lck* expression is largely confined to T cells, and its overexpression may contribute to certain T-cell tumours (Perlmutter *et al.*, 1988; Abraham *et al.*, 1991). Thus, selective inhibition of *lck* function may preferentially inhibit the replication of T cells, including those of the tumour. Other replicating normal cells, which do not express *lck*, should be relatively unaffected.

Altered regulation of oncogene transcription may provide opportunities for preferential inhibition of selected oncogenes

The regulation of oncogene expression may be altered in certain cancers. For example, translocations of c-*myc* are frequently seen in Burkitt's lymphoma and, although these abnormalities do not change the protein, alterations in the regulation of c-*myc* expression are evident (Cory, 1986). Transcription may be driven by an immunoglobulin enhancer located near the breakpoint of the recipient chromosome. Additionally, the first exon of c-*myc*, which has important transcriptional regulation domains (Hay *et al.*, 1987), is frequently altered in these tumours. Thus, an inhibitor of c-*myc* transcription in tumour cells may have a target that does not control c-*myc* transcription in normal cells. As a consequence, down-regulation of c-*myc* in key normal tissues may be avoided and a degree of tumour selectivity may be obtained.

What would be the consequences of inhibition of an oncogene?

A potential disadvantage of therapy based on inhibition of oncogene function is that it may produce only a temporary growth arrest. Thus such therapy would have to be continually applied without hope of a cure by eradication of the tumour cells. Although such a prospect is not necessarily prohibitive if the agents are otherwise of low toxicity, the need for chronic continuous treatment places severe constraints on the drugs. Fortunately there is some evidence that inhibition of an oncogene function can lead to 'terminal differentiation' of some tumour cells or even programmed cell death (apoptosis, see Chapter 2).

Experiments with antisense sequences have provided much of the evidence for differentiation upon inhibition of oncogene expression. HL-60 cells can be induced to differentiate in response to down-regulation of c-*myc* by antisense (Yokoyama & Imamato, 1987; Holt *et al.*, 1988). Similarly, antisense to *myc* can down-regulate *myc* expression and produce differentiation of F9 teratocarcinoma cells (Griep & Westphal, 1988).

It is likely that one important consequence of oncogene-induced cell proliferation is reduced responsiveness to normal signals for differentiation. For example the PA-1 human teratocarcinoma cell line, transformed with N-*ras*, has reduced responsiveness to retinoic acid as a differentiation inducer (Buettner *et al.*, 1991). It is possible that even intermittent treatment with an inhibitor of *ras* would permit differentiation of such cells in the presence of normal retinoid concentrations or in combination with pharmacological levels of retinoids.

Inhibition of an oncogene might be expected to produce only a reduction of the percentage of cycling cells and not cytotoxicity; it is therefore interesting that there is evidence that cell death may also result. The *bcl*-2 oncogene is frequently overexpressed in human B-cell lymphomas as a result of translocation (Reed *et al.*, 1988). Antisense oligonucleotides specific for *bcl*-2 produce not only inhibition of replication but also cell death in leukaemic cells (Reed *et al.*, 1990). Although *bcl*-2 may be a special case, directly linked to control of apoptosis, there is also evidence that depriving cells of stimulus from growth factor pathways can lead to cell death. Depriving fibroblasts of PDGF (Scher *et al.*, 1982), depriving prostate cells of androgen (see Chapter 13), depriving mature T lymphocytes of interleukin-2 (IL-2) (Duke & Cohen, 1986) or blocking oestrogen effects in breast tumour cells with tamoxifen (Lippman *et al.*, 1976) have all been reported to produce cell death. Oncogenes are often components of growth factor pathways, therefore inhibitors of these oncogenes may also induce cell death in some instances.

Ras as an example of an oncogene to target for chemotherapy

Since the discovery that c-*ras* is activated to a transforming form by single point mutations (Reddy *et al.*, 1982; Tabin *et al.*, 1982), *ras* (p21) has offered an attractive target for chemotherapy. Mutations of *ras* are found in a substantial percentage of three of the most frequent and lethal human cancers—colon, lung and pancreatic cancer (Bos, 1989), and in a subset of melanomas, acute myelogenous leukaemias and thyroid tumours. As summarized above, there is evidence that a continued action of mutant *ras* is necessary to drive the malignancy. Most importantly, mutant *ras* protein is present only in the tumour and not in the normal tissues of the patient. Thus, in contrast to standard chemotherapy, toxicity resulting from effects on normal cellular function or replication would not be limiting—if a mutant-specific agent could be identfied.

Only a compound that binds specifically to the mutant form of p21^{ras} will completely satisfy the promise of absolute tumour selectivity for a *ras* inhibitor. Unfortunately the mutations found in human cancer are point mutations that result in only a single amino acid substitution, usually at the twelfth or thirteenth amino acid, and produce only small changes in the three-dimensional structure of p21^{ras} (Milburn *et al.*, 1989; Krengel *et al.*, 1990; Schlichting *et al.*, 1990). The discovery of a mutant-specific inhibitor either by design or screening is therefore likely to be very difficult. The less daunting task of finding an inhibitor of p21^{ras} without specificity for the mutant form is also less attractive because it is likely that the cellular *ras* proteins play some important role in normal cell replication and function, although this role is currently unknown.

The *ras* oncogene was originally identified by genetic techniques rather than biochemical techniques and our knowledge of the biochemical function of p21^{ras} remains incomplete. A substantial body of evidence suggests that p21^{ras} operates as a component of a signal transduction pathway, and that it is active when bound to guanosine triphosphate (GTP) and inactivated when bound to guanosine diphosphate (GDP) (Bourne *et al.*, 1991). However, the identity of both the input signals and the output signals (effectors) in mammalian cells are unknown. Despite these difficulties and uncertainties, a number of different approaches to discovery of a 'ras inhibitor' can be considered and some of these have been pursued. These various approaches illustrate the obstacles to the use of our knowledge of oncogenes to guide the discovery of a therapeutic agent.

Approaches based on inhibition of nucleotide binding or activation of guanosine triphosphatase (GTPase) activity

The fundamental defect of the mutant p21^{ras} is a failure to revert to the inactive GDP-bound form by action of GTPase. Although the inherent

GTPase activity of most mutant p21s is lower than the wild type, the inability to respond productively to GTPase-activating proteins (GAP or NF1) and thereby down-regulate (McCormick, 1989) appears more important. This defect results in a higher proportion of the mutant p21^{ras} in the GTP-bound (active) form intracellularly (Hoshino *et al.*, 1988; Satoh *et al.*, 1988). A straightforward approach to a *ras* inhibitor, therefore, is to shift the mutant p21^{ras} back to a primarily GDP-bound form by either blocking the binding of GTP or restoring the GTPase activity of the mutant p21^{ras} to normal levels.

Although it would seem difficult to restore or enhance an enzyme activity of a protein by addition of a small molecule, such an activation of a GTPase has been reported for the antibiotic kirromycin (Parmeggiani & Swart, 1985; Sigal *et al.*, 1987). An activation of the GTPase could perhaps be achieved by a small molecule that binds so as to properly orient key functional groups in p21^{ras} to enhance hydrolysis, but no such compound has yet been reported.

An inhibitor of GTP binding to p21^{ras} would be expected to block p21^{ras} function, because specific conformational changes induced by GTP are required for activation (Milburn *et al.*, 1989; Krengel *et al.*, 1990; Schlichting *et al.*, 1990). A competitive inhibitor of GTP binding would have to be of extraordinary affinity, however, because GTP and GDP bind tightly to p21^{ras}, with an affinity of about 10^{11} M^{-1}, and the concentration of GTP in cells is near 1 mM (Bourne *et al.*, 1991). The structural determinants for nucleotide binding to p21^{ras} are rather strict and a number of small alterations lead to striking loss of affinity. Furthermore, GTP suffers from several problems as a starting point for synthesis; it is labile biologically, highly charged and a substrate for a variety of key enzymes. Analogues of GTP with improved affinity and even modest preference for binding to a mutant versus normal p21^{ras} have been synthesized recently (Noonan *et al.*, 1991), but at present these appear unlikely to be effective on intact cells.

Approaches based on disruption of the effector/p21^{ras} interaction

The mechanism by which *ras* transforms cells or performs its normal function in mammalian cells remains unknown, but presumably involves interaction of the active (GTP-bound) form with an 'effector' molecule that transmits the signal. The identification of this effector(s) remains the central problem of *ras* research. Several candidates, including GAP and NF1 are now under intense investigation, but an unambiguous link between any 'effector' and transformation has not been established. Nonetheless, an inhibitor of the interaction of p21^{ras} and its 'effector' should prevent its transforming action.

Genetic evidence suggests that a disruption of the p21/effector interaction may reverse the transformed phenotype; transfection of the K-*rev*-1 gene into *ras*-transformed fibroblasts restored the flat morphology and reduced soft-agar colony formation (Kitayama *et al.*, 1989). The K-*rev*-1 gene product has an 'effector binding region' sequence that is identical to that of p21^{ras} and can bind at least one potential effector of p21^{ras}, GAP (Frech *et al.*, 1990; Zhang *et al.*, 1990). Thus reversal of transformation by K-*rev*-1 may result from interference of the interaction of p21^{ras} and its effector, and a pharmacological agent which blocks this interaction may produce similar effects on transformed cells.

Site-directed mutagenesis studies have identified key residues (aa 32–40) that are necessary for transformation and for interaction of p21^{ras} with GAP. A synthetic peptide corresponding to residues 17–44 of p21 competes with p21 for binding to GAP (Schaber *et al.*, 1989) and a synthetic peptide corresponding to residues 35–47 of p21^{ras} was able to block the p21-induced increase in pinocytosis of 3T3 cells (Lee *et al.*, 1990). Conversely, peptides derived from the region of GAP that may bind p21^{ras} were shown to prevent GAP activation of p21^{ras} GTPase, possibly by binding to p21^{ras} (Rubinfeld *et al.*, 1991). These peptides may therefore serve as model compounds for the design of inhibitors, although the synthetic modification of a peptide to a form capable of robust intracellular activity may be a formidable task.

This approach at present is limited by lack of certainty about the effector; this makes design of appropriate screens as well as analysis of the biochemical effects of putative inhibitors difficult. Furthermore, because both normal and mutant p21^{ras} probably bind the same effector and the mutation is not in the 'effector region' of p21^{ras}, the possible adverse effects of inhibiting normal p21^{ras} function remains a concern.

Approaches based on blocking p21^{ras} post-translational processing

p21^{ras} must be modified post-translationally by addition of a farnesyl group at the C-terminus in order to be transforming; thus inhibition of this process has been proposed as an approach to *ras* inhibition (Schafer *et al.*, 1989; Der & Cox 1991; Gibbs, 1991). Initial efforts focused on lovastatin, an inhibitor of isoprenoid biosynthesis that would be expected to inhibit p21^{ras} farnesylation by blocking the synthesis of the farnesyl donor. Lovastatin has been shown to inhibit p21 processing and block *ras*-dependent processes in several cellular systems (Schafer *et al.*, 1989; Mendola & Backer, 1990; Defeo-Jones *et al.*, 1991); but the inhibition of cell replication by lovastatin has recently been shown to be independent of its effects on *ras* (DeClue *et al.*, 1991). This result is not surprising in view of the diversity of processes that involve isoprenoids—in addition a large number of proteins other than *ras* are modified by addition of isoprenoid-derived groups and may play essential roles in normal cells.

The monoterpene limonene inhibits the isoprenylation of p21^{ras} and other 21–26 kDa proteins in cultured cells, without inhibition of cholesterol synthesis (Crowell *et al.*, 1991). Interestingly, isoprenylation of several other proteins including nuclear laminins is not inhibited. This is of interest in view of the reported chemotherapeutic activity of limonene, although high (mM) concentrations are required for the inhibition of isoprenylation. Similarly, although the adrenal steroid, dehydroepiandosterone, has recently been found to decrease the association of p21^{ras} with the cell membrane, the relation of this biochemical effect to the anticancer effects of dehydro-epiandosterone is unclear (Schulz & Nyce, 1991). More specific and potent inhibitors of the farnesyltransferases will probably be needed to clarify the potential of inhibition of farnesylation of p21^{ras} for chemotherapy.

Recently, the enzyme responsible for addition of the farnesyl group to p21^{ras} in mammalian cells has been identified, the genes for both subunits cloned, and the enzyme expressed (Manne *et al.*, 1990; Reiss *et al.*, 1990; Chen *et al.*, 1991a,b). This should enable pursuit of more specific inhibitors of p21^{ras} farnesylation, although other key proteins such as transducin and nuclear lamins may also be modified by this enzyme. Mutant and normal p21^{ras} are equally recognized by the farnesyltransferase (Manne *et al.*, 1990); therefore inhibitors of farnesylation would probably not be selectively effective against cells with mutant p21^{ras}, although Gibbs has recently presented an argument for this possibility (Gibbs, 1991). Even without selective inhibition of the mutant p21^{ras}, a partial inhibition of *ras* farnesy-lation may produce antitumour effects without unacceptable toxicity.

Following addition of a farnesyl group, p21^{ras} is further modified by proteolytic clipping of the three C-terminal amino acids and methylation of the resulting terminal cysteine. Inhibitors of these steps may also block the transforming action of p21^{ras}, because p21^{ras} that is farnesylated but not methylated does not bind well to membranes (Hancock *et al.*, 1991). If these reactions are catalysed by enzymes specific for *ras* they may be attractive targets, but this remains to be determined.

An interesting alternative approach to inhibition of the enzyme responsible for farnesylation is the incorporation of fraudulent analogues of the modifying lipid. The substitution of a modified myristate moiety markedly reduces membrane associated pp60^{src} levels (Heuckeroth & Gordon, 1989), but similar studies with *ras* have not yet been reported.

Inhibition of *ras* transcription

An alternative to directly targeting the p21^{ras} protein is to identify compounds that block transcription of *ras* genes. The success of this approach will depend in part on the presence of promoter control elements or transactivating factors unique to the *ras* genes. The transcriptional control of *ras* gene expression is under investigation, but the feasibility of this approach for drug discovery remains to be established. Berberine, a plant alkaloid, has been reported to decrease selectively the expression of the c-Ki-*ras* proto-oncogene and produce differentiation of a human teratocarcinoma cell line (Chang *et al.*, 1990), but the mechanism of action and degree of selectivity of this effect need further investigation.

Ras-induced vulnerability

A pragmatic approach to *ras*-directed chemotherapy is to look for compounds that selectively inhibit *ras*-transformed cells versus cells transformed by other oncogenes or proliferating normal cells (Merriman *et al.*, 1990). This approach is based on the assumption that *ras*-transformation may generate some (undefined) vulnerability. A related approach is to look for compounds that reverse the *ras*-induced morphologically transformed phenotype (Itoh *et al.*, 1989; Ogawara *et al.*, 1989; Shindo-Okada *et al.*, 1989; Suzukake-Tauchiya, 1990). Both of these approaches may prove useful, but because they do not focus on a specific molecular target, an understanding of the action of a compound emanating from such efforts will require extensive further investigation. Any compound found in such a screening programme may ultimately be found to target a protein unrelated to p21^{ras}.

Antisense oligonucleotides

Transfection of a gene encoding antisense RNA complementary to K-*ras* mRNA has been shown to inhibit the replication of a lung tumour cell line with mutant K-*ras* both *in vivo* and *in vitro* (Mukhopadhyay *et al.*, 1991). Transfection of this same antisense into a cell line expressing only the normal K-*ras* did not affect its growth rate. A reduction in the expression of K-*ras* in all tissues, rather than exclusively in the tumour cells as in this study, may be toxic, and therefore a mutant-specific antisense could be more selective.

A modified antisense oligonucleotide complementary to mutant H-*ras* has been shown to selectively induce ribonuclease cleavage of the mutant mRNA versus the normal H-*ras* mRNA in an *in vitro* assay, to reduce *ras* expression in cells, and to inhibit selectively the growth of a *ras*-transformed cell line (Saison-Behmoaras *et al.*, 1991). Similarly, a psoralen-derivatized antisense oligonucleotide inhibited mutant p21^{ras} expression by 96% at 15 μM with only a 15% inhibition of expression of normal p21^{ras} (Chang *et al.*, 1991). The selectivity shown in these studies is impressive, because the mutant *ras* differs from the normal *ras* gene by only a single nucleotide. If the problems of stability, delivery and supply common to the antisense approaches can be resolved, the promise of mutant-specific antisense will certainly become very attractive.

Conclusion

The explosive growth in research on oncogenes and tumour-suppressor genes has triggered extensive discussion of the oncogenes as targets for chemotherapy. Recent reviews have addressed approaches to inhibition of oncogenes (Huber, 1989) and the probability of reversing transformation with an inhibitor of a single oncogene (Klein, 1990). This review has attempted a critical evaluation of the advantages and drawbacks of onco- genes as targets for chemotherapy. We have not attempted to be com- prehensive in our examples, but rather have selected only a few to illustrate our points—where possible we have indicated reference reviews. New opportunities for therapeutic intervention will be suggested as our knowl- edge of oncogenes expands.

The deletion and mutation of tumour-suppressor genes appears to be at least as important as the activation of oncogenes in human cancer (Stanbridge, 1990; Marshall, 1991), and therefore approaches to the res- toration of normal function of these genes deserves careful consideration as an approach to chemotherapy. The replacement of the tumour-suppres- sor genes p53 or RB by transfection or infection with a recombinant retrovirus encoding the suppressor protein can reduce or eliminate the tumorigenicity of diverse types of tumour cells (Baker *et al.*, 1990; Bookstein *et al.*, 1990; Chen *et al.*, 1990a,b, 1991; Diller *et al.*, 1990; Sumegi *et al.*, 1990; Takahashi *et al.*, 1990; Issacs *et al.*, 1991; Johnson *et al.*, 1991; Shaulsky *et al.*, 1991; Cheng *et al.*, 1992). These studies validate the view that the renewed expression of these tumour-suppressor genes would slow or block tumour growth. At present such functional restoration in the clinic would seem difficult and may require a form of 'gene therapy' for success. There should be an increasing amount of effort in this area in the near future.

Current cytotoxic chemotherapy, although of vital value to many patients, suffers inherently from the identity of targets in normal replicat- ing cells and in the tumour cells. The result is toxicity to bone marrow, gut and skin. Elucidation of the fundamental genetic changes in carcinogene- sis has identified essential proteins and genes unique to tumour cells as targets for chemotherapy, and continued rapid progress in this area can be expected. A major challenge for medicinal chemists and pharmacologists is to exploit these targets for new chemotherapeutic drugs. Inhibitors of oncogenes may have the efficacy and selectivity needed to make a quantum advance in cancer chemotherapy.

Acknowledgements

The authors would like to thank Penny Miller and Drs M. Morin and J. Beebe for their suggestions regarding this manuscript.

References

Abraham, K.M., Levin, S.D., Marth, J.D., Forbush, K.A. & Perlmutter, R.M. (1991). Thymic tumorigenesis induced by overexpression of p56^{lck}. *Proceedings of the National Academy of Sciences USA* **88**, 3977–3981.

Baker, S.J., Markowitz, S., Fearon, E.R., Willson, J.K. & Vogelstein, B. (1990). Suppression of human colorectal carcinoma cell growth by wild-type p53. *Science* **249**, 912–915.

Basler, K. & Hafen, E. (1988). Control of photoreceptor cell fate by the *sevenless* protein requires a functional tyrosine kinase domain. *Cell* **54**, 299–311.

Bishop, J.M. (1987). The molecular genetics of cancer. *Science* **235**, 305–311.

Bishop, J.M. (1989). Oncogenes and clinical cancer. In Weinberg, R.A. (ed.) *Oncogenes and the Molecular Origins of Cancer*, pp. 327–358. Cold Spring Harbor Laboratory Press, Cold Spring Harbor.

Bishop, J.M. (1991). Molecular themes in oncogenesis. *Cell* **64**, 235–248.

Bolen, J.B., Viellette, A., Schwartz, A.M., DeSeau, V. & Rosen, N. (1987). Activation of pp60 c-src protein kinase activity in human colon carcinoma. *Proceedings of the National Academy of Sciences USA* **84**, 2251–2255.

Bookstein, R., Shew, J-Y., Chen, P-L., Scully, P. & Lee, W-H. (1990). Suppression of tumorigenicity of human prostate carcinoma cells by replacing a mutated RB gene. *Science* **247**, 712–715.

Bos, J.L. (1989). *Ras* oncogenes in human cancer: a review. *Cancer Research* **49**, 4682–4689.

Bourne, H.R., Sanders, D.A. & McCormick, F. (1991). The GTPase superfamily: conserved structure and molecular mechanism. *Nature* **349**, 117–127.

Brysch, W., Kneba, M. & Schlingensiepen, K.H. (1991). Inhibition of c-*erb*B-2 overexpression in SK-BR-3 carcinoma cells reduces kinases and DNA synthesis and arrest cell proliferation. *Proceedings of the American Association for Cancer Research* **32**, A2574.

Buettner, R., Yim, S.O., Hong, Y.S., Bonicinelli, E. & Tainsky, M.A. (1991). Alteration of homobox gene expression by N-ras transformation of PA-1 human teratocarcinoma cells. *Molecular and Cellular Biology* **11**, 3573–3583.

Cantley, L.C., Auger, K.R., Carpenter, C., Duckworth, B., Graziani, A., Kapeller, R. & Soltoff, S. (1991). Oncogenes and signal transduction. *Cell* **64**, 281–302.

Cesarman, E., Dalla-Favera, R., Bentley, D. & Groudine, M. (1987). Consistent mutations in a region of the first exon are associated with altered transcription of the c-*myc* oncogene in Burkitt's lymphoma. *Science* **238**, 1272–1275.

Chang, E.H., Miller, P.S., Cushman, C., Devadas, K., Pirollo, K.F., Ts'o, P.O. & Yu, Z.P. (1991). Antisense inhibition of *ras* p21 expression that is sensitive to a point mutation. *Biochemistry* **30**, 8283.

Chang, K.S.S., Gao, C. & Wang, I.-C. (1990). Berberine-induced morphologic differentiation and down-regulation of c-Ki-*ras*2 protooncogene expression in human teratocarcinoma cells. *Cancer Letters* **55**, 103–108.

Chen, W.-J., Andres, D.A., Goldstein, J.L., Russel, D.W. & Brown, M.S. (1991a). cDNA cloning and expression of the peptide-binding β subunit of rat p21^{ras} farnesyltransferase, the counterpart of yeast DPR1/RAM1. *Cell* **66**, 327–334.

Chen, W.-J., Andres, D.A., Goldstein, J.L., Russel, D.W. & Brown, M.S. (1991b). Cloning and expression of a cDNA encoding the α subunit of rat p21^{ras} protein farnesyltransferase. *Proceedings of the National Academy of Sciences USA* **88**, 11368–11372.

Chen, Y., Chen, P-L., Arnaiz, N., Goodrich, D. & Lee, W-H. (1991c). Expression of wild-type p53 in human A673 cells suppresses tumorigenicity but not growth rate. *Oncogene* **5**, 1799–1805.

Cheng, J., Yee, J-K., Yeargin, J., Friedmann, T. & Haas, H. (1992) Suppression of acute lymphoblastic leukemia by the human wild-type p53 gene. *Cancer Research* **52**, 222–226.

Cory, S. (1986). Activation of cellular oncogenes in hematopoietic cells by chromosome translocation. *Advances in Cancer Research* **47**, 189–234.

Crowell, P.L., Chang, R.R., Ren, Z., Elson, C.E. & Gould, M.N. (1991). Selective inhibition of isoprenylation of 21–26 kDa proteins by the anticarcinogen d-limonene and its metabolites. *Journal of Biological Chemistry* **266**, 17679–17685.

Daaka, Y. & Wickstrom, E. (1990) Target dependence of antisense oligodeoxynucleotide inhibition of c-Ha-*ras* p21 expression and focus formation in T24-transformed NIH3T3 cells. *Oncogene Research* **5**, 267–275.

DeClue, J.E., Vass, W.C., Papageorge, A.G., Lowy, D.R. & Willumsen, B.M. (1991). Inhibition of cell growth by lovastatin is independent of *ras* function. *Cancer Research* **51**, 712–717.

Defeo-Jones, D., McAvoy, E.M., Jones, R.E., Vuocolo, G.A., Haskell, K.M., Wegrzyn, R.J. & Oliff, A. (1991). Lovastatin selectively inhibits *ras* activation of the 12-O-tetradecanoylphorbol-13-acetate response element in mammalian cells. *Molecular and Cellular Biology* **11**, 2307–2310.

DePinho, R., Mitsock, L., Hatton, K., Ferrier, P., Zimmerman, K., Legouy, E., Tesfaye, A., Collum, R., Yancopoulos, G., Nisen, P., Kriz, R. & Alt, F. (1987). *Myc* family of cellular oncogenes. *Journal of Cellular Biochemistry* **33**, 257–266.

Der, C.J. & Cox, A.D. (1991). Isoprenoid modification and plasma membrane association: critical factors for *ras* oncogenicity. *Cancer Cells* **3**, 331–340.

Diller, L., Kassel, J., Nelson, C.E., Gryka, M.A., Litwak, G., Gebhardt, M., Bressac, B., Ozturk, M., Baker, S.J., Vogelstein, B. & Friend, S.H. (1990). p53 functions as a cell cycle control protein in osteosarcomas. *Molecular and Cellular Biology* **10**, 5772–5781.

Drebin, J.A., Link, V.C. & Greene, M.I. (1988a). Monoclonal antibodies reactive with distinct domains of the *neu* oncogene encoded p185 molecule exert synergistic anti-tumor effects *in vivo*. *Oncogene* **2**, 273–277.

Drebin, J.A., Link, V.C. & Greene, M.I. (1988b). Monoclonal antibodies specific for the *neu* oncogene product directly mediate anti-tumor effects *in vivo*. *Onogene* **2**, 387–394.

Drebin, J.A., Link, V.C., Stern, D.F., Weinberg, R.A. & Greene, M.I. (1985). Down-modulation of an oncogene protein product and reversion of the transformed phenotype by monoclonal antibodies. *Cell* **41**, 695–706.

Drebin, J.A., Link, V.C., Weinberg, R.A. & Green, M.I. (1986). Inhibition of tumor growth by a monoclonal antibody reactive with an oncogene-encoded tumor antigen *Proceedings of the National Academy of Sciences USA* **83**, 9129–9133.

Duke, R.C. & Cohen, J.J. (1986). IL-2 addiction: withdrawal of growth factor activates a suicide program in dependent T cells. *Lymphokine Research* **5**, 289–299.

Fearon, E.R. & Vogelstein, B. (1990). A genetic model for colorectal tumorigenesis. *Cell* **61**, 759–767.

Frech, M., John, J., Pizon, V., Chardin P., Tavitian, A., Clark, R., McCormick, F. & Wittinghofer, A. (1990). Inhibition of GTPase activating protein stimulation of *ras*-p21 GTPase by the K-*rev*-1 gene product. *Science* **249**, 169–171.

Gazit, A., Osherov, N., Posner, I., Yaish, P., Poradosu, E., Gilon, C. & Levitzki, A. (1991). Tyrphostins. 2. Heterocyclic and α-substituted benzylidenemalononitrile tyrphostins as potent inhibitors of EGF receptor and *erb*B2/*neu* tyrosine kinases. *Journal of Medicinal Chemistry* **34**, 1896–1907.

Gibbs, J.B. (1991). *Ras* C-terminal processing enzymes—new drug targets? *Cell* **65**, 1–4.

Griep, A.E. & Westphal, H. (1988). Antisense *myc* sequences induce differentiation of F9 cells. *Proceedings of the National Academy of Sciences USA* **85**, 6806–6810.

Hancock, J.F., Cadwallader, K. & Marshall, C.J. (1991). Methylation and proteolysis are essential for efficient membrane binding of prenylated p21-K-*ras*(B). *EMBO Journal* **10**, 641–646.

Hay, N., Bishop, J.M. & Levens, D. (1987). Regulatory elements that modulate expression of human c-*myc*. *Genes and Development* **3**, 293–303.

Heuckeroth, R.O. & Gordon, J.I. (1989). Altered membrane association of p60v-src and a murine 63-kDA *N*-myristoyl protein after incorporation of an oxygen-substituted analog of myristic acid. *Proceedings of the National Academy of Sciences USA* **86**, 5262–5266.

Holt, J.T., Redner, R.L. & Niehuis, A.W. (1988). An oligomer complementary to c-*myc* mRNA inhibits proliferation of HL60 promyelocytic cells and induces differentiation. *Molecular and Cellular Biology* **8**, 963–973.

Hoshino, M., Kawakita, M. & Hattori, S. (1988). Characterization of a factor that stimulates hydrolysis of GTP bound to *ras* gene product p21 (GTPase-activating protein) and correlation of its activity to cell density. *Molecular and Cellular Biology* **8**, 4169–4173.

Huang, A.L., Ostrowski, M.C., Berard, D. & Hager, G.L. (1981). Glucocorticoid regulation of the Ha-MuSV p21 gene conferred by sequences from mouse mammary tumor virus. *Cell* **27**, 245–255.

Huber, B.E. (1989). Therapeutic opportunities involving cellular oncogenes: novel approaches fostered by biotechnology. *FASEB Journal* **3**, 5–13.

Hudziak, R.M., Lewis, G.D., Winget M., Fendly, B.M., Shepard, H.M. & Ullrich, A. (1989). p185^{HER2} monoclonal antibody has antiproliferative effects *in vitro* and sensitizes human breast tumor cells to tumor necrosis factor. *Molecular and Cellular Biology* **9**, 1165–1172.

Hunter, T. (1991). Cooperation between oncogenes. *Cell* **64**, 249–270.

Ingvarsson, S. (1990). The *myc* family proteins and their role in transformation and differentiation. *Seminars in Cancer Biology* **1**, 359–369.

Issacs, W.B., Carter, B.S. & Ewing, C.M. (1991). Wild-type p53 suppresses growth of human prostate cancer cells containing mutant alleles. *Cancer Research* **51**, 4716–4720.

Itoh, O., Kuroiwa, S., Atsumi, S., Umezawa, K., Taekuchi, T. & Hori, M. (1989). Induction by the guanosine analogue oxanosine toward the normal phenotype of Ki-*ras*-transformed rat kidney cells. *Cancer Research* **49**, 996–1000.

Jacobovits, E.B., Majors, J.E. & Varmus, H.E. (1984). Hormonal regulation of the Rous sarcoma *src* gene via a heterologous promoter defines a threshold dose for cellular transformation. *Cell* **38**, 757–765.

Johnson, P., Gray, D., Mowat, M. & Benchimol, S. (1991). Expression of wild-type p53 is not compatible with continued growth of p53-negative tumor cells. *Molecular and Cellular Biology* **11**, 1–11.

Kitayama, H., Sugimoto, Y., Matsuzaki, T., Ikawa, Y. & Noda, M. (1989). A *ras*-related gene with transformation suppressor activity. *Cell* **56**, 77–84.

Klein, G. (1990). Multistep emancipation of tumors from growth control: can it be curbed in a single step? *BioEssays* **12**, 347–350.

Krengel, U., Schlichting, I., Scherer, A., Schumann, R., Frech, M., John, J., Kabsch, W., Pai, E.F. & Wittinghofer, A. (1990). Three-dimensional structures of H-*ras* p21 mutants: molecular basis for their inability to function as signal switch molecules. *Cell* **62**, 539–548.

Krystal, G., Birrer, M., Way, J., Nau, M., Sausville, E., Thompson, C., Minna, J. & Battey, J. (1988) Multiple mechanism for transcriptional regulation of the *myc* gene family in small cell cancer. *Molecular and Cellular Biology* **8**, 3373–3381.

Lee, G., Ronai, Z.A., Pincus, M.R., Murphy, R.B., Delohery, T.M., Nishimura, S.,

Yamaizumi, Z., Weinstein, I.B. & Brandt-Rauf, P.W. (1990) Inhibition of *ras* oncogene encoded p21 protein-induced pinocytotic activity by a synthetic peptide corresponding to an effector domain of the protein. *Medical Science Research* **18**, 771–772.

Lerner, L.J. & Jordan, V.C. (1990). Development of antiestrogens and their use in breast cancer: eighth Cain Memorial Award Lecture. *Cancern Research* **50**, 4177–4189.

Libermann, T.A., Nusnaum, H.R., Razon, N., Kris, R., Lax, I., Soreq, H., Whittle, N., Waterfield, M.D., Ullrich, A. & Schlessinger, J. (1985). Amplification, enhanced expression and possible rearrangement of EGF receptor gene in primary human brain tumors of glial origin. *Nature* **313**, 144–147.

Lippman, M., Bolan, G. & Huff, K. (1976). The effects of estrogens and anti-estrogens on hormone-responsive human breast cancer in long-term tissue culture. *Cancer Research* **36**, 4595–4601.

Lupu, R., Colomer, R., Zugmaier, G., Sarup, J., Shepard, M., Slamon, D. & Lippman, M. (1990). Direct interaction of a ligand for the *erb*B2 oncogene product with the EGF receptor and p185-*erb*B2. *Science* **249**, 1552–1555.

McCormick, F. (1989). *ras* GTPase activating protein: signal transmitter and signal terminator. *Cell* **56**, 5–8.

Manne, V., Roberts, D., Tobin, A. O'Rourke, E., De Virgilio, M., Meyers, C., Ahmed, N., Kurz, B., Resh, M., Kung, H-F. & Barbacid, M. (1990). Identification and preliminary characterization of protein-cysteine farnesyltransferase. *Proceedings of the National Academy of Sciences USA* **87**, 7541–7545.

Marshall, C.J. (1991). Tumor suppressor genes. *Cell* **64**, 313–326.

Mendelsohn, J. (1990). The epidermal growth factor receptor as a target for therapy with antireceptor monoclonal antibodies. *Seminars in Cancer Biology* **1**, 339–344.

Mendola, C.E. & Backer, J.M. (1990). Lovastatin blocks N-*ras* oncogene induced neuronal differentiation. *Cell Growth and Differentiation* **1**, 499–502.

Merlino, G.T. (1990). Epidermal growth factor receptor regulation and function. *Seminars in Cancer Biology* **1**, 277–284.

Merriman, R.L., Tanzer, L.R., Schakelford, K.A., Matsumoto, K., Robison, P.M. & Swift, R.A. (1990). Differential cytotoxic action of ovalicin and fumagillin against epithelial cells transformed by *ras* oncogenes. *Proceedings of the American Association for Cancer Research* **31**, 411.

Millburn, M.V., Tong, L., de Vos, A.M., Brunger, A., Yamaizumi, Z., Nishimura, S. & Kim, S-H. (1989). Molecular switch for signal transduction: structural differences between active and inactive forms of protooncogenic *ras* proteins. *Science* **247**, 939–945.

Mukhopadhyay, T., Tainsky, M., Cavender, A.C. & Roth, J.A. (1991). Specific inhibition of K-*ras* expression and tumorigenicity of lung cancer cells by antisense RNA. *Cancer Research* **51**, 1744–1748.

Noonan, T., Brown, N., Dudycz, L. & Wright, G. (1991). Interaction of GTP derivatives with cellular and oncogenic *ras*-p21 proteins. *Journal of Medicinal Chemistry* **34**, 1302–1307.

Ogawara, H., Hasumi, Y., Higashi, K., Ishii, Y., Saito, T., Watanabe, S-I., Suzuki, K-I., Kobori, M., Tanaka, K-I. & Akiyama, T. (1989). Acetoxycycloheximide and cycloheximide convert transformed morphology of *ras*-transformed cells to normal morphology. *Journal of Antibiotics* **42**, 1530–1533.

Parmeggiani, A. & Swart, G.W.M. (1985). Mechanism of action of kirromycin-like antibiotics. *Annual Review of Microbiology* **39**, 557–577.

Patterson, J.S., Battersley, L.A. & Edwards, D.G. (1981). Review of the clinical pharmacology and international experience with tamoxifen in advanced breast cancer. *Endocrine Treatment Reviews* **9**, 563–582.

Perlmutter, R.M., Marth, J.D., Ziegler, S.F., Garvin, A.M., Pawar, S., Cooke, M.P. & Abraham, K.M. (1985). Specialized protein tyrosine proto-oncogenes in hematopoietic cells. *Biochimica Biophysica Acta* **948**, 245–262.

Prochovnik, E.V., Kukowska, J. & Rodgers, C. (1988). c-*myc* antisense transcripts accelerate differentiation and inhibit G1 progression in murine erythroleukemia cells. *Molecular and Cellular Biology* **8**, 3683–3695.

Ramakrishnan, L. & Rosenberg, N. (1989). *abl* genes. *Biochimica Biophysica Acta* **989**, 209–224.

Reddy, E.P., Reynolds, R.K., Santos, E. & Barbacid, M. (1982). A point mutation is responsible for the acquisition of transforming properties by the T24 human bladder carcinoma oncogene. *Nature* **300**, 149–152.

Reed, J.C., Cuddy, M., Slabiak, T., Croce, C.M. & Nowell, P.C. (1988). Oncogenic potential of *bcl*-2 demonstrated by gene transfer. *Nature* **336**, 259–261.

Reed, J.C., Stein, C., Subasinghe, C., Haldar, S., Croce, C.M., Yum, S. & Cohen, J. (1990). Antisense-mediated inhibition of *BCL2* protooncogene expression and leukemic cell growth and survival: comparisons of phosphodiester and phosophorothioate oligodeoxynucleotides. *Cancer Research* **50**, 6565–6570.

Reiss, Y., Goldstein, J.L., Seabra, M.C., Casey, P.J. & Brown, M.S. (1990). Inhibition of purified p21ras farnesyl : protein transferase by *cys*-AAX tetrapeptides. *Cell* **62**, 81–88.

Rozengurt, E. (1986). Early signals in the mitogenic response. *Science* **234**, 161–166.

Rubinfeld, B., Wong, G., Bekesi, E., Wood, A., Heimer, E., McCormick, F. & Polakis, P. (1991). Asynthetic peptide corresponding to a sequence in the GTPase activating protein inhibits p21*ras* stimulation and promotes guanine nucleotide exchange. *International Journal of Protein Research* **38**, 47–53.

Saison-Behmoaras, T.B., Rey, I., Chassignol, M., Thuong, N.T. & Helene, C. (1991). Short modified antisense oligonucleotides directed against Ha-*ras* point mutation induce selective cleavage of the mRNA and inhibit T24 cell proliferation. *EMBO Journal* **10**, 1111–1118.

Satoh, T., Endo, M., Nakamura, S. & Kaziro, Y. (1988). Analysis of guanine nucleotide bound to *ras* protein in PC12 cells. *FEBS Letters* **236**, 185–189.

Schaber, M.D., Garsky, V.M., Boylan, D., Hill, W.S., Skolnick, E.M., Marshall, M.S., Sigal, I.S. & Gibbs, J.B. (1989). *Ras* interaction with the GPTase-activating protein (GAP). *Proteins* **6**, 306–315.

Schafer, W.R., Kim, R., Sterne, R., Thorner, J., Kim, S.-H. & Rine, J. (1989). Genetic and pharmacological suppression of oncogenic mutations in *ras* genes of yeast and humans. *Science* **245**, 379–385.

Scher, C.D., Young, S.A. & Locatell, K.L. (1982). Control of cytolysis of *BALB*/c-3T3 cells by platelet-derived growth factor: a model system for analyzing cell death. *Journal of Cellular Physiology* **113**, 211–218.

Schlichting, I., Almo, S.C., Rapp, G., Wilson, K., Petratos, K., Lentfer, A., Wittinghoffer, A., Kabsch, W., Pai, E.F., Petsko, G.A. & Goody, R.S. (1990). Time-resolved X-ray crystallographic study of the conformational change in Ha-*ras* p21 protein on GTP hydrolysis. *Nature* **345**, 309–315.

Schulz, S. & Nyce, J.W. (1991). Inhibition of protein isoprenylation and p21*ras* membrane association by dehydroepiandrosterone in human colonic adenocarcinoma cells *in vitro*. *Cancer Research* **51**, 6563–6567.

Shaulsky, G., Goldfinger, N. & Rotter, V. (1991). Alterations in tumor development *in vivo* mediated by expression of wild-type or mutant p53 proteins. *Cancer Research* **51**, 5232–5237.

Shindo-Okada, N., Makabe, O., Nagahara, H. & Nishimura, S. (1989). Permanent conversion of mouse and human cells transformed by activated *ras* or *raf* genes to apparently normal cells by treatment with the antibiotic azatyrosine. *Molecular Carcinogenesis* **2**, 159–167.

Sigal, I.S., Smith, G.M., Jurnak, F., Marsico-Ahern, J.D., D'Alonzo, J.S., Scolnick, E.M. & Gibbs, J.B. (1987). Molecular approaches towards an anti-*ras* drug. *Anti-Cancer Drug Design* **2**, 107–115.

Sklar, M.D., Thompson, E., Welsh, M.J., Liebert, M., Harney, J., Grossman, H.B., Smith, M. & Prochownik, E.V. (1991). Depletion of c-*myc* with specific antisense sequences reverses the transformed phenotype in *ras* oncogene-transformed NIH 3T3 cells. *Molecular and Cellular Biology* **11**, 3699–3710.

Smith, M.R., DeGudicibus, S.J. & Stacey, D.W. (1986). Requirement for c-*ras* protein during viral oncogene transformation. *Nature* **320**, 540–543.

Soriano, P., Montgomery, C., Geske, R. & Bradley, A. (1991). Targeted disruption of the c-*src* proto-oncogene leads to osteopetrosis in mice. *Cell* **64**, 693–702.

Stacey, D.W., DeGudicibus, S.R. & Smith, M.R. (1987). Cellular *ras* activity and tumor cell proliferation. *Experimental Cell Research* **171**, 232–242.

Stanbridge, E.J. (1990). Human tumor suppressor genes. *Annual Review of Genetics* **24**, 615–657.

Stanbridge, E.J. & Cavenee, W.J. (1989). Heritable cancer and tumor suppressor genes: a tentative connection. In Weinberg, R.A. (ed.) *Oncogenes and the Molecular Origins of Cancer*, pp. 281–306. Cold Spring Harbor Laboratory Press, Cold Spring Harbor.

Sumegi, J., Uzvolgyi, E. & Klein, G. (1990). Expression of the RB gene under the control of MuLV-LTR suppresses tumorigenicity of WERI-Rb-27 retinoblastoma cells in immunosuppressive mice. *Cell Growth and Differentiation* **1**, 247–250.

Suzuke-Tauchiya, K., Moriya, Y., Kawai, H., Hori, M., Uehara, Y., Iinuma, H., Naganawa, H. & Taekuchi, T. (1991). Inhibition of pinocytosis by hygrolidin family antibiotics/ possible correlation with their selective effects on oncogene-expressed cells. *Journal of Antibiotics* **44**, 344–348.

Suzukake-Tauchiya, K., Moriya, Y., Yamzaki, K., Hori, M., Hosokawa, N., Sawa, T., Iinuma, H., Naganawa, H., Imada, C. & Hamada, M. (1990). Screening of antibiotics preferentially active against *ras* oncogene expressed cells. *Journal of Antibiotics* **43**, 1489–1496.

Szczylik, C., Skorski, T., Nicolaides, N.C., Manzella, L., Malaguarnera, L., Ventuelli, D., Gewirtz, A.M. & Calabretta, B. (1991). Selective inhibition of leukemia cell proliferation by BCR-ABL antisense oligonucleotides. *Science* **253**, 562–565.

Tabin, C.J., Bradley, S.M., Bargemann, C.I., Weinberg, R.A., Papageorge, A.G., Scolnick, E.M., Dhar, R., Lowy, D.R. & Chang, E.H. (1982). Mechanism of activation of a human oncogene. *Nature* **300**, 143–149.

Takahashi, R., Hashimoto, T., Xu, H-J., Hu, S-X, Matsui, T., Miki, T., Bigo-Marshall, H., Aaronson, S.T. & Benedict, W.F. (1991). The retinoblastoma gene functions as a growth and tumor suppressor in human bladder carcinoma cells. *Proceedings of the National Academy of Sciences USA* **88**, 5257–5261.

Weinberg, R.A. (ed.) (1989a) *Oncogenes and the Molecular Origins of Cancer*. Cold Spring Harbor Laboratory Press, Cold Spring Harbor.

Weinberg, R.A. (1989b) Oncogenes and multistep carcinogenesis. In Weinberg, R.A. (ed.) *Oncogenes and the Molecular Origins of Cancer*, pp. 307–326. Cold Spring Harbor Laboratory Press, Cold Spring Harbor.

Yokoyama, K. & Imamoto, F. (1987). Transcriptional control of the endogenous *myc* protooncogene by antisense RNA. *Proceedings of the National Academy of Sciences USA* **84**, 7363–7367.

Zhang, K., Noda, M., Vass, W.C., Papageorge, A.G. & Lowy, D.R. (1990). Identification of small clusters of divergent amino acids that mediate the opposing effects of *ras* and *Krev*-a. *Science* **249**, 162–164.

Chapter 2
Apoptosis and cancer chemotherapy

Caroline Dive and Andrew H. Wyllie

Introduction

In recent decades, emphasis within cancer research has focused on understanding the cellular mechanisms which regulate tumour cell proliferation. This research emphasis is mirrored by the number of antiproliferative drugs used in the clinic today. Generally, antiproliferative agents are ineffectual against the low growth potential carcinomas which beleaguer our society. A phase of diminishing returns within drug development has ensued as we search for new cellular targets which will facilitate novel and rational drug design.

This chapter aims to direct the readers' attention to tumour cell death, the opposing side of the 'cell gain–cell loss' balance which dictates tumour progression. Two modes of cell death, necrosis and apoptosis*, are reviewed with respect to morphology, incidence and the current understanding of their mechanisms. Attention is then concentrated on the subject of apoptosis in tumours. We consider the relevance of this to the long-standing problem of tumour recurrence after initial sensitivity to chemotherapy. Hypotheses are proffered which relate the expression of key genes to the susceptibility of the tumour cell to undergo apoptosis, and hence we argue, to its drug sensitivity or resistance. An approach to cancer

*Apoptosis, derived from the ancient Greek meaning the falling of leaves from trees or petals from flowers.

21

chemotherapy which focuses on the process of tumour cell death rather than cessation of tumour cell proliferation is discussed. In particular, the potential applications of research into the molecular mechanisms of both the induction and suppression of tumour cell apoptosis are described.

Cell death, a panoramic view

Although the processes which culminate in cell death are undoubtedly important and intrinsic to every normal cell, they have not evoked the global interest generated by other cellular processes such as differentiation and proliferation. Cell death is usually considered fleetingly as a degenerative phenomenon caused by tissue injury. But, throughout embryogenesis and development in birds and mammals, and metamorphosis in insects, the utmost precision in the regulation of cell death is crucial (Saunders, 1966; Hinchliffe, 1981; Nishikawa *et al.*, 1989; Pierce *et al.*, 1989). In these circumstances cell death is spontaneous and physiological. Massive cell death is involved in the fashioning of limbs and elimination of redundant larval organs. For example, disregulated cell death during mammalian development is liable to result in cleft palate, deformed limbs or webbed digits (Fallon & Cameron, 1977; Goldman *et al.*, 1983; Alles & Sulik, 1989). Tightly controlled cell death occurs in hormone-sensitive tissues in response to changes within the physiological range of the appropriate trophic hormones (Ferguson & Anderson, 1981a,b). Selective cell death regulates B cell (Liu *et al.*, 1989), T cell (Williams *et al.*, 1990; Cohen, 1991) and erythrocyte production (Koury & Bondurant, 1990) and occurs in immune target cell killing (Cohen *et al.*, 1985). In healthy adults, tissue size is maintained via the balance between cell proliferation and cell death. Pathological states result where too many cells die, as in atrophy and in the degenerative diseases of the central nervous system (CNS). Rather than describing cancer merely as uncontrolled cell proliferation, it can be equally argued that the process of carcinogenesis includes disregulation of cell death. The vast field of toxicology has traditionally focused on toxicant and environmental insults which precipitate cell death, although the nature of the death itself has received scant attention.

There are many unanswered but fundamental questions. Do all these examples of cell death result from one death process? Does cell death in one cell type such as a neurone, have common features to that in another cell type such as an epithelial cell, or do cells die in fundamentally different ways? Do toxic agents cause death simply because they interact with vital cellular components in such a way that continuing life is impossible, or might some engage physiological death mechanisms that exist in some cells but not others?

Two modes of cell death have been described, namely necrosis and apoptosis, which differ in incidence, morphology and mechanism (Wyllie,

1981; Duval & Wyllie, 1986; Potten, 1987; Boobis *et al.*, 1989; Williams, 1991). In brief, whereas necrosis is almost invariably the result of severe perturbation of the cellular environment, apoptosis has many features indicative of an internally regulated process. Through detailed study of these, and apoptosis in particular, an attempt is made in this chapter to approach the answers to these questions.

Necrosis

Incidence

Necrosis is a thermodynamically downhill process which can be summarized as cellular metabolic collapse followed by cell disintegration (Trump *et al.*, 1973; Trump & Mergner, 1974; Jennings *et al.*, 1975; Wyllie, 1981). With few exceptions, necrosis is inflicted when circumstances diverge from physiological normality. It is caused by membrane disruptants, respiratory poisons, severe hypoxia and wide deviations of physiological temperature. *In vivo,* the pattern of necrotic cell death is often dictated by vasculature, for example necrotic cells are found in the hypoxic centre of solid tumours at a distance from blood vessels that reflects the diffusion distance for oxygen (Denekamp *et al.*, 1982). Typically, contiguous sheets of cells are affected *in vivo* and necrosis is accompanied by exudative inflammation. Tumour necrosis factor (TNF) has been reported to invoke both necrosis and apoptosis (Laster *et al.*, 1988; Flieger *et al.*, 1989). It is important to note, however, that if an agent stimulates apoptosis in endothelial cells, necrosis will follow in those adjacent cells deprived of oxygen.

Morphology

Necrosis is an irreversible process but is often preceded by reversible changes (Fig. 2.1). Early indications that a cell is about to undergo necrosis are slight swelling of cytoplasm and mitochondria, dilation of the endoplasmic reticulum and plasma membrane blebbing. Removal of the injurious stimulus at this point would result in the recovery and survival of the cell. Persistence of damage leads to high amplitude swelling of mitochondria with rupture of internal cristae. This is followed by extensive cytoplasmic oedema, dissolution of internal organelles, increased nuclear volume and ultimately the bursting apart of the plasma membrane resulting in the appearance of cell ghosts (karyolysis).

Mechanism

Although the precise sequence of cellular events is not fully defined in

'Point of no return'

Reversible changes

Dilatation of organelles
Ribosome disaggregation
Blebbing

Mitochondrial high
amplitude swelling
Mitochondrial matrix
densities
Violent blebbing

Irreversible changes

Membrane rupture
Dispersal of organelles

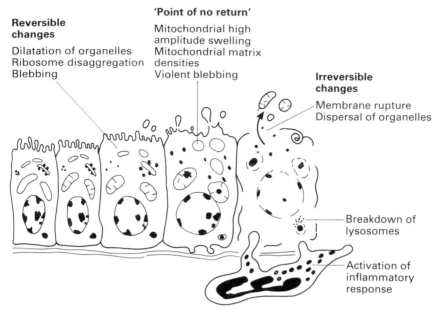

Breakdown of
lysosomes

Activation of
inflammatory
response

Fig. 2.1. A generalized representation of the key morphological features of necrosis.

necrosis, several major changes in cell homeostasis are recognized (Fig. 2.2). A fall in adenosine triphosphate (ATP) below a critical threshold precedes fatal disruption of ionic homeostasis. Sodium and water enter and potassium leaves the cell. Calcium influx is probably responsible for mitochondrial damage. Cellular pH is decreased, and protein and RNA synthesis are depressed. Calcium imbalance may also be responsible for the activation of phospholipases which hydrolyse membrane phospholipids, and proteases which cleave cytoskeletal or integral membrane proteins. Reactive oxygen intermediates also appear to play a significant role in necrosis (Dean, 1987). For this reason, agents which depress cellular glutathione and other free radical scavenging mechanisms precipitate necrosis. Finally, release of lysosomal enzymes from ruptured organelles causes digestion of intracellular components and rupture of the plasma membrane mediates an inflammatory reaction in surrounding tissue. Membrane damage leading to necrosis can be direct (e.g. by complement) or secondary to energy depletion (e.g. hypoxia or iodoacetate). Other than removing the necrotic stimulus, and with the current mechanistic understanding of necrosis, it is difficult to see room for delicate pharmacological manoeuvre to modulate this type of cell death. The application of drugs which alter tissue vasculature might be an exception (Denekemp *et al.*, 1982). Should the aim be to induce tumour cell death, this type of death with its associated inflammatory response is clearly not favourable.

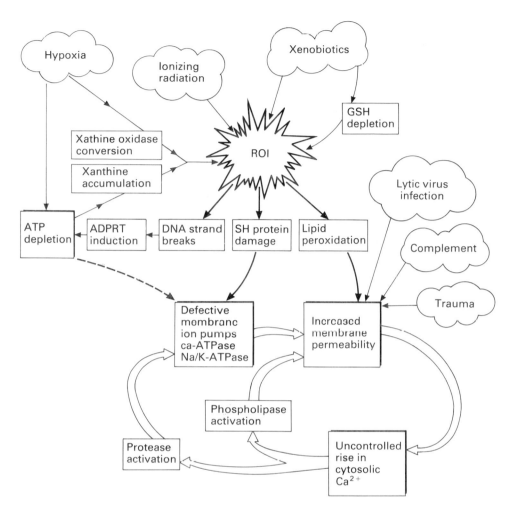

Fig. 2.2. A generalized representation of the key biochemical pathways involved in precipitating necrosis. ADPRT, poly ADP ribosyltransferase; ATP, adenosine triphosphate: GSH, glutathione; ROI, reactive oxygen intermediates; SH, thiol.

Apoptosis

The term apoptosis was first introduced in 1972 to describe a morphologically distinct form of cell death (Kerr *et al.*, 1972). Many recent reports use the term apoptosis synonymously with that of programmed cell death (PCD). Strictly speaking, however, apoptosis is currently identifiable by morphological and biochemical features, rather than proof of a genetic programme. For this reason, before we address questions concerning genetic control and associated ramifications of apoptosis in tumours, it is pertinent to first consider the morphological features, the overall incidence of apoptosis and what is known of the biochemistry of this process.

Incidence

The great majority of the physiologically regulated cell death alluded to in the introduction of this chapter has been described as internally controlled and called apoptosis. Apoptosis is also the mode of death seen in pathological scenarios. For instance, apoptosis has been reported in many tumour types (see below) and inappropriate induction of apoptosis in the T-cell repertoire is possibly implicated in the qualitative and quantitative T-cell defects of human immunodeficiency virus (HIV) infected patients (Amiesen & Capon, 1991; Terai *et al.*, 1991). The most studied cell system with respect to apoptosis is that of the immature rodent thymocyte (Wyllie, 1980) and as such deserves a mention. Autoreactive thymocytes are deleted within the thymus before what would be a catastrophic release into the general circulation. This vital removal of defective cells is via apoptosis. *In vitro*, studies of apoptosis in the immature thymocyte follow induction by glucocorticoid treatment.

Incidence of apoptosis in tumours

It has been apparent to tumour kineticists for decades that tumour size is dictated by a balance between cell gain (proliferation) and cell loss (cell differentiation and cell death, see Steel, 1977; Dive & Hickman, 1991). Kinetic data indicate that a high rate of cell loss is typical in most experimental, and in almost all human, tumours (Wyllie, 1985). Some of this cell loss is accounted for by zones of necrosis, but in tumours where necrosis is scarce and mitotic indices are high (such as basal cell carcinomas), the cell loss rate is also curiously high (Kerr & Searle, 1981). Apoptosis occurs widely in tumours with enhanced rate during spontaneous regression (Kerr *et al.*, 1972). Moreover, the regression of malignant neoplasms that initially follows apparently successful chemotherapy must clearly be accompanied by loss of cells. A graphic example of this is the initial regression within a 2-week period of treatment with cyclophosphamide, vincristine and methotrexate, of the often massive facial tumours of children with endemic Burkitt's lymphoma (BL) (Olweny *et al.*, 1980) (Fig. 2.3). How do these tumour cells die?

Apoptosis has been identified in many tumour types encompassing embryonal carcinomas, hepatic neoplasms, ascites tumours, sarcomas, small cell lung carcinoma, and tumours of the breast, prostate and colon (Wyllie, 1985; Potten, 1987; Sarraf & Bowen, 1988; Bowen & Bowen, 1990; Harmon *et al.*, 1991; Kyprianou *et al.*, 1991b; Martikainen *et al.*, 1991). Indeed, the histology of very few human malignant tumours is free from apoptosis. Leukaemias and lymphomas seem particularly sensitive to the induction of apoptosis by multiple stimuli (Blewitt *et al.*, 1983; Baxter *et al.*, 1989; Collins *et al.*, 1989, 1991; Kaufmann, 1989; Bansal

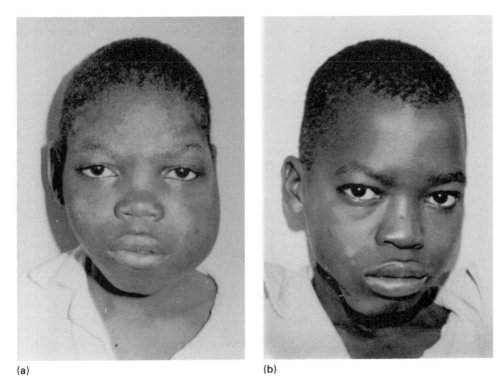

(a)   (b)

Fig. 2.3. A Ugandan child with endemic Burkitt's lymphoma with typical jaw
swelling before (a) and 2 weeks after chemotherapy with methotrexate, vincristine
and cyclophosphamide (b).

et al., 1990; Gregory *et al.*, 1991; Lucas *et al.*, 1991; Martin & Cotter,
1991), including the application of a monoclonal antibody anti-APO-1 to
a specific surface receptor (Trauth *et al.*, 1989; Debatin *et al.*, 1990).
Hormone-dependent tumours of the breast and prostate also show a
propensity to undergo apoptosis. Antiandrogens and androgen ablation
evoke apoptosis in prostate cancer (Kyprianou *et al.*, 1990), and apoptosis
is induced in breast tumours following oestrogen ablation (Kyprianou
et al., 1991b), or treatment with analogues of luteinizing hormone-releasing hormone (LHRH) and with somatostatin (Szende *et al.*, 1989a). The
latter is thought to influence levels of steroid hormones and possibly exert
a direct effect. LHRH analogues and somatostatin also trigger apoptosis
in pancreatic carcinomas (Szende *et al.*, 1989b).

Several theories have been put forward to explain the occurrence of
apoptosis in tumours, both spontaneous and induced (reviewed by Wyllie,
1985). Firstly, it has been argued that tumour cell populations are so
abnormal that they are unduly susceptible to induction of apoptosis by
mildly injurious stimuli. Secondly, tumour cell apoptosis may result from
activities of cytotoxic T, K, or natural killer (NK) cells, though there is

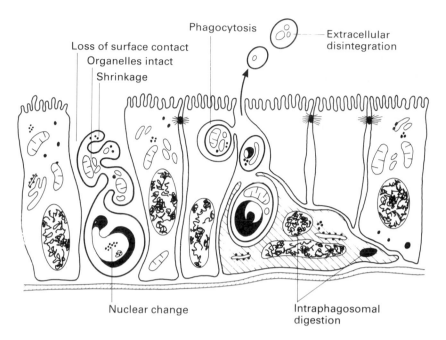

Phagocytosis

Extracellular disintegration

Loss of surface contact
Organelles intact
Shrinkage

Nuclear change

Intraphagosomal digestion

Fig. 2.4. A generalized representation of the key morphological features of apoptosis.

little morphological evidence to support this idea. Thirdly, a change in the local concentration of cytokines or other trophic factors may increase apoptosis levels (for example, TNF has been shown to induce apoptosis). Fourthly, tumour cell apoptosis may represent a residual autoregulation within an expanding cell population. Confirmation of any of these four theories has not as yet been forthcoming. There may be cellular hierarchies which determine propensity for this type of cell death (Ijiri & Potten, 1983). Since both spontaneous and provoked apoptosis seem so prevalent in tumours, then surely a more pertinent question addresses the converse situation of why some tumour cells do not die via apoptosis, but survive to repopulate tumours in relapsing patients, or metastasize. One can speculate that they either do not receive an apoptotic stimulus or that they are in some way defective in the programme of apoptotic cell death. This is discussed at length below.

Morphology

A series of coordinate structural changes occur in apoptosis regardless of the affected cell type (Figs 2.4–2.7) (Wyllie *et al.*, 1980; Wyllie, 1988; Cotter *et al.*, 1990). The most characteristic changes are of condensation within the nucleus (Arends *et al.*, 1990). Initially, a dense band of granular heterochromatin underpins the nuclear membrane-forming aggregates in

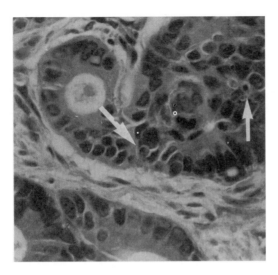

Fig. 2.5. Apoptosis in a human colorectal carcinoma. The arrow on the left shows a single apoptotic cell with a nuclear fragment, while the right-hand arrow points to a cluster of small apoptotic bodies. A cell in anaphase lies between.

hemilunar caps. Subsequently, the nuclear membrane undergoes bizarre convolutions and the condensed nucleus fragments to form spheres of dense granular material. Cytoplasmic features of apoptosis include the aggregation of organelles which are otherwise morphologically intact and normal but disordered in their orientation to each other. The endoplasmic reticulum dilates (a feature in common with necrosis) and forms expanded vesicles, some of which fuse with the plasma membrane giving it a pitted appearance when viewed by scanning electron microscopy. The cell's shape eventually becomes distorted and membrane-bound apoptotic bodies form of various sizes with or without condensed chromatin contained. These apoptotic bodies can be seen to bud off the major mass of the cell. *In vivo*, apoptotic cells and bodies are rapidly recognized and engulfed by phagocytes wherein they progressively disintegrate (Savill *et al.*, 1989). *In vitro*, in the absence of phagocytosis, a terminal phase of cell disintegration occurs often confusingly called secondary necrosis (and most likely often mistaken for primary necrosis). In stark contrast to necrosis, apoptosis affects single cells and is not associated with an inflammatory response. In most documented cases, apoptosis in mammalian tumour cells takes on the classical apoptotic cell death morphology seen in the immature thymocyte.

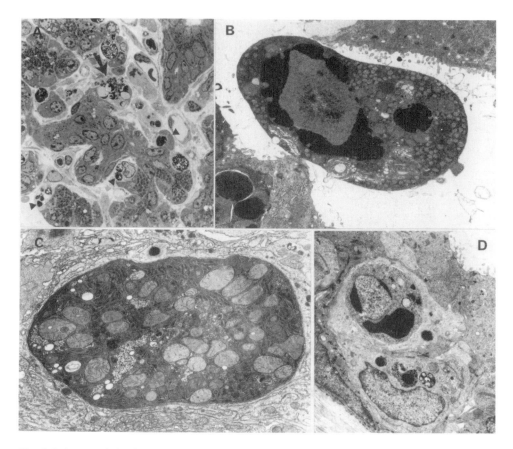

Fig. 2.6. Apoptosis in the rat salivary gland during atrophy induced by duct
ligation. (A) Overview, through the light microscope showing several apoptotic cells
that have undergone phagocytosis within a macrophage (large arrow), and many
other apoptotic cells (arrowheads) within the epithelium of the gland. (B) Many
characteristic ultrastructural features of apoptosis are indicated: the cell surface is
smooth (contrasting with the microvillus surface of adjacent viable epithelial cells),
peripheral condensation of nuclear chromatin, and nucleolar disaggregation are
obvious, and the cell has lost contact with its neighbours. (C) The compacted
organelles. (D) The phagocytosis of apoptotic cells. (By courtesy of Dr N. Walker,
Brisbane, Australia.)

Mechanism

The molecular mechanism of apoptosis is incompletely defined. However,
an increasingly clear picture is emerging of the cell biology underlying the
morphological changes described above. Several distinct coordinated
effector events are now recognized.

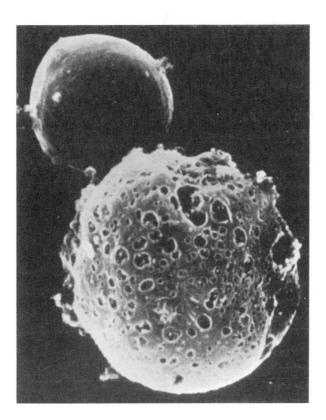

Fig. 2.7. The pitted surface of a thymocyte, undergoing apoptosis following gluco-corticoid treatment, viewed with the scanning electron microscope.

Endonuclease activation

The most precisely defined biochemical event in apoptosis is the activation of an endonuclease which results in the characteristic chromatin condensation described above. This endonuclease(s) is dependent on calcium and magnesium (Cohen & Duke, 1984; Duke *et al.*, 1986), but inhibited by zinc (Flieger *et al.*, 1989). It cleaves DNA at internucleosomal linker sites and this double strand cutting yields 180 bp DNA integer oligonucleosomes (Fig. 2.8) (Arends *et al.*, 1990). Concomitant exonuclease activity appears unlikely since 185 bp is the length of mononucleosomal DNA and cleavage results in integers closely similar to this length. Chromatin remaining attached to the nuclear structure is incompletely digested by the endo-nuclease and is seen as long oligonucleosomal chains associated with histone H1 but not HMG1 or -2 proteins, consistent with transcriptionally inactive DNA. Mononucleosomal DNA yielded by endonuclease activity is deficient in H1 but enriched in HMG1 and -2 suggesting origin from transcriptionally active DNA. Attempts to purify this endonuclease have

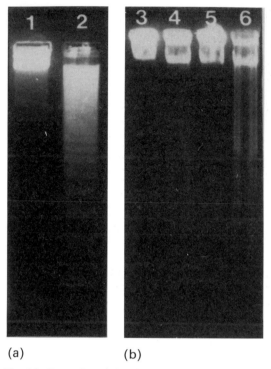

(a)   (b)

Fig. 2.8. Examples of the characteristic DNA 'ladders' which imply that apoptosis has occurred. DNA was extracted from immature rat thymocytes and L1210 mouse leukaemia cells and subjected to gel electrophoresis using the method of Smith *et al.* (1989). Gel a, lane 1: untreated control immature rat thymocytes prepared as described by Wyllie (1980) showing high mol. wt DNA consistent with cell viability. Lane 2: immature thymocytes treated for 4 h with methylprednisolone at 10^{-5} M showing apoptotic DNA fragmentation. Gel b, lanes 3 and 5: control L1210 cells showing high mol. wt DNA consistent with cell viability. Lane 4: L1210 cells treated for 40 h with ionomycin at 1 μg/ml. Lane 6: L1210 cells 6 h after treatment with 10 μM nitrogen mustard both exhibiting apoptotic DNA fragmentation indicative of endonuclease activation. (Unpublished data, courtesy of Tom Fisher and Rachel Chapman, Manchester, UK.)

not yet met with success. Whether the enzyme is constitutive or synthesized on stimulation is a matter for debate and this may depend on cell type (see later). It would seem, however, that endonuclease activity might occur relatively late within the process of apoptosis. It is conceivable, but unlikely, that this type of internucleosomal cleavage is a reversible step.

Tissue transglutaminase and membrane rigidity

Apoptotic hepatocytes become insoluble in chaotropic agents, urea, guanidine hydrochloride and reducing agents (Fig. 2.9) (Fesus *et al.*, 1989). This observation is consistent with the activation of tissue transgluta-

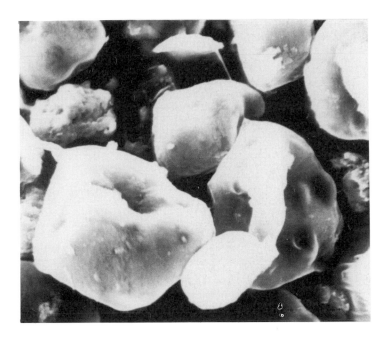

Fig. 2.9. Insoluble (transglutaminated) cellular residues obtained after extraction of apoptotic hepatocytes with strong ionic detergent (Fesus *et al.*, 1989). (By courtesy of Dr M. Piacentini, Rome, Italy.)

minase (EC 2.3.2.13) concomitant with the induction of apoptosis (Piacentini *et al.*, 1991). The enzyme forms membrane–protein crosslinks which are resistant to proteases and increase rigidity of the plasma membrane (Fesus *et al.*, 1987). It is an attractive speculation that this transglutaminase-induced, protein-crosslinked scaffold is needed to keep degradative enzymes and DNA tightly confined until the final phases of apoptosis are complete and a safe haven within a phagocyte is accomplished.

Shrinkage

The abrupt discontinuous rise in cell density, accompanied by loss of cell volume occurs in apoptosis (Wyllie & Morris, 1982). The rise in density can be accounted for by the loss of aqueous and solute volume, but the mechanism is not known.

Recognition

In vivo, apoptotic cells are swiftly recognized by phagocytes presumably due to cell surface alterations. The recognition of apoptotic thymocytes by isologous peritoneal macrophages has been studied *in vitro* (Morris *et al.*, 1984; Duvall *et al.*, 1985). Macrophages bound preferentially to apoptotic cells. Binding occurred in the absence of serum and was inhibited by

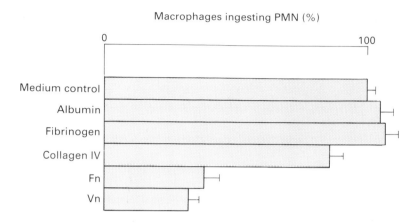

Macrophages ingesting PMN (%)

Fig. 2.10. Recognition of apoptotic aged polymorphonuclear neutrophils (PMN) by macrophages is inhibited by prior attachment of macrophages to surfaces coated for 2 h with fibronectin (Fn) and vitronectin (Vn) but not collagen IV, fibrinogen or albumin at 80 μg/ml as described by Saville *et al.* (1990). (Redrawn from Saville *et al.*, 1990, by courtesy of Dr C. Haslett, London, UK.)

several polysaccharides. The results suggested that lectin-like molecules on the macrophage surface recognized changes in the cell-surface car-bohydrate of the apoptotic cell. In separate studies on neutrophils and lymphocytes undergoing apoptosis, both treatment with antivitronectin monoclonal antibody and the prior coating of macrophages with vitronec-tin inhibited 70% interaction between macrophages and apoptotic aged neutrophils (Fig. 2.10) (Savill *et al.*, 1990). This demonstrates a novel and direct role for the vitronectin receptor in macrophage recognition of apoptosis. A full understanding of this recognition process might pave the way for modulation of tumour cell membrane character which evokes a phagocytosis. From the point of view of a therapeutic strategy in tumours, the entrapment and destruction of the dead tumour cell within a phagocyte has obvious attractions in avoiding inflammatory responses.

Signal pathways to trigger apoptosis

Although the effector mechanisms described above have been observed in many cell types, it is not clear which signalling pathways are employed to trigger them in response to physiological, pathological or pharmacological stimuli. Several pieces of evidence implicate a rise in cellular free calcium as a critical event for apoptosis. A moderate but sustained increase in intracellular calcium has been demonstrated to precede both endonuclease activation and cell death in glucocorticoid-treated immature thymocytes (Fig. 2.11) (McConkey *et al.*, 1989b). In this cell system, both removal of extracellular calcium, and intracellular calcium buffering prevented DNA fragmentation and death, and calcium ionophores stimulated apoptosis.

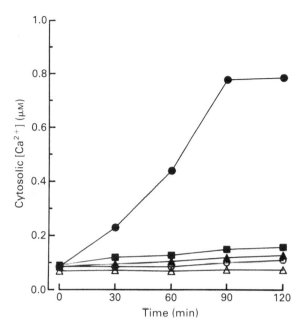

Fig. 2.11. The effect of methylprednisolone (MP) on cytosolic calcium in immature rat thymocytes. Quin-2 loaded cells were loaded with MP in the absence of presence of various inhibitors as described by McConkey *et al.* (1989b). Treatments (○) control, (●) 10^{-5} M MP; (△) 10^{-5} M MP plus the glucocorticoid receptor antagonist RU-486 10^{-5} M; (▲) 10^{-5} M MP plus the protein synthesis inhibitor cycloheximide 10^{-5} M; (■) 10^{-5} M MP plus the inhibitor of mRNA synthesis actinomycin D 1 µg/ml. (From McConkey *et al.*, 1989b, by courtesy of Professor S. Orrenius, Stockholm, Sweden, with permission from Academic Press, Inc.)

Calmidazolium did not affect the calcium rise seen but did prevent DNA fragmentation and death, suggesting a role for calmodulin in activating the endonuclease. The calcium channel blocker flunarizine inhibited the neuronal cell death induced by withdrawal of nerve growth factor (NGF) (Rich & Hollowell, 1990). Its mode of action was suggested to be intracellular possibly by inhibition of calmodulin and thus supporting a role for calcium in apoptosis. Since calcium is implicated in signalling for a multitude of cellular activities including proliferation and differentiation, it seems unlikely that a simple influx of calcium from outside the cell activates a specific pathway for apoptotic death. Nor is it clear how a sustained calcium rise permits maintenance of membrane integrity typical of an apoptotic cell. In direct conflict with the situation described for thymocytes, it has been shown that protection of interleukin-3 (IL-3) dependent haemopoietic progenitor cells from apoptosis is afforded by calcium ionophores (Rodriguez-Tarduchy *et al.*, 1990). Moreover, a lack of early calcium involvement has been observed in dexamethasone-induced killing of human lymphoid cells of T-cell derivation CEM-C7

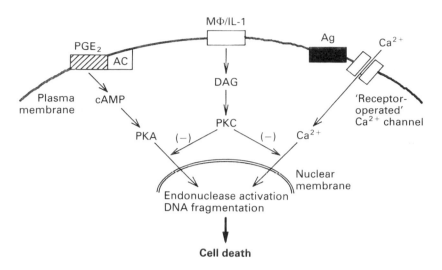

Fig. 2.12. Theoretical model for regulatory signals in the induction of programmed cell death. AC, adenylate cyclase; Ag, antigen; DAG, diacylglycerol; IL-1, interleukin-1; PGE$_2$, prostaglandin E$_2$; PKA, protein kinase A; PKC, protein kinase C. (From McConkey *et al.*, 1990b, by courtesy of Professor S. Orrenius, Stockholm, Sweden, with permission from Elsevier.)

(Bansal *et al.*, 1990). Furthermore, it is not obvious how topoisomerase II inhibitors, which have been shown to induce apoptosis in various tumour cells could effect a sustained moderate calcium rise. Although an important role for calcium in the signalling pathway leading to apoptosis seems possible, experiments with ionophores may mask the complexity of this signal transduction. Extracellular calcium influx can be initiated by release of inositol 1,5,5-trisphosphate (Ins(1,4,5)P$_3$)-sensitive intracellular calcium stores (calcium-activated calcium-influx; Berridge & Irvine, 1989), and it has been reported recently that IP$_3$ levels increase when apoptosis is triggered in thymocytes (Conroy *et al.*, 1991).

A model for thymocyte apoptosis based on unbalanced signalling has been proposed, whereby there is 'cross talk' between protein kinase A (PKA) and protein kinase C (PKC, Fig. 2.12) (McConkey *et al.*, 1990b). In the absence of second signals, sustained calcium or cyclic adenosine monophosphate (cAMP) stimulate endonuclease activation and death (McConkey *et al.*, 1989a, 1990a). Evidence for a possible role of PKC as the second signal which prevents apoptosis is summarized below. Treatment of thymocytes with an activator of this enzyme, the phorbol ester 12-O-tetradecanoylphorbol 13-acetate (TPA), inhibits glucocorticoid-induced apoptosis and inhibitors of PKC such as H7 induce apoptosis (McConkey *et al.*, 1989a, 1990b; Lanotte *et al.*, 1991). Phorbol ester protected endothelial cells from apoptosis due to serum depletion (Araki *et al.*, 1990) and polymixin B treatment of serum withdrawal induced apoptosis in mature lymphocytes which was counteracted by TPA (Lucas *et al.*, 1991). Direct measurements of PKC levels and cellular location were not performed in any of these reports and since both H7 and polymixin B are non-specific inhibitors, their activation of apoptosis is clearly not direct proof of PKC involvement. It is possible that intracellular calcium and PKC may play different signalling roles in different cell types. Despite present uncertainty surrounding what must be precise and complex signal transduction in apoptosis, the potential for modulation of the signals in this pathway is an alluring prospect.

Measurement of cell death

The uncertainties regarding the triggers of apoptosis have implications for the ways in which the processes of cell death may be recognized and quantitated. It appears possible that common signalling components may be employed in both apoptosis and fundamentally different biological processes such as cell proliferation. In addition, the external stimuli alone need not be specific to apoptosis, necrosis or other processes. Some agents may cause either apoptosis or proliferation depending on the target cell type. Many others cause necrosis at high concentration but apoptosis when the concentration is lower. Therefore, the methodology for the measurement of cell death must rely heavily on detection of the effector phenomena.

The obvious differences in the morphology of apoptosis and necrosis can be seen using light and electron microscopy (Potten, 1987), which has been the mainstay technique of the early research characterizing cell death. However, the short half-life of apoptotic cells before rapid phagocytosis and removal, and the usual heterogeneity seen where apoptotic cells are surrounded and outnumbered by viable cells, has probably led to underestimation of apoptosis. Traditional assays for cytotoxicity fall into two categories; those which measure increased membrane permeability in cells interpreted as irreversibly damaged, and those which assess functional activities attributed to living cells alone. Into the first category fall trypan blue exclusion, propidium uptake, and release of fluorescein or lactate dehydrogenase, to mention a few. Immunologists particularly favour release of radiolabelled chromium. Whilst these methods readily identify necrotic cells they will not identify all apoptotic cells. Thymocytes, hepatocytes and cultured tumour cells in the first recognizable stages of apoptosis exclude both trypan blue and propidium. *In vitro*, in the absence of phagocytosis, only the later phase of apoptosis, i.e. disintegration, will be recognized by the above techniques. Measurement of functional capabilities of living cells such as the methylthiazotetrazolium (MTT) assay, or uptake of neutral red give negative results for metabolically exhausted

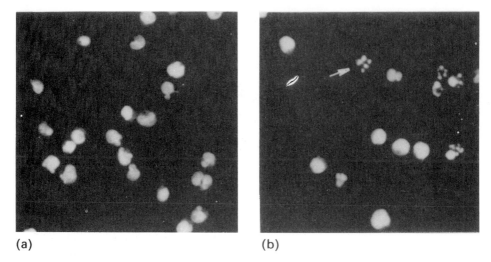

(a)   (b)

Fig. 2.13. Typical acridine orange–staining patterns for Burkitt's lymphoma group I cells (Gregory *et al.*, 1991). (a) Untreated control cells show regular diffuse nuclear staining, in contrast to (b) the markedly condensed and fragmented nuclei seen following 24 h treatment with ionomycin at 1 μg/ml (marked with the arrow). (Unpublished data, courtesy of Dr C.D. Gregory & Dr A. Milner, Birmingham, UK.)

necrotic cells, but it is as yet unclear how apoptotic cells behave in this type of cytotoxicity test.

Several techniques are currently used to assess apoptosis. Fluorescence microscopy using acridine orange allows identification and quantitation of apoptotic cells by illuminating characteristic chromatin condensation patterns (Fig. 2.13) (McConkey *et al.*, 1988; Gregory *et al.*, 1991). Gel electrophoresis of apoptotic cell DNA yields a classical DNA ladder indicative of endonuclease activity (Fig. 2.8) (Wyllie, 1980), whereas the degraded DNA of necrotic cells yields a nondescript smear on the gel. This technique is qualitative but masks heterogeneity. Flow cytometric assays which rapidly discriminate and quantitate viable, necrotic and apoptotic cells are now emerging (Afanas'ev *et al.*, 1986; Compton *et al.*, 1988; Nicoletti *et al.*, 1991; Swat *et al.*, 1991; Dive *et al.*, 1992) (Fig. 2.14). Here, DNA-binding fluorochromes report chromatin changes and simultaneous light scatter measurements report changes in cell granularity and cell size. Improvements in measurement such as these will undoubtedly facilitate mechanistic studies of apoptosis.

Is apoptosis dependent on gene expression?

Genes directly responsible for a 'programme of cell death' in mammalian cells have not yet been conclusively identified. However, it is not unreasonable to suspect that a process as utterly fundamental as apoptotic cell death should be exquisitely conserved. A blueprint of gene expression

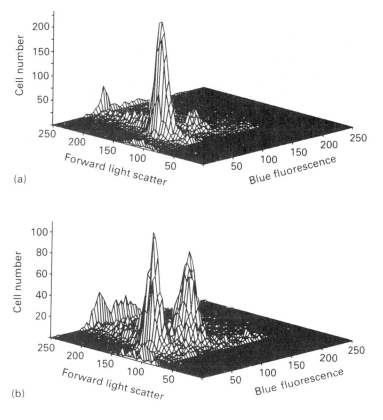

(a)

(b)

Fig. 2.14. Flow cytometric analysis of apoptosis in immature rat thymocytes following treatment with glucocorticoids. Cells were isolated and treated with methylprednisolone (MP) at 10^{-5} M as described by Wyllie (1980). After 4 h untreated control cells (a) and those treated with MP (b) were stained with Hoechst 33342 and analysed by flow cytometry as described by Dive *et al.* (1992). Comparison of the isometric plots shows an increase in the high blue (Hoechst 33342) fluorescence cell subpopulation in plot b which represents the increase in apoptotic cell number induced by MP.

involved in a programmed cell death has emerged from studies of normal development of the nematode. In *Caenorhabditis elegans* 11 genes have been identified that function in this programmed cell death (Fig. 2.15) (Ellis & Horvitz, 1986; Yuan & Horvitz, 1990; Ellis *et al.*, 1991). These genes encode for three general processes, death, engulfment of the dying cell by its neighbours and degradation of cellular debris. The genes *ced-3* and *ced-4* act cell autonomously to cause programmed cell death. The genes *ced-1,2,5,6,7,8* and *-10*, direct the process of phagocytosis and *nuc-1* encodes a deoxyribonuclease that degrades DNA in dead cells. Of pivotal importance is the recently discovered *ced-9* gene which is thought to act by preventing cell death. Intriguing parallels exist in mammalian cells (see later). Morphologically this programmed cell death has similarities to the

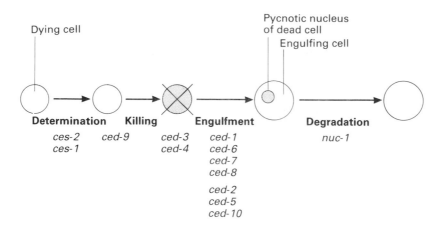

Fig. 2.15. The genes involved in the programmed cell death of two pharyngeal cells of *C. elegans*. (Courtesy of Dr R. Horvitz, Massachusetts, USA.)

mammalian apoptosis in that the nucleus is condensed and the affected cells are swiftly recognized by phagocytes. In addition, this type of death is different from that seen in degenerative neuronal cell death where *ced-3* and *ced-4* are not involved (Ellis *et al.*, 1991). Another example of pro-grammed cell death in development is the removal of the feeding muscles of caterpillars during metamorphosis (Schwartz *et al.*, 1990). Polyubiqui-tin gene expression is thought to play a role in this programme of cell death which may differ from mammalian apoptosis.

There are many candidates for the genes involved in programmed cell death in mammalian cells. Several laboratories have reported the induc-tion of a gene in cells undergoing programmed cell death induced by trophic hormone-removal from sensitive tissues such as the prostate and the breast. This gene was named testosterone-repressed prostate-message 2 (TRPM-2, Fig. 2.16) (Monpetit *et al.*, 1986; Buttyan *et al.*, 1989; Bandyk *et al.*, 1990; Kyprianou *et al.*, 1990, 1991b). Sequence analysis of a partial cDNA encoding TRPM-2 revealed close homology with sulphated glyco-protein-2 gene (SGP-2 or clusterin gene) which is expressed in Sertoli and epididymal rodent cells (Bettuzi *et al.*, 1991). In addition to increased expression of TRPM-2 coordinated with the onset of apoptosis is an enhanced expression of transforming growth factor beta (TGF-β), a potent inhibitor of cell proliferation (Kyprianou *et al.*, 1990, 1991b). Expression of these two genes is also enhanced during the onset of apop-tosis following removal of oestrogen ablation in human breast and prostate tumours (Kyprianou *et al.*, 1990, 1991a). A cascade induction of c-*fos*, c-*myc* and heat shock protein 70 (*hsp70*) transcripts have been observed during apoptosis in the regressing rat ventral prostate gland

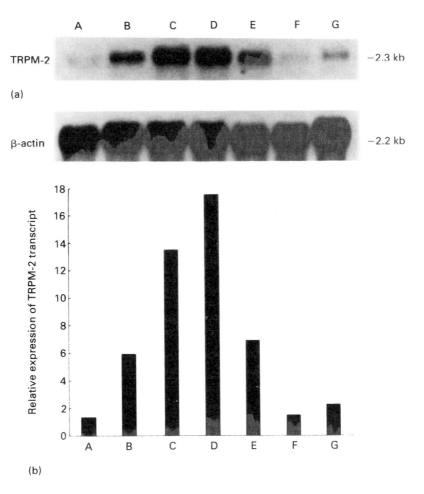

Fig. 2.16. Induction of testosterone-repressed prostate message-2 (TRPM-2).
(a) Expression of TRPM-2 and β-actin mRNA, and (b) relative expression of
TRPM-2 transcripts following androgen ablation. Samples were isolated from PC-
82 tumours of (A) intact mice, (B) 1-day, (C) 3-day, (D) 7-day and (E) 14-day
castrated mice, and of 7-day castrated mice given (F) 7 days or (G) 14 days exogenous testosterone treatment.

following castration (Buttyan *et al.*, 1988). In this system, most of the
acinar epithelial cells die during the first 5 days after androgen ablation.
The c-*fos*, c-*myc*, *hsp70* reactive cascade described mimicks the molecular
events which occur during proliferative stimulation. The authors of this
work suggest that these two basic cellular processes of proliferation and
death may share common signals. In rodent thymocytes two newly discovered mRNAs (RP-2 and RP-8) appear within 2 h of irradiation, a
stimulus known to result in apoptosis in these cells (Owens *et al.*, 1991).

The role of these 'death message' transcripts is not yet defined and their sequence is not homologous to known genes.

Protein synthesis, a requirement for apoptosis?

Many reports emphasize the role of protein synthesis in apoptosis. Cyclo-heximide (and many other protein synthesis inhibitors) completely block apoptosis in several cell types when applied coincidentally with, or even shortly after, the lethal stimulus (e.g. Cohen & Duke, 1984; McConkey *et al.*, 1988). This effect is not universal, however, and there are good examples of apoptosis, defined both morphologically and by DNA cleavage in which cycloheximide has the opposite effect and stimulates apoptosis in the target cell (Cotter *et al.*, 1990; Collins *et al.*, 1991). This paradox is not difficult to resolve. As with other inhibitors, it is not clear that the machinery for protein synthesis is the only target for cyclo-heximide action. Furthermore, what we have shown above indicates that two classes of process are involved in apoptosis. The first requires gene expression, where protein synthesis is presumably responsible for generat-ing the effector molecules of apoptosis. The second requires only the transduction of a lethal stimulus and the activation of preformed effectors. We call the first step 'priming' or 'induction' and it is clearly sensitive to inhibitors of protein synthesis, whereas the second step, which we call 'triggering', is not.

To die or not to die . . .

A central issue in tumour chemotherapy is whether all cells contain the effectors of apoptosis and therefore require only to be triggered in order to enter the process. Conversely, the effector molecules may themselves need to be synthesized before apoptosis can be executed at all (priming). The implications of this second scenario are great. Cells without effector molecules would be unable to enter apoptosis even if exposed to the appropriate triggering stimuli. Although such cells could no doubt be killed by suitably violent perturbations of their environment, they do not possess the means to enter the physiological death programme. Induction of the effectors of apoptosis in such cells would therefore be expected to alter their probability of death in response to a variety of stimuli, including anticancer agents. From studies of two of the effectors mentioned above —the transglutaminase and the Ca^{2+}/Mg^{2+} endonuclease—it is clear that the second scenario is the correct one: not all cells possess the effectors of apoptosis, and in at least one situation, the effectors appear within cells as they become susceptible to apoptosis (Fig. 2.17) (Wyllie *et al.*, 1986). If this process is a general phenomenon, the induction of apoptotic effectors could become a major focus in the search for new anticancer agents. It is

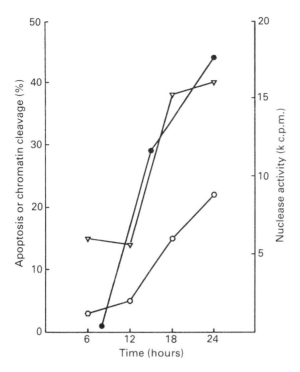

Fig. 2.17. Induction of the morphology of apoptosis (O), endogenous chromatin cleavage (▲) and extractable endonuclease activity (●) in glucocorticoid-treated murine S49 thymoma cells. (Redrawn from Wyllie *et al.*, 1986, with permission from Plenum Press.)

probable that many of the drugs now in use are effective because they trigger apoptosis; they merely activate apoptosis in the subpopulation of tumour cells susceptible to the process in any case. The critical question is whether resistant cells (responsible for tumour repopulation and patient relapse) can be made sensitive by induction of the effectors of apoptosis.

We know little of the induction process, but the presently available clues are of singular interest. One physiological situation provides direct insight into the way in which cells move to and from a state in which they are particularly susceptible to apoptosis (Fig. 2.18). During B-cell maturation within the germinal follicles of lymph nodes, three cellular states can be identified. In the first, cells are out of cycle, but may be activated to proliferate by mitogenic stimuli in the environment of the germinal follicle. Virgin B cells trafficking through the lymph node are in this state which we call **growth arrest**. The second state is characterized by rapid proliferation accompanied by profuse cell death by apoptosis. We call this the **high turnover** state and it is characteristic of the cycling cells within the germinal follicle. Most of these cells die. In the third state cells are selected to provide long-term memory. They proliferate without apoptosis and a

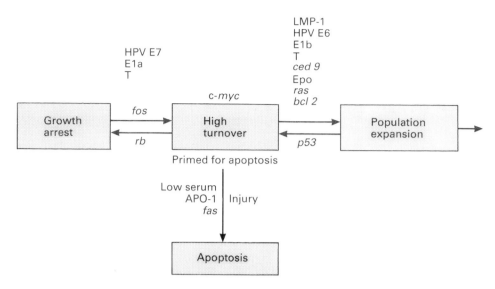

Fig. 2.18. A hypothetical scheme, in which data from many different cell systems are compounded, to illustrate how many critical gene products regulate cell transit to and from the states of growth arrest, high population turnover (with susceptibility to apoptosis) and population expansion. Although the diagram related to proliferating populations, high c-*myc* expression may also induce apoptosis in non-proliferating cells. Abbreviations are as in the text, with the addition of Epo, for erythropoietin, relevant in erythroid precursors of bone marrow (Koury & Bondurant, 1990) and *fas*, a protein identical to the surface receptor APO-1 (Trauth *et al.*, 1989; Itoh *et al.*, 1991).

rapid increase in the size of the selected population occurs. We call this the **population expansion** state.

The regulation of cell movement between these three states is quite well understood. Exit from growth arrest in lymphocytes and other cells requires specific growth factor stimuli (e.g. IL-1–IL-6) and is associated with expression of the immediate early growth response genes such as c-*fos*, *egr-1* and c-*myc* (Sukhatme *et al.*, 1988; Waters *et al.*, 1990, 1991). Whereas *egr-1* and c-*fos* expression is transient, c-*myc* expression persists. Recent evidence is consistent with the view that down-regulation of c-*myc* is a critical signal in returning cells to growth arrest whilst continuous c-*myc* expression commits cells to the high turnover state (Askew *et al.*, 1991; Evan *et al.*, 1992). Movement from the high turnover state to the population expansion state is dependent upon engagement of surface immunoglobulin with the appropriate cognate antigen, and is signalled intracellularly by expression of the proto-oncogene *bcl-2* (Vaux *et al.*, 1988; Tsujimoto, 1989; Hockenbery *et al.*, 1990, 1991).

Detailed analysis of the cultured cell lines derived from BL shows that they can be aligned with this pattern (Gregory *et al.*, 1991; Henderson *et al.*, 1991). Two types of cell line are recognized. Group I cells are closely similar to BL *in vivo*, and behave as if they were in the high turnover state. They show high proliferation and high death rates. They are sensitive to culture conditions, being highly susceptible to apoptosis in response to serum deprivation and other adverse conditions. Due to the well known translocation of c-*myc* to the vicinity of one of the immunoglobulin enhancers, they show constitutive high expression of c-*myc* (Gregory *et al.*, 1990). In contrast, group III cells proliferate without apoptosis, are resistant to adverse growth conditions, and cannot be induced to enter apoptosis by stimuli such as calcium ionophore. They thus exhibit the features of the population expansion state. Significantly, group III cells express genes of the infecting Epstein–Barr virus (EBV) which are silent in group I cells. One of these, *LMP-1*, codes for a membrane protein known to associate with neoplastic transformation, and to be responsible for *bcl-2* induction (Henderson *et al.*, 1991).

It is clear that the proliferative status of the cell is not always inextricably linked to the susceptibility or resistance of the cell to apoptosis. In evidence, non-proliferating thymocytes are acutely susceptible to apoptosis induced by a plethora of agents (McConkey *et al.*, 1988, 1989b, 1990a) and non-proliferating androgen-insensitive prostatic cells undergo apoptosis after ionomycin treatment (Martikainen *et al.*, 1991), whereas other non-proliferating cells, for example in the gut crypt, have been shown to be resistant (Ijiri & Potten, 1983). Recently, expression of *bcl-2* has been demonstrated elsewhere in a number of tissue locations: bone marrow; thymus medulla; CNS neurones; the epithelia of breast ducts, thyroid, prostate and pancreas; and the lower portion of the crypts of large and small intestine (Hockenbery *et al.*, 1991). In all these situations which involve both non-proliferating and proliferating cells, a role for *bcl-2* in prolonging lifespan may reasonably be supposed.

It appears probable that other critical genes may substitute for some of those mentioned above to regulate transition between growth arrest, high turnover and population expansion states in particular cell types. Thus myeloid leukaemia cells expressing a conformationally altered form of *p53* switch to a high apoptotic state on conversion of the *p53* expression by means of a temperature-sensitive mutation to the wild type (Yonish-Rouach *et al.*, 1991). Agents which affect the concentration of wild type *p53* within cells are well known, and include the transforming genes of other DNA viruses—the T antigen of papova viruses, papilloma virus E6 and the adenovirus E1b. Presumably these viral products are acting as surrogates for physiological molecules normally concerned with switching between the susceptibility and resistance to apoptosis. Similarly, *ras* expression appears to hold cells in the resistant population expression state (Wyllie *et al.*, 1987; Sklar, 1988).

One of the key molecules involved in reversion to growth arrest appears to be the retinoblastoma protein RB. Defective RB expression (as occurs in retinoblastoma cells) is associated with persistently raised expression of c-*myc*, whilst transfection of cells with RB under control of a constitutive expression signal leads to growth arrest (Huang *et al.*, 1988). TGF-β appears to induce growth arrest through activation of RB (Moses *et al.*, 1990). Once again, DNA virus-transforming genes appear to have 'tapped into' this mechanism. The RB protein has strong binding affinities for the T antigen, the papilloma E7 product and the adenovirus EIa protein.

Much in the scheme described above derives from observations restricted to one cell type, and the evidence of the states of apoptotic effector molecules is incomplete. Even so, the hypothetical scheme offered here and in Fig. 2.18 has much to offer our concepts of tumour progression and tumour cell drug sensitivity. Firstly, it offers a clear explanation for the selection processes in carcinogenesis that couple together genes that mediate the growth arrest to high turnover transition and the high turnover to population expansion transition, as occurs in DNA-transforming DNA viruses. Presumably, the association of high c-*myc* expression with other genetic abnormalities (e.g. *ras* mutation) which occurs almost universally in malignant tumours reflects the same phenomenon. Whereas entry to a high turnover state might not lead to recognizable tumour growth in every case, addition of a rescuing gene effects the transition to population expansion and the loss of susceptibility to apoptosis. Secondly, this hypothesis rationalizes the otherwise paradoxical clinical observation that some tumours that show high proliferation rates are exquisitely sensitive to chemotherapeutic agents and prone to recurrence in drug-resistant form. Such tumours comprise a high proportion of high turnover cells, all of them ready to undergo apoptosis if exposed to a suitable trigger. The resistant variants are presumably the homologues of group III BL cell lines and represent the persistence of cells in the population expansion state or perhaps their evolution through rescue from the high turnover state. Thirdly, it emphasizes the importance of genes such as *ras*, *bcl-2* and perhaps *p53* in conferring resistance to a wide variety of agents through removal of the susceptibility to undergo apoptosis. Significantly, such pleotropic resistance need not be associated with cell proliferation. It might be expected to be associated with poor prognosis, since the affected cells will be insensitive to both endogenous and pharmaceutical triggers of apoptosis. There is some evidence that colorectal carcinomas with structural abnormalities involving *p53* do indeed carry a poorer prognosis (Kern *et al.*, 1989).

Response to anticancer agents

Some tumour cells appear to be sensitive to the induction of apoptosis in response to anticancer agents which interact with widely disparate primary cellular targets. For example, human promyclocytic leukaemia cells (HL-60) are triggered into apoptosis by etoposide (VP16), campotothecin, cisplatin, methotrexate (MTX), *N*-propargyl-5,8-dideazafolic acid (CB3717), vinblastine, chlorambucil, antinomycin-D (Kaufmann, 1989; Cotter *et al.*, 1990; Walker *et al.*, 1991). Ultraviolet irradiation also results in apoptosis in these cells (Martin & Cotter, 1991). A series of human lymphoid cell lines also exhibit this sensitivity to apoptosis in response to multiple cytotoxic agents including vincristine, 5-fluorouracil (5FU), 1,3-*bis*(2-chloroethyl)-1-nitrosourea (BCNU), melphalan and methylprednisolone (Dyson *et al.*, 1986). Glucocorticoids also induce apoptosis in CCRF-CEM T-lymphoblastoid cells (Yuh & Thompson, 1989).

Not all reports where apoptosis is induced by cytotoxic agents involve haemopoietic cells. Chinese hamster ovary (CHO) cells undergo apoptosis after treatment with MTX, 5FU, VP16, dexamethasone and cisplatin (Barry *et al.*, 1990). Rat hepatoma cells are also triggered into apoptosis by cisplatin (Evans *et al.*, 1991). It appears likely that the death induced in mouse mammary FM3A cells by 5FU and in M14 human melonoma cells by CB3717 and MTX are also effected by apoptosis, although in these cases morphological evidence was not provided (Yoshioka *et al.*, 1987; Lorico *et al.*, 1988). Actinomycin D, mitomycin C, cytosine arabinoside and cycloheximide all induced apoptosis in murine sarcoma (Searle *et al.*, 1975).

Much is known about the primary drug targets in the cell of most of the agents mentioned above, and the interactions of the drugs with their targets are often well characterized. Yet, the events which follow drug–target interaction and precipitate apoptosis are largely unknown. We have speculated that the cell phenotype may be a major determinant of the outcome of drug–target interaction (Dive & Hickman, 1991). We suggest that the critical phenotype is determined by either the existence of the primed (high turnover) state or the ability of the cell to enter it.

In order for a cell to undergo apoptosis after drug insult, it must first sense damage. It must then signal this damage, effect any necessary alterations in gene transcription or translation, and acquire appropriate concentrations and locations of the effector molecules for apoptosis (Fig. 2.19). These stages in this adaptive response of the cell to drugs may vary according to both the cell type and the damaging agent. The ability of the cell to repair damage, or to exclude drug and hence avoid damage, must clearly be taken into consideration. One can envisage 'a race' between damage repair and irreversible commitment for apoptosis. Slow repair may be inconsequential in cells primed for apoptosis. In contrast, the death process may be aborted in cells that can complete adequate repair before achieving transit between states or synthesis of effector molecules for apoptosis. To test these hypotheses we require evidence relating to

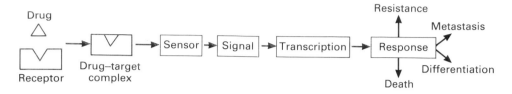

Fig. 2.19. Outline of some of the events described as a cellular response to the formation of a drug–receptor complex. The initiation of the response might be due to the drug–receptor complex *per se*, or to a limited repertoire of metabolic changes which ensue from the drug–receptor complex. (From Dive & Hickman (1991) with permission from Macmillan Press Ltd.)

both the key genes involved in the transit of cells to and from high turnover and population expansion states, and to the presence or absence of effector molecules at the time of drug treatment.

Another consideration is the relevance of the position of the cell in the cell cycle to the onset of apoptosis. Several studies of cycling cells might imply that the initiation of apoptosis is intimately entwined with the regulation of the cell cycle (Eastman, 1990; Kung *et al.*, 1990). Perturbations of normally integrated cell cycle events may present a stimulus to initiate apoptosis. Recent experiments to study apoptosis in CHO cells with differing repair capabilities treated with cisplatin suggest that repair-deficient cells progress through S phase at a normal rate following exposure to the drug, then cells were arrested in G2 and subsequently died via apoptosis (Eastman, 1990). Repair-competent cells transiently arrested in G2 and dependent on cisplatin concentration could eventually recover and survive. The implication of this study was that events determining the fate of the cell occur during G2. This obviously cannot be universally applied as an apoptosis-initiating hypothesis since immature thymocytes rapidly triggered to undergo this process by glucocorticoid are not in cell cycle.

Clearly, several important questions remain with regard to drug-induced apoptosis. Is there a single pathway leading to apoptotic cell death? How do disparate drug-induced cell lesions encompassing direct DNA modulating agents such as cisplatin, enzyme inhibitors such as MTX, and agents like dexamethasone which bind to membrane-bound receptors, all cause the cell to traverse the pathway leading to apoptosis. How is drug-induced damage sensed by the cell? What are the signalling events which follow? If calcium is a central signal involved in activating the endonuclease(s) in apoptosis, do all the above agents provoke this calcium change? What are the critical differences between cells like fibroblasts in which c-*myc* expression appears to specify the high turnover state (Evan *et al.*, 1992), and lymphoid cell lines in which down-regulation of c-*myc* precedes, and is an apparent pre-requisite of apoptosis (Yuh & Thompson, 1989)?

Conclusion

The central hypothesis of this chapter is that both normal tissues and tumours comprise cell populations that differ in their capacity to undergo both proliferation and apoptosis. These differences are conceived as depending upon expression of certain key genes, of which certain proto-oncogenes and tumour-suppressor genes are important examples. Maximum sensitivity to a wide variety of potentially lethal stimuli occurs only when cells are in a state in which physiological apoptosis is also possible, by virtue of the presence of effector molecules (e.g. endonuclease and transglutaminase). Whilst in this state, the cells are liable to proliferate if growth factors are present, but to enter apoptosis if these factors are withdrawn, or if their environment is rendered hostile for other reasons. Hence we have called this the high turnover state. Cells may leave the high turnover state by reversion to a growth arrest (if for instance, c-*myc* expression is down-regulated), or by transition to a second state in which proliferation is possible but apoptosis is improbable. This transition results in expanding cell populations, and is effected by expression of genes such as *bcl-2* or *ras* in appropriate cell types. In this population expansion state, cells are liable to be resistant to many drugs regardless of their primary cellular target, that are effective in the high turnover state where the capacity to undergo apoptosis is restored. The effectiveness of such drugs is liable to be particularly sensitive to temporal factors since the transition between states and the accumulation of the effector molecules of apoptosis are reversible.

Answers to the fundamental questions of why and how a cell dies may provide clues regarding which avenues beckon for improved cancer chemotherapy. Many cancers currently resistant to chemotherapy may be so because their access to the endogenous mechanism of death is suppressed. New therapeutic strategies may profitably be directed against suppression of apoptosis.

Acknowledgements

We would like to acknowledge John Hickman, Chris Gregory, Gerard Evan and Catherine Waters, all of whom made major contributions to the structure of this chapter and the ideas within it, and to the Cancer Research Campaign for our funding.

References

Afanas'ev, V.N., Korol, B.A., Mantsygin, Y.S.A., Nelipovich, P.A., Pechatnikov, V.A.

& Umansky, S.R. (1986). Flow cytometry and biochemical analysis of DNA degradation characteristic of two types of cell death. *FEBS Letters* **194**, 347–350.

Alles, A.J. & Sulik, K.K. (1989). Retinoic-acid-induced limb-reduction defects: perturbation of zones of programmed cell death as a pathogenic mechanism. *Teratology* **40**, 163–171.

Amiesen, J.C. & Capon, A. (1991). Cell dysfunction and depletion in AIDS: the programmed cell death hypothesis. *Immunology Today* **12**, 102–105.

Araki, S., Simada, Y., Kaji, K. & Hirashi, H. (1990). Role of protein kinase C in the inhibition by fibroblast growth factor of apoptosis in serum-depleted endothelial cells. *Biochemical and Biophysical Research Communications* **172**, 1081–1085.

Arends, M.J., Morris, R.J. & Wyllie, A.H. (1990). Apoptosis: the role of the endonuclease. *American Journal of Pathology* **136**, 593–608.

Askew, D.S., Ashmun, R.A., Simmons, B.C. & Cleveland, J.L. (1991). Constitutive *c-myc* expression in an IL-3 dependent myeloid cell line suppresses cell cycle arrest and accelerates apoptosis. *Oncogene* **6**, 1915–1922.

Bandyk, M.G., Sawczuk, I.S., Olsson, C.A., Katz, A.E. & Buttyan, R. (1990). Characterisation of the products of a gene expressed during androgen-withdrawal induced programmed cell death and their potential use as a marker or urogenital injury. *Journal of Urology* **143**, 407–413.

Bansal, N., Houle, A.G. & Melnykovych, G. (1990). Dexamethasone-induced killing of neoplastic cells of lymphoid derivation: lack of early calcium involvement. *Journal of Cellular Physiology* **143**, 105–109.

Barry, M.A., Benke, C.A. & Eastman, A. (1990). Activation of programmed cell death (apoptosis) by cisplatin and other anticancer drugs, toxins and hyperthermia. *Biochemical Pharmacology* **40**, 2352–2362.

Baxter, G.D., Collins, R.J., Harmon, B.V., Kumar, S., Prentice, R.L., Smith, P.J. & Lavin, M.F. (1989). Cell death by apoptosis in acute leukaemia. *Journal of Pathology* **158**, 123–129.

Berridge, M.J. & Irvine, R.F. (1989). Inositol phosphates and cell signalling. Review. *Nature* **341**, 197–205.

Bettuzzi, S., Toriano, L., Davalli, P., Tropea, F., Grassilli, E., Monti, A., Corti, A. & Franceschi, C. (1991). *In vivo*, accumulation of sulfated glycoprotein 2 mRNA in rat thymocyte upon dexamethasone-induced cell death. *Biochemical and Biophysical Research Communications* **175**, 810–815.

Blewitt, R.W., Abbott, A.C. & Bird, C.C. (1983). Mode of cell death induced in human lymphoid by high and low dose of glucocorticoid. *British Journal of Cancer* **47**, 477–486.

Boobis, A.R., Fawthrop, D.J. & Davies, D.S. (1989). Mechanisms of cell death. *Trends in Pharmacological Sciences* **10**, 279–280.

Bowen, I.D. & Bowen, S.M. (1990). *Programmed Cell Death in Tumours and Tissues*, Chapman and Hall, London.

Buttyan, R., Olsson, C.A., Pintar, J., Chang, C., Bandyk, M., Ng, P.Y. & Sawczuk, I.S. (1989). Induction of the TRPM-2 gene in cells undergoing programmed cell death. *Molecular and Cellular Biology* **9**, 3473–3481.

Buttyan, R., Zakeri, Z., Lockshin, R. & Wolgemuth, D. (1988). Cascade induction of *c-fos*, *c-myc* and heat shock protein 70K transcripts during regression of rat ventral prostate gland. *Molecular Endocrinology* **11**, 650–656.

Cohen, J.J. (1991). Programmed cell death in the immune system. *Advances in Immunology* **50**, 55–85.

Cohen, J.J. & Duke, R.C. (1984). Glucocorticoid activation of a calcium-dependent endonuclease in thymocyte nuclei leads to cell death. *Journal of Immunology* **132**, 38–42.

Cohen, J.J., Duke, R.C., Chervenak, R., Sellins, I.S. & Olsson, L.K. (1985). DNA fragmentation in targets of CTL: an example of programmed cell death in the immune system. *Advances in Experimental and Medical Biology* **184**, 493–508.

Collins, R.J., Harmon, B.V., Souvlis, T., Pope, J.H. & Kerr, J.F.R. (1991). Effects of cycloheximide on B-chronic lymphocytic leukaemic and normal lymphocytes *in vitro*: induction of apoptosis. *British Journal of Cancer* **64**, 518–522.

Collins, R.J., Verschuer, L.A., Harmon, B.V., Prentice, R.L., Pope, J.H. & Kerr, J.F.K. (1989). Spontaneous programmed cell death (apoptosis) in B-chronic lymphocytic leukaemia cells following their culture *in vitro*. *British Journal of Haematology* **71**, 353–350.

Compton, M.M., Haskill, S.J. & Cidlowski, J.A. (1988). Analysis of glucocorticoid actions on rat thymocyte deoxyribonucleic acid by fluorescence-activated flow cytometry. *Endocrinology* **122**, 2158–2164.

Conroy, L.A., Jenkinson, E.J., Owen, J.J.T. & Mitchell, R.H. (1991). The role of inositol lipid hydrolysis in the selection of immature thymocytes. *Biochemical Society Transactions* **19**, 90S.

Cotter, T.G., Lennon, S.V. & Martin, S.J. (1990). Apoptosis: programmed cell death. *Journal of Biomedical Science* **1**, 72–80.

Dean, R.T. (1987). Free radicals, membrane damage and cell-mediated cytolysis. *British Journal of Cancer* **55**, 39–45.

Debatin, K., Goldmann, C.K., Bamford, R., Walsman, T.A. & Krammer, P.H. (1990). Monoclonal antibody-mediated apoptosis in adult T-cell leukaemia. *Lancet* **335**, 497–500.

Denekamp, J., Hill, S.A. & Hibson, B. (1982). Vascular occlusion and tumour death. *European Journal of Cancer and Clinical Oncology* **19**, 271–278.

Dive, C. & Hickman, J.A. (1991). Drug-target interactions: only the first step in the commitment to a programmed cell death? Review. *British Journal of Cancer* **64**, 192–196.

Dive, C., Gregory, C.D., Phipps, D.J., Evans, D.L., Milner, A. & Wyllie, A.H. (1992). Analysis and discrimination of necrosis and apoptosis (programmed cell death) by multiparameter flow cytometry. *Biochemica Biophysica Acta* **1133**, 275–285.

Duke, R.C., Cohen, J.J. & Chervenak, R. (1986). Endogenous endonuclease-induced DNA fragmentation: an early event in cell-mediated cytolysis. *Proceedings of the National Academy of Sciences USA* **80**, 6361–6365.

Duvall, E. & Wyllie, A.H. (1986). Death and the cell. *Immunology Today* **7**, 115–119.

Duvall, E., Wyllie, A.H. & Morris, R.G. (1985). Macrophage recognition of cells undergoing programmed cell death (apoptosis). *Immunology* **56**, 351–358.

Dyson, J.E.D., Simmons, D.M., Daniel, J. McLaughlin, J.M., Quirke, P. & Bird, C.C. (1986) Kinetic and physical studies of cell death induced by chemotherapeutic agents or hyperthermia. *Cell and Tissue Kinetics* **19**, 311–324.

Eastman, A. (1990). Activation of programmed cell death by anticancer agents: cisplatin as a model system. *Cancer Cells* **2**, 275–280.

Ellis, H.M. & Horvitz, H.R. (1986). Genetic control of programmed cell death in the nematode *C. elegans*. *Cell* **44**, 817–829.

Ellis, R.E., Yuan, J. & Horvitz, H.R. (1991). Mechanisms and functions of cell death. *Annual Review of Cell Biology* **7**, 663–698.

Evan, G., Wyllie, A.H., Gilbert, C.S., Littlewood, T.D., Land, H., Brooks, M., Waters, C.M., Penn, L.Z. & Hancock, D.C. (1992). Induction of apoptosis in fibroblasts by c-myc protein. *Cell* **69**, 119–128.

Evans, D.L., Gescher, A. & Dive, C. (1991). Cisplatin triggers apoptotic cell death in JB1 rat hepatoma cells (abstract). *British Journal of Cancer* **63**, 41.

Fallon, J.F. & Cameron, J.A. (1977). Interdigital cell death during limb development of the turtle and lizard with an interpretation of evolutionary significance. *Journal of Embryology* **40**, 285–289.

Ferguson, D.J.P. & Anderson, T.J. (1981a). Morphological evaluation of cell turnover in relation to the menstrual cycle in the 'resting' human breast. *British Journal of Cancer* **44**, 177–181.

Ferguson, D.J.P. & Anderson, T.J. (1981b). Ultrastructural observations on cell death by apoptosis in the 'resting' human breast. *Virchows Archives (Pathological Anatomy)* **393**, 193–201.

Fesus, L., Thomazy, V., Autori, A., Ceru, M.P., Tarsca, E. & Piacentini, M. (1989). Apoptotic hepatocytes become insoluble in detergents and chaotropic agents as a result of transglutaminase action. *FEBS Letters* **245**, 150–154.

Fesus, L., Thomazy, V. & Falus, A. (1987). Induction and activation of tissue trans-glutaminase during programmed cell death. *FEBS Letters* **224**, 104–108.

Flieger, D., Reithmuller, G. & Zielger-Heitbrock, H.W. (1989). Zn^{2+} inhibits both tumour necrosis factor-mediated DNA fragmentation and cytolysis. *International Journal of Cancer* **44**, 315–319.

Goldman, A.S., Baker, M.K., Piddington, R. & Herold, R. (1983). Inhibition of programmed cell death in mouse embryonic palate *in vitro* by cortisol and phenytoin. Receptor involvement and requirement for protein synthesis. *Proceedings of the Society for Experimental Biological Medicine* **174**, 239–243.

Gregory, C.D., Dive, C., Henderson, S., Smith, C.A., Williams, G.T., Gordon, J. & Rickinson, A.B. (1991). Activation of Epstein–Barr virus latent genes protects human B cells from death by apoptosis. *Nature* **349**, 612–614.

Gregory, C.D., Rowe, M. & Rickinson, A.B. (1990). Different Epstein–Barr virus–B cell interactions in phenotypically distinct clones of a Burkitt's lymphoma cell line. *Journal of General Virology* **71**, 1481–1495.

Harmon, B.V., Takano, Y.S., Winterford, C.M. & Gobe, G.C. (1991). The role of apoptosis in the response of cells and tumours to mild hyperthermia. *International Journal of Radiation Biology* **59**, 489–501.

Henderson, S., Rowe, M., Gregory, C.D., Croom-Carter, D., Wang, F., Longnecker, R., Kieff, E. & Rickinson, A.B. (1991). Induction of *bcl-2* expression by Epstein–Barr virus latent membrane protein 1 protects infected B cells from programmed cell death. *Cell* **65**, 1107–1115.

Hinchliffe, J.R. (1981). Cell death in embryogenesis. In Bowen, I.D. & Lockshin, R.A. (eds) *Cell Death in Pathology and Biology*, pp. 35–48. Chapman and Hall, London.

Hockenbery, D.M., Nunez, G., Schreiber, R.D. & Korsmeyer, S.J. (1990). *Bcl-2* is an inner nitochondrial membrane protein that blocks programmed cell death. *Nature* **348**, 334–336.

Hockenbery, D.M., Zutter, M., Hickey, W., Nahm, M. & Korsmeyer, S.J. (1991). *Bcl-2* protein is topographically restricted in tissues characterized by apoptotic cell death. *Proceedings of the National Academy of Sciences USA* **88**, 6961–6965.

Huang, H-J.S., Yee, J-K., Shew, J-Y., Chen, P-L., Brookstein, R., Friedmann, T., Lee, E.Y-H. & Lee, W-H. (1988). Suppression of the neoplastic phenotype by replacement of the *RB* gene in human cancer cells. *Science* **242**, 1563–1566.

Ijiri, K. & Potten, C.S. (1983). Response of intestinal cells of differing topographical and hierarchical status to ten cytotoxic drugs and five sources of radiation. *British Journal of Cancer* **47**, 175–185.

Itoh, N., Yonehara, S., Ishii, A., Yonehara, M., Mizushima, S-I., Sameshima, M., Itase, A., Yoshiyuki, S. & Negata, S. (1991). The polypeptide encoded by the cDNA of human cell surface antigen *fas* can modulate apoptosis. *Cell* **66**, 233–243.

Jennings, R.B., Ganote, C.E. & Reimer, K.A. (1975). Ischaemic tissue injury. *American Journal of Pathology* **81**, 179–198.

Kaufmann, S.H. (1989). Induction of endonucleolytic DNA cleavage in human acute myelogenous leukaemia cells by etoposide, camptothecin, and other cytotoxic anticancer drugs; a cautionary tale. *Cancer Research* **49**, 5870–5878.

Kern, S.E., Fearon, E.R., Tersmette, K.W.F., Enterline, J.P., Leppert, M., Nakamura, Y., White, R., Vogelstein, B. & Hamilton, S.R. (1989). Allelic loss in colorectal carcinoma. *Journal of the American Medical Association* **261**, 3099–3103.

Kerr, J.F.K. & Searle, J. (1981). A suggested explanation for the paradoxically slow rate of growth of basal cell carcinomas that contain numerous mitotic figures. *Journal of Pathology* **107**, 41–47.

Kerr, J.F.K., Wyllie, A.H. & Currie, A.H. (1972). Apoptosis, a basic biological phenomenon with wider implications in tissue kinetics. *British Journal of Cancer* **26**, 239–245.

Koury, M.J. & Bondurant, M.C. (1990). Erythropoietin retards DNA breakdown and prevents programmed cell death in erythroid progenitor cells. *Science* **248**, 378–381.

Kung, A.L., Zetterberg, A., Sherwood, S.W. & Schimke, R.T. (1990). Cytotoxic effects of cell cycle phase specific agents: result of cell cycle perturbation. *Cancer Research* **50**, 7307–7317.

Kyprianou, N., Alexander, R.B. & Isaacs, J.T. (1991a). Activation of programmed cell death by recombinant human tumour necrosis factor plus topoisomerase II-targeted drugs in L929 tumour cells. *Journal of the National Cancer Institute* **83**, 346–350.

Kyprianou, N., English, H.F., Davidson, N.E. & Isaacs, J.T. (1991b). Programmed cell death during regression of the MCF-7 human breast cancer following oestrogen ablation. *Cancer Research* **51**, 162–166.

Kyprianou, N., English, H.F. & Isaacs, J.T. (1990). Programmed cell death during regression of PC-82 human prostate cancer following androgen ablation. *Cancer Research* **50**, 3748–3753.

Lanotte, M., Rivere, J.B., Hermouuet, S., Houge, G., Vintermyr, O.K., Gjertson, B.T. & Doskeland, S.O. (1991). Programmed cell death (apoptosis) is induced rapidly and with positive cooperativity by activation of cyclic adenosine monophosphate-kinase I in a myeloid leukaemia cell. *Journal of Cellular Physiology* **146**, 73–80.

Laster, S.M., Wood, J.G. & Gooding, L.R. (1988). Tumour necrosis factor can induce both apoptotic and necrotic forms of cell lysis. *Journal of Immunology* **141**, 2629–2634.

Liu, Y.J., Joshua, D.E., Williams, G.T., Smith, C.A., Gordon, J. & McClennan, I.C.M. (1989). The mechanisms of antigen-driven selection in germinal centres. *Nature* **342**, 929–931.

Lorico, A., Toffoli, G., Biochhi, M., Broggini, M., Rappa, G. & D'Incalci, M. (1988). Accumulation of DNA strand breaks in cells exposed to methotrexate or *N*-10-propargyl-5,8-dideazafolic acid. *Cancer Research* **48**, 2036–2041.

Lucas, M., Solano, F. & Sanz, A. (1991). Induction of programmed cell death (apoptosis) in mature lymphocytes. *FEBS Letters* **279**, 19–20.

McConkey, D.J., Hartzell, P., Duddy, S.K., Hakasson, H. & Orrenius, S. (1988). 2,3,7,8-tetrachlorobenzo-*p*-dioxin kills immature thymocytes by calcium mediated endonuclease activation. *Science* **242**, 256–259.

McConkey, D.J., Hartzell, P., Jondal, M. & Orrenius, S. (1989a). Inhibition of DNA fragmentation in thymocytes and isolated thymocyte nuclei by agents that stimulate protein kinase C. *Journal of Biological Chemistry* **264**, 13399–13402.

McConkey, D.J., Nicotera, P., Hartzell, P., Bellomo, G., Wyllie, A.H. & Orrenius, S. (1989b). Glucocorticoids activate a suicide process in thymocytes through an elevation of cytosolic calcium concentration. *Archives of Biochemistry and Biophysics* **269**, 365–370.

McConkey, D.J., Orrenius, S. & Jondal, M. (1990a). Agents that elevate cAMP stimulate DNA fragmentation in thymocytes. *Journal of Immunology* **145**, 1227–1230.

McConkey, D.J., Orrenius, S. & Jondal, M. (1990b). Cellular signalling in programmed cell death (apoptosis). *Immunology Today* **11**, 120–121.

Martikainen, P., Kyprianou, N., Tucker, R.W. & Isaacs, J.T. (1991). Programmed cell death of nonproliferating androgen-independent prostatic cancer cells. *Cancer Research* **51**, 4693–4700.

Martin, S.J. & Cotter, T.G. (1991). Ultraviolet B irradiation of human leukaemia cells *in vitro*, induces apoptosis. *International Journal of Radiation Biology* **59**, 1001–1016.

Monpetit, M.L., Lawless, K.R. & Tenniswood, M. (1986). Androgen-repressed messages in the rat ventral prostate. *The Prostate* **8**, 25–30.

Morris, R.G., Hargreaves, A.D., Duvall, E. & Wyllie, A.H. (1984). Hormone induced cell death. Surface changes in thymocytes undergoing apoptosis. *American Journal of Pathology* **115**, 426–436.

Moses, H.L., Yuang, E.Y. & Pietenpot, J.A. (1990). TGF-β stimulation and inhibition of cell proliferation: new mechanistic insights. *Cell* **63**, 245–247.

Nicolettei, I., Miglioratti, G., Pagliacci, M.C. & Riccardi, C. (1991). A rapid and simple method for measuring thymocyte apoptosis by propidium iodide staining and flow cytometry. *Journal of Immunological Methods* **139**, 271–279.

Nishikawa, A., Kaiho, M. & Yoshizato, K. (1989). Cell death in the anuran tadpole tail: thyroid hormone induces keratinization and tail-specific growth inhibition of epidermal cells. *Developmental Biology* **131**, 337–344.

Olweny, C.L.M., Katongole-Mbidde, E., Otim, D., Lwanga, S.K., Magrath, I.T. & Ziegler, J.L. (1980). Long-term experience with Burkitt's lymphoma in Uganda. *International Journal of Cancer* **26**, 261–266.

Owens, G.P., Hahn, W. & Cohen, J.J. (1991). Identification of mRNAs associated with programmed cell death in immature thymocytes. *Molecular and Cellular Biology* **11**, 4177–4188.

Piacentini, M., Fesus, L., Farrace, M.G., Ghibelli, L. & Peredda, L. (1991). The expression of tissue transglutaminase in two human cancer cell lines is related with the programmed cell death (apoptosis). *European Journal of Cell Biology* **54**, 246–254.

Pierce, G.B., Lewellyn, A.L. & Parchment, R.E. (1989). Mechanism of programmed cell death in the blastocyst. *Proceedings of the National Academy of Sciences USA* **86**, 3654–3658.

Potten, C.S. (1987). *Perspectives on Mammalian Cell Death*. Oxford University Press, Oxford.

Rich, K.M. & Hollowell, J.P. (1990). Flunarizine protects neurones from death after axotomy and nerve growth factor deprivation. *Science* **248**, 1419–1426.

Rodriguez-Tarduchy, G., Collins, M. & Lopez-Rivas, A. (1990). Regulation of apoptosis in interleukin-3-dependent haemopoietic cells by interleukin 3 and calcium ionophores. *EMBO Journal* **9**, 2997–3002.

Sarraf, C.E. & Bowen, I.D. (1988). Proportions of mitotic and apoptotic cells in a range of untreated experimental tumours. *Cell and Tissue Kinetics* **21**, 45–49.

Saunders, J.W. (1966). Death in embryonic systems. *Science* **154**, 605–612.

Savill, J.S., Dransfield, I., Hogg, N. & Haslett, C. (1990). Vitronectin receptor-mediated phagocytosis of cells undergoing apoptosis. *Nature* **343**, 170–173.

Savill, J.S., Wyllie, A.H., Henson, J.E., Walport, M.J., Henson, P.M. & Haslett, C. (1989). Macrophage phagocytosis of aging neutrophil inflammation. Programmed cell death in the neutrophil leads to recognition by macrophage. *Journal of Clinical Investigation* **83**, 865–875.

Scwartz, L.M., Myer, A., Kosz, L., Engelstein, M. & Maier, C. (1990). Activation of polyubiquitin gene expression during developmentally programmed cell death. *Neuron* **5**, 411–419.

Searle, J., Lawson, T.A., Abbott, P.J., Harmon, B.V. & Kerr, J.F.R. (1975). An electron microscopy study of the mode of cell death induced by cancer-chemotherapeutic agents in populations of proliferating normal and neoplastic cells. *Journal of Pathology* **116**, 129–138.

Sklar, M. (1988). The *ras* oncogene increases the intrinsic resistance of NIH 3T3 cells to ionizing radiation. *Science* **239**, 645–647.

Smith, C.A., Williams, G.T., Kingston, R., Jenkinson, E.J. & Owen, J.J.T. (1989). Antibodies to CD3/T receptor complex induce cell death by apoptosis in immature thymic cultures. *Nature* **337**, 181–184.

Steel, G.G. (1977). *Growth Kinetics of Tumours*. Oxford University Press, Oxford.

Sukhatme, V.P., Cao, X., Chang, L.C. *et al.* (1988). A zinc finger-encoding gene co-regulated with *c-fos* during growth and differentiation and after depolarization. *Cell* **53**, 37–43.

Swat, W., Ignatowicz, L. & Kisielow, P. (1991). Detection of apoptosis of immature CD4+, CD8+ thymocytes by flow cytometry. *Journal of Immunological Methods* **137**, 79–87.

Szende, B., Lapis, K., Redding, T.W., Srkalovic, G. & Schally, A.V. (1989a). Growth inhibition of MXT mammary carcinoma by enhancing programmed cell death (apoptosis) with analogs of LH-RH and somatostatin. *Breast Cancer Research and Treatment* **14**, 307–314.

Szende, B., Zalatini, A. & Schally, A.W. (1989b). Programmed cell death (apoptosis) in pancreatic cancers of hamsters after treatment with analogs of both luteinizing hormone-releasing hormone and somatostatin. *Proceedings of the National Academy of Sciences USA* **86**, 1643–1647.

Terai, G., Kornbluth, R.S., Pauza, D., Richman, D.D. & Carson, D.A. (1991). Apoptosis as a mechanism of cell death in cultured T lymphoblasts acutely infected with HIV. *Journal of Clinical Investigation* **87**, 1710–1715.

Trauth, B.C., Klas, C., Peters, A.M., Matzku, S., Moller, P., Falk, W., Debatin, K.M. & Kramer, P.H. (1989). Monoclonal antibody-mediated tumour regression by induction of apoptosis. *Science* **245**, 301–305.

Trump, B.F. & Mergner, W.J. (1974). Cell injury. In Zweifach, B.W., Grant, L. & McCluskey, R.T. (eds) *The Inflammatory Process*, 2nd edn, Vol. 1, pp. 115–257. Academic Press, London.

Trump, B.F., Valigorsky, J.M., Dees, J.M., Mergner, W.J., Kim, K.M., Jones, R.T., Pendergrass, R.E., Garbus, J. & Cowley, R.A. (1973). Cellular change in human disease. A new method of pathological analysis. *Human Pathology* **4**, 89–109.

Tsujimoto, Y. (1989). Stress-resistance conferred by high levels of *bcl-2* protein in human B lymphoblastoid cell. *Oncogene* **33**, 1131–1136.

Vaux, D.L., Cory, S. & Adams, J.M. (1988). *Bcl-2* gene promotes haemopoietic cell survival and cooperates with *c-myc* to immortalise pre-B cells. *Nature* **335**, 440–442.

Walker, P.R., Smith, C., Youdale, T., Whitfield, J.F. & Sikorska, M. (1991). Topisomerase II-reactive chemotherapeutic drugs induce apoptosis in thymocytes. *Cancer Research* **51**, 1078–1085.

Waters, C.M., Hancock, D.C. & Evan, G.I. (1990). Identification and characterisation of the *egr-1* gene product as an inducible, short-lived, nuclear phosphoprotein. *Oncogene* **5**, 669–674.

Waters, C.M., Littlewood, D., Hancock, D.C., Moore, J.P. & Evan, G.I. (1991). *c-myc* protein expression in untransformed fibroblasts. *Oncogene* **6**, 797–805.

Williams, G.T. (1991). Programmed cell death: apoptosis and oncogenesis. mini review. *Cell* **65**, 1–20.

Williams, G.T., Smith, C.A., Spooncer, E., Dexter, T.M. & Taylor, D.R. (1990). Haemopoietic colony stimulating factors promote cell survival by suppressing apoptosis. *Nature* **343**, 76–78.

Wyllie, A.H. (1980). Glucocorticoid-induced thymocyte apoptosis is associated with endogenous endonuclease activation. *Nature* **284**, 555–556.

Wyllie, A.H. (1981). Cell death: a new classification separating apoptosis from necrosis. In Bowen, I.D. & Lockshin, R.A. (eds) *Cell Death in Biology and Pathology*, Chapman and Hall, London.

Wyllie, A.H. (1985). The biology of cell death in tumours. *Anticancer Research* **5**, 131–136.

Wyllie, A.H. (1988). Apoptosis. *ISI Atlas of Immunology* **0894-3745**, 192–196.

Wyllie, A.H. & Morris, R.G. (1982). Hormone-induced cell death. Purification and properties of thymocytes undergoing apoptosis after glucocorticoid treatment. *American Journal of Pathology* **109**, 78–87.

Wyllie, A.H., Kerr, J.F.R. & Currie, A.R. (1980). Cell death: the significance of apoptosis. *International Review of Cytology* **68**, 251–306.

Wyllie, A.H., Morris, R.G. & Arends, M.J. (1986). Nuclease activation in programmed cell death. In Clayton, R.M. & Truman, D.E.S. (eds) *Coordinated Regulation of Gene Expression*, pp. 33–44. Plenum Press, London.

Wyllie, A.H., Rose, K.A., Morris, R.G., Steel, C.M., Foster, E. & Spandidos, D.A. (1987). Rodent fibroblast tumours expressing *myc* and *ras* genes. Growth, metastasis and endogenous oncogene expression. *British Journal of Cancer* **56**, 251–259.

Yonish-Rouach, E., Resnitsky, D., Lotem, J., Sachs, K., Kimchi, A. & Oren, M. (1991). Wild-type *p53* induces apoptosis of myeloid leukaemic cells that is inhibited by interleukin-6. *Nature* **352**, 345–347.

Yoshioka, A., Tanaka, S., Ossamu, H., Koyama, Y., Hirota, Y., Ayusawa, D., Seno, T., Garrett, C. & Wataya, Y. (1987). Deoxyribonucleoside triphosphate imbalance. 5-fluorodeoxyuridine-induced DNA double strand breaks in mouse FM3A cells and the mechanism of cell death. *Journal of Biological Chemistry* **262**, 8235–8241.

Yuan, J. & Horvitz, H.R. (1990). The *Caenorhabditis elegans* genes *ced-3* and *ced-4* act cell autonomously to cause programmed cell death. *Developmental Biology* **138**, 33–41.

Yuh, Y.S. & Thompson, E.B. (1989). Glucocorticoid effect on oncogene/growth gene expression in human T lymphoblastic cell line CCRF-CEM. Specific c-*myc* RNA suppression by dexamethasone. *Journal of Biological Chemistry* **264**, 10904–10910.

Chapter 3
The cytoskeleton as a chemotherapeutic target

Lisa A. Speicher and Kenneth D. Tew

Cytoskeletal structure

The cell's internal architecture or cytoskeleton consists of a complex network of filamentous proteins which are involved in a plurality of functions including: (i) regulation of cell shape, adhesion and cell–cell interactions; (ii) cell division (Fig. 3.1); (iii) cell motility; and (iv) intracellular organelle movement and protein synthesis. The three principle components of the cytoskeleton are actin microfilaments (MFs), intermediate filaments (IFs) and microtubules (MTs). A number of accessory or filament-associated proteins serve to link these components together as well as to other cellular structures. In addition, accessory proteins play an important role in the regulation of actin and MT polymerization and depolymerization. Although the individual components of the cytoskeleton will be discussed separately, it is important to realize the complexity and interrelations of this system.

Cytoskeleton as a target for cancer chemotherapy

Most of the anticancer agents currently employed that target the cytoskeleton, do so through interactions with the MTs. While a great number of both natural and synthetic compounds are effective MT poisons, the number of agents affecting either actin or IFs are quite sparse. This could indicate a more important role of functioning MTs with respect to cell viability and proliferation as compared to the MFs/IFs. However, this does raise an interesting question as to why a protein as abundant as actin is such a poor target for anticancer agents. Because actin is so well conserved throughout the various phyla, it is unlikely that a significant

57

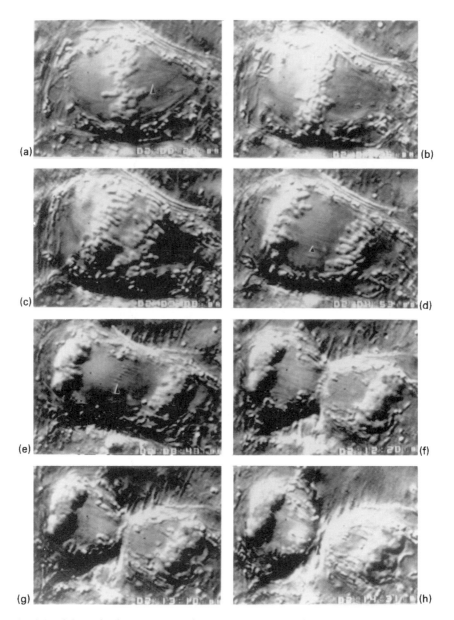

Fig. 3.1. Living mitotic prostate carcinoma (DU 145) cell visualized with video-enhanced differential interference contrast (DIC) optics. Time is displayed in lower right (hour, minute, second, hundredth of a second). (a) Metaphase, showing spindle fibres (arrowhead). (b–d) Anaphase, interzonal microtubule bundles in d indicated by arrowhead. (e) Telophase, stembodies indicated by arrowhead. (f–h) Cytokinesis, midbody indicated in h by arrowhead (bar = 10 μm).

therapeutic advantage could be gained through tumour–normal cell differences in actin expression. Although similar arguments could be applied to tubulin, heterogeneity of expression and the presence of multiple isoforms serves to broaden the 'target base' for antitubulin drugs. In addition, the reduced role of actin in mitotic spindle formation presumably serves to make it a less critical target in dividing cells.

Cytoskeleton of tumour cells

Although the components of the cytoskeleton will be discussed as separate entities, these proteins are linked together and their functions must somehow be coordinated in order to mediate changes in cell shape and resulting cellular functions. Thus, any alterations of one of the many cytoskeletal proteins could have a major impact on the total cellular organization and subsequent functions. The basis of this chapter is to understand the role that the cytoskeleton can play as a target for cancer chemotherapy. While the descriptions given of the individual skeletal components will be for 'normal'-functioning cells, the reader must be reminded that the targets of cancer drugs, neoplastic cells, do not exhibit an entirely 'normal' cellular composition. As an example, normal growth control is an anchorage-dependent phenomenon, while tumorigenicity is correlated with anchorage-independent growth (Shin et al., 1975; Wright et al., 1977; Kahn & Shin, 1979). Studies by Folkman and Moscana (1978) demonstrated a relationship between cell shape and proliferation, such that DNA synthesis decreased as a function of reduction in cell spreading. Because changes in cell shape result in altered macromolecular metabolism and the cytoskeleton is responsible for maintaining cellular morphology, it was hypothesized that the cytoskeletal elements transmit signals of shape changes and surface interactions to the nucleus resulting in biochemical responses (Buckley & Porter, 1967; Albrecht-Buehler, 1977; Puck, 1977). The cell's extracellular matrix also has an impact on phenotypic expression through its modulation of shape in vivo. Resulting changes of even a single cytoskeletal element can effect that cell's response to growth factors through an alteration in the cytoskeletal-regulated signal transduction to the nucleus (Teng et al., 1977).

Neoplastic cell growth is less sensitive to changes in cell shape than that of normal cells, which exhibit a growth control tightly coupled to morphology. Tumour progression is hypothesized to be correlated to altered cellular morphology through a failure of the cytoskeleton to transduce cell shape and surface signals (Wittelsberger et al., 1981). In addition, the metastatic ability of malignant cells is greatly increased when they are grown on non-adhesive surfaces and lose their 'well-spread' morphology (Raz & Ben-Ze'ev, 1981). Thus, it is highly probable that the morphology of a cell is somehow involved in expression of the malignant phenotype.

With respect to alterations in individual cytoskeletal components of neoplastic cells, the most apparent are in the actin MFs and their associated proteins. Numerous studies have demonstrated that transformed cells exhibit a loss of MFs, as well as membrane–MF complexes. In addition, polymerized actin was found to form aggregates near the ventral surface of the cell and a reduction in stress fibres was seen (Mautner & Hynes, 1977; Carley et al., 1981). The disorganization of adhesion plaques, cell substrate contact areas, leads to a loss of fibronectin from the surface and subsequent rounding up of many cells. This is accompanied by loss of adhesion and inability to link actin to the membrane. Recent evidence indicates that tyrosine kinase products of oncogenes (pp60^{src}, yes, abl) (Willingham et al., 1979; Rohrschneider & Najita, 1984) can induce changes in the cytoskeleton through phosphorylation of elements of the adhesion plaque, thus changing the organization of normal cellular function. A better understanding of the mechanism of action of these oncogene proteins could help elucidate the factors responsible for destruction of the signal transduction pathway of normal growth control that occurs during neoplastic transformation.

Controversy surrounds the subject of MT organization in transformed cells. Demonstrations of either altered MT organization or reduction in MT number/tubulin content in transformed cells have come from numerous groups (Fonte & Porter, 1974; Brinkley et al., 1975; Fuller et al., 1975; Ostlund & Pastan, 1975; Edelman & Yahara, 1976). In contrast, no differences in tubulin content of normal versus transformed cells could be detected using a radioimmunoassay technique (Hiller & Weber, 1978). Although transformed cells have disrupted MT–IF interactions, they continue to maintain well-developed MT and IF systems.

In contrast to MTs and MFs, IFs maintain their ultrastructural and immunological characteristics during neoplastic transformation (Osborn & Weber, 1983). In addition, metastatic cells from solid tumours retain the IFs characteristic of the primary tumour. Thus, IF identification of tumour cells has proven to be an invaluable tool in both the classification and diagnosis of tumours.

An understanding of the mechanisms of action of chemotherapeutic agents which target cytoskeletal components requires knowledge of the structure and function of these constituents. Towards this purpose, a review of the individual cytoskeletal proteins is provided; followed by details of what is currently known about anticytoskeletal agents, with emphasis placed on MT poisons.

Actin

Actin, the most abundant protein found in virtually all eukaryotic cells, is a major contractile and structural protein playing a role in cell structure, motility and the generation of contractile force in both muscle and non-muscle cells. It is also one of the most highly conserved proteins in nature with over 80% of the amino acid sequence being shared amongst species ranging from amoeba to humans (Vandekerckhove & Weber, 1978). The widespread distribution and evolutionary stability of actin are indicative of its biological importance. The actin molecule (G-actin) is a bilobed single polypeptide chain (42 kDa) 375 amino acids long (Suck *et al.*, 1981; Korn, 1982), and is associated with one molecule of non-covalently bound adenosine triphosphate (ATP) (Oosawa & Asakura, 1976). Although ATP is hydrolysed during actin polymerization, energy is not required for this process. Actin filaments (F-actin) are polar structures, 8 nm in width with actin monomers uniformly arranged in a tight helix. Actin is distributed throughout the cytoplasm; however, a concentration of actin filaments and associated proteins is found in the periphery of the cell just below the plasma membrane (Bray *et al.*, 1986). This cell cortex provides the surface of the cell with mechanical strength and allows cell movement and shape change.

The polymerization of actin occurs in four reversible steps (Pollard, 1986; Korn *et al.*, 1987):

1 Initially, a slow nucleation of three actin monomers occurs, which is followed by step 2.

2 A bidirectional elongation phase. Elongation ceases when the number of monomers decreases to a concentration such that the rates of loss and addition of monomers at both ends of the filament are equal.

3 Once actin subunits are incorporated into the polymer ends their non-covalently bound ATP molecules are hydrolysed to adenosine diphosphate (ADP) and inorganic phosphate. Although ATP is not resynthesized when F-actin depolymerizes, the ADP bound to the G-actin that dissociates from the filament and exchanges with free ATP and G-ATP-actin is regenerated. Thus, a continual hydrolysis of ATP occurs as a result of actin polymerization and depolymerization (Korn, 1982).

4 Lastly, filaments can fragment in the middle and two filaments can anneal end to end (Oosawa & Asakura, 1976).

Actin filaments exhibit a structural polarity resulting in different kinetics of polymerization at the two ends such that during assembly one end of the filament (plus end) grows faster than the other (minus end). The rate of actin subunit addition to the polymer is proportional to the number of free monomers; however, subunit loss occurs at a fixed rate. As assembly proceeds, the concentration of free monomers decreases until a 'critical concentration' is reached where filament growth ceases due to the equal rates of subunit addition and loss (Bonder *et al.*, 1983). Actin filaments are not static at steady-state because of the different critical concentrations at each end of the filament. This results in a 'treadmilling' effect where the filament continues to grow at one end and shorten at the other, while the total concentration of F-actin remains unaltered.

Numerous actin-binding proteins, capable of interacting with a large number of accommodating binding sites on actin, are responsible for altering the MFs during cell movement, division or differentiation (Stossel *et al.*, 1985; Pollard, 1986; Way & Weeds, 1990). Although the activities of these proteins seen *in vitro* do not necessarily reflect their cellular effects, an understanding of their interactions is critical for the elucidation of MF functions and dynamics. Proteins such as profilin act to sequester actin monomers (G-actin) which prevents the spontaneous nucleation of actin and thus ensures an adequate pool of G-actin monomers for subsequent filament formation. A second class of proteins (i.e. B-actinin and acumentin) regulates filament growth and the equilibrium between F- and G-actin by promoting nucleation and end-blocking of actin filaments. In addition, several proteins which are regulated by calcium concentrations can sever actin filaments into fragments. These include gelsolin, villin fragmin and severin. Other classes include proteins that crosslink actin filaments into bundles or gels (a-actinin, fimbrin, filamin and gelation factor), and those that link actin filaments to the plasma membrane (vinculin and talin). Actin-binding proteins are capable of mediating rapid changes in cytoskeletal organization. Because actin can interact with numerous proteins simultaneously, the balance of actin-associated proteins may be crucial for regulation of actin-dependent processes. Therefore, studies of these actin-binding proteins will prove invaluable for assessing the motile processes occurring in the cells.

Intermediate filaments (IFs)

IFs represent a large and diverse family of insoluble cytoplasmic filaments whose dimensions (8–10 nm diameter) fall between those of MTs and actin filaments. Using biochemical, immunological and molecular biological techniques, at least five distinct subclasses of IF proteins have been identified (Geiger, 1987; Steinert & Roop, 1988). The largest of these are the keratin heteropolymers comprising at least 20 different polypeptides with M_r ranges of 40 000–70 000. These IFs are distinguished by their relative insolubility and are found mainly in epithelial cells. Vimentin (a homopolymer M_r 54 000–58 000) is a major structural protein found in mesenchymal cells such as fibroblasts (Steinert *et al.*, 1984). The morphology of vimentin networks is dependent upon MTs (Goldman, 1985) and in many cells MT depolymerization can result in a collapse of the IF array (Aubin *et al.*, 1980). Other IF classes include those found in muscle (desmin), neurofilaments and glial filaments (glial fibrilar acidic protein) (Small & Sobieszek, 1977; Bignami *et al.*, 1980; Shaw *et al.*, 1981).

IFs are quite distinct from MTs and MFs in that they do not go through an assembly/disassembly process and exhibit half-lives in excess of cell-cycle times. Studies indicate that IFs play a more mechanical and less dynamic role in cells. Their associations with numerous cellular components including the nucleus, mitochondria, plasma membrane and other cytoskeletal elements has led to the idea of IFs being mechanical integrators of cell space (Lazarides, 1980). However, the cellular function of IFs has yet to be clearly defined.

Microtubules (MTs)

MTs are long cytoplasmic cylinder-like fibres, 25 nm in diameter, composed of 13 protofilaments assembled from the 100 000 mol. wt protein, tubulin (Dustin, 1984). Tubulin is a highly conserved heterodimer, consisting of α- and β-subunits, each 50 000 Da, which contains two guanosine triphosphate (GTP) binding sites important in the regulation of polymerization. Tubulin consists of many isoforms (Feit et al., 1977) and expression of these multigene family products is subjected to several post-translational modifications including phosphorylation (Hargreaves et al., 1986) and tyrosination (Gundersen et al., 1984). The reasons for the existence of such a diversity of highly conserved α- and β-tubulin isotypes are not clear but may reflect a functional relationship to specific interactions with MT-associated proteins (MAPs). In order to understand the intracellular functions of MTs and their propensity to act as a target for drugs, the dynamics and control of the MT assembly process must first be considered (for reviews see Kirschner & Mitchison, 1986a; Cassimeris et al., 1988; Engelborghs, 1990).

MT polymerization occurs in three distinct phases: nucleation, elongation and steady-state (Avila, 1990). The nucleation step is believed to occur differently in vitro than in vivo, where in the latter case, nucleation is organized by the centrosome. The polymerization of MTs in vitro requires a minimum concentration of tubulin monomers and some type of oligomer or nucleation centre, where elongation can proceed in both longitudinal and lateral directions (Erickson & Voter, 1986). Oosawa and Asakura (1975) proposed a mechanism for elongation in which the rate of polymerization is determined by the following equation:

$$-dc/dt \;=\; (mck_+) - (mck_-)$$

where c is the tubulin (monomer) concentration, t is time, m is the number of MTs and k_+ and k_- are the rate constants for MT polymerization and depolymerization, respectively. At steady-state or equilibrium, a critical concentration of tubulin is reached where the net incorporation into polymers is zero, and although there is no net change in MT length, there is a continual addition and loss of tubulin from the MT ends. Oosawa and Asakura's equation did explain the mechanism of MT polymerization, however, experimental observations that MTs exhibit a more dynamic nature than predicted needed an explanation (Kirschner & Mitchison, 1986b). The role of GTP hydrolysis may provide such an answer. *In vitro* tubulin polymerization is known to require the presence of GTP (Weisenberg & Deery, 1976). There are two guanine nucleotide binding sites on tubulin: the exchangeable (E) site on the β-subunit non-covalently binds one guanine nucleotide molecule which can readily exchange with free GTP; the non-exchangeable site (N) of the α-subunit does not exchange with exogenous GTP nor is it hydrolysed during MT assembly (Penningroth & Kirschner, 1977). When tubulin becomes incorporated into the growing MT, the GTP bound to the E site is hydrolysed to guanosine diphosphate (GDP) and becomes non-exchangeable (Weisenberg *et al.*, 1976; Carlier & Pantaloni, 1981). This GTP hydrolysis is not coupled to tubulin incorporation into polymer, nor is it necessary for the assembly process. However, the presence of bound GDP serves to destabilize MTs.

How do MTs assemble? Prior to the current 'dynamic instability' theory of MT dynamics, both a treadmilling and capping model had been proposed. The treadmilling model described by Margolis and Wilson (1981) suggested that during steady-state, the plus end of the MT (requiring a lower tubulin concentration for incorporation) incorporated tubulin at the same rate as was released from the minus end. This model hypothesized that GTP hydrolysis was directly coupled to MT assembly and a polymer with defined polarity was formed. Once a tubulin monomer/polymer equilibrium was reached, the average size and net number of assembled MTs did not change. The demonstration by Carlier and Pantaloni (1981) that GTP hydrolysis was not directly coupled to tubulin polymerization argued against the treadmilling model and led to their hypothesis of GTP capping. In this model, which was theoretically described by Hill and Chen in 1984, the GTP–tubulin subunits are at the polymer's ends, whereas the GDP–tubulin is internal. Later studies by Mitchison and Kirschner (1984) showed that MTs of varying lengths existed under *in vitro* conditions where no net polymer changes were occurring. In addition, with longer incubation periods, the number of MTs decreases as their average sizes increases, suggesting the presence of interchangeable growing and shrinking MT populations. These studies and observations led to the currently accepted theory of MT dynamics. MT dynamic instability describes a growing MT assembly and shrinking MT disassembly phase, characterized by the presence or absence of GTP-bound tubulin at the polymer's end. Stable, slow-growing MTs have a GTP cap at their end, while the presence of GDP-bound tubulin at the end leads to rapid and complete depolymerization. The role that tubulin concentration plays in the dynamics of MT polymerization is described as follows (Mitchison & Kirschner, 1984). Incorporation of the subunit into the polymer results in a change in its configuration that triggers the first-order reaction of GTP hydrolysis. The subsequent formation of GDP tubulin occurs at a fixed probability per unit time of hydrolysis. In contrast, GTP–tubulin subunits add to the MT following second-order rate kinetics dependent upon the concentration of monomers. This implies that GTP–tubulin incorporation into the polymer will increase or decrease depending on the presence of high or low tubulin concentrations, and MT will either continue to grow or rapidly depolymerize. The following equation defines the incorporation of monomeric tubulin into the MT polymer within a cell (Mitchison & Kirschner, 1987):

$$\frac{dCp}{dCt} = \frac{(\gamma + 1)(Ct - Cp)^{\gamma}}{(\gamma + 1)(Ct - Cp)^{\gamma} + \eta\Omega_{\gamma}V/NK}$$

where Cp and Ct represent the amount of polymerized tubulin and total tubulin, respectively, exponential γ is an arbitrary number, Ω is the first-order rate constant of growing to shrinking, V is the volume of the cell, η is Avogrado's number, N is number of nucleating MT sites and K is the on-rate constant.

Earlier studies which were not explainable by any previously hypothesized MT dynamic models, are quite compatible with the predictions of the dynamic instability model. These include light microscopic observations of *in vitro* MT behaviour (Horio & Hotani, 1986) and intracellular observations of microinjected fluorescently-labelled tubulin (Salmon *et al.*, 1984).

Other factors to be considered when trying to understand the dynamics of MTs in an *in vivo* system include post-translational modifications and the presence of different MAPs. Specific MAPs may be significant in the differential stabilities of MTs that occur within an individual cell or amongst a variety of cells. In addition, it has been suggested that MAPs may have a role in the enhancement of nucleotide triphosphate affinity for the exchangeable tubulin binding-site (Hamel *et al.*, 1983).

Microtubule-associated proteins (MAPs)

MAPs represent a collection of protein molecules defined by their ability to copurify with tubulin through repeated cycles of assembly and disassembly. These proteins play a crucial role in the regulation of MT polymerization and turnover, and hence in many fundamental cellular events, including mitosis. Although some of these proteins have been well characterized, many remain less well defined. Mammalian brain is a rich source of MTs, which has led to extensive studies of brain MAPs (for review see Olmsted, 1986). The MAPs originally described fell into three categories based on size. These included the high molecular weight MAPs (MAP1 and 2) which were shown to form projections (mol. wt 55–68 kDa). The MAP1 family, consisting of three unrelated polypeptides (MAP1A, 1B and 1C) ranging in mol. wt from 300 to 350 kDa, are heat labile proteins widely distributed throughout a variety of cell and tissue types (Wiche *et al.*, 1984; Bloom *et al.*, 1984, 1985; Koska *et al.*, 1985). MAP1C has since been demonstrated to be dynein, and to function as a retrograde transport motor (Paschal & Vallee, 1987; Vallee *et al.*, 1988). In contrast to MAP1, the heat stable MAP2 family (mol. wt 270 kDa) is restricted to neuronal tissue. Tau was the first MAP identified to exhibit heterogeneity. A single gene is responsible for the numerous tau isoforms (12 currently cloned) occurring through alternative RNA splicing (Himmler *et al.*, 1989). Recently, the determination of the primary structure of tau and MAP2 (Lee *et al.*, 1988; Lewis *et al.*, 1988) revealed that these proteins share two distinguishable, functional domains: (i) a tubulin-binding domain of three (or four) imperfect 18 amino acid residue repeats, each separated by 13 or 14 amino acids; and (ii) a short α helical sequence on the C terminus which through hydrophobic zipper interactions crosslinks MTs into dense, stable bundles (Lewis *et al.*, 1989). In addition, Aizawa *et al.* (1989) demonstrated that an adrenal MAP (190 kDa) contains an MT assembly-promoting sequence homologous to the repetitive sequence in tau and MAP2. It is tempting to speculate that this repeated sequence is a general characteristic of MT binding proteins; however, this domain is absent from the newly discovered kinesin MAP (Yang *et al.*, 1989) as well as the tubulin-binding domain of MAP1B (Nobel *et al.*, 1989).

Other MAPs identified include: 125 and 210 kDa proteins purified from HeLa cells (Bulinski & Borisy, 1979; Weatherbee *et al.*, 1982); the novel brain MAP, MAP3 (mol. wt 180 kDa) (Matus *et al.*, 1983); MAP4 (220–240 kDa) isolated from MT preparations of murine neuroblastoma cells (Olmsted & Lyon, 1981), believed to be the species-specific homologue of the HeLa 210 kDa MAP (Olmsted *et al.*, 1986); stable tubule only peptides (STOPS), found in neuronal tissue and capable of sliding along the MT (Pabion *et al.*, 1984); chartins (Magendantz & Solomon, 1985); and dynamin (100 kDa), which is capable of inducing MT bundling and categorized with MAP1C and kinesin as being a mechanochemical enzyme, able to exert force on the MT (Sheptner & Vallee, 1989).

As mentioned above, different MAP subspecies have been shown *in vitro* to play various roles in the regulation of MT assembly, stability and spatial organization. Although the physical association of MAPs with MTs has been confirmed through electron microscopy and immunofluorescent studies, little is known about the dynamics of their *in vivo* interactions. As MAPs are an integral part of microtubular arrays, it is important to understand their potential role in linking MTs not only to one another, but also to other components of the cytoskeletal system.

Drugs which affect the cytoskeleton: mechanisms of action

MT poisons

Drugs interacting with the colchicine binding-site on tubulin

Colchicine. Colchicine, an alkaloid isolated from the plant *Colchicum autumnale* (meadow saffron), is an anti-inflammatory agent that has been used for centuries in the treatment of gout (Hartung, 1954). It is also the oldest and probably the best known antimitotic agent and serves as a prototype of the spindle poisons. Experimental data demonstrated that colchicine inhibits mitosis in a substoichiometric manner (Taylor, 1965) and blocks the *in vitro* polymerization of MTs (Olmsted & Borisy, 1973). Colchicine binding to tubulin is non-covalent, site-specific and essentially irreversible over a short period of time (Wilson, 1975). Various studies have shown that tubulin dimers have one high-affinity binding-site for colchicine (Shelanski & Taylor, 1967; Margolis *et al.*, 1980) and that the binding reaction kinetics are temperature-dependent (Wilson, 1975). The rate of colchicine–tubulin binding is augmented by anions, which increase the accessibility of the binding site of colchicine's C ring to the tubulin molecule (Bhattacharyya & Wolf, 1976b).

It is hypothesized that colchicine inhibits MT assembly through a sequential binding to, and formation of, a complex with soluble tubulin. This colchicine–tubulin complex binds tightly, but reversibly, to the growing end of MTs, thereby inhibiting further polymerization (Margolis & Wilson, 1977). The detailed molecular methods of colchicine–tubulin binding and events leading to inhibition of MT growth remain controversial. A capping model has been proposed where the tubulin–colchicine complex binds to the net assembly end of a steady-state MT, 'capping' the end and preventing further assembly. The continuing net disassembly at the opposite end of the MT results in depolymerization (Margolis & Wilson, 1978). The binding of colchicine to tubulin is a complex process which has been shown to occur in two steps; a faster, reversible binding followed by a slow conformational change in the protein (Garland, 1978). In addition, colchicine itself undergoes some conformational alterations when binding to tubulin. Colchicine has also been found to inhibit the alkylation and intrapolypeptide crosslinking of β-tubulin by sulphhydryl reactive agents (Luduena & Roach, 1981b), suggesting the presence of a sulphhydryl residue at the colchicine binding-site on tubulin.

The high toxicity level of colchicine limits its clinical value as an antineoplastic agent. This has led to the development of numerous colchicine analogues with improved therapeutic properties. The identification of the active parts of the colchicine molecule (the tropolone and trimethoxy

Benzyl-1,3-benzodioxole backbone

Podophyllotoxin

Steganacin

R = COCH₃ colchicine
R = CH₃ colcemid

phenol rings) has aided this process. There have been few reports of modifications in either the A or C rings of the molecule, whereas modifications of colchicine's B ring have resulted in numerous active derivatives. However, both the A and C ring play critical roles in colchicine's binding to tubulin.

Chalcones. Chalcones are a novel class of antimitotic agents modelled after colchicine. The basic structure of these compounds is a benzalacetophenone (1,3-diphenyl-2-propen-1-one) molecule that contains a trimethoxyphenyl group in addition to a group with the potential to interact with sulphhydryl residues. The prototypical chalcone, when appropriately substituted, acts as a powerful antimitotic agent. Substitutions on the trimethoxyphenyl ring do not significantly alter activity compared to the parent compound. However, 4-dimethylamino or diethylamino substitutions on the acetamido-substituted ring produce enhanced *in vitro* antimitotic activity in HeLa cells, while meta substitution diminishes activity. Other modifications of the compound resulting in diminished biological activity include heterocyclic ring substitution of the dimethyl-aminobenzene ring, and reduction of the carbonyl group or the double bond (Edwards *et al.*, 1990). Some of these compounds exhibit antiproliferative activity comparable to that of vinblastine and greater than colchimide in both animal tumour models and *in vitro*. In addition, one

Vinblastine

Combretastatin

Chalcones

analogue with dramatic *in vitro* antiproliferative activity (Sunkara *et al.*, 1987), acts as a powerful inhibitor of *in vitro* tubulin polymerization and has a greater affinity for tubulin in PtK2 cells than the vinca alkaloids (Peyrot *et al.*, 1986).

Colcemid. Colcemid (*N*-deacetyl-*N*-methylcolchicine, for structure see above) has anti-MT effects at lower concentrations than colchicine. In addition, shorter drug-incubation periods are necessary to produce the same anti-MT effects both *in vitro* and in cells (Serpinskaya *et al.*, 1981). In contrast to colchicine, both the bonding of colcemid to tubulin and the drug-induced MT depolymerization are freely reversible (Banerjee & Bhattacharyya, 1979). The rate of colcemid uptake is fast with evidence of mitotic arrest after only 2 h, compared to 24 h for colchicine. Colcemid also demonstrates much higher rates of binding to and dissociation from tubulin than colchicine, factors which contribute to the differential effects of the two drugs.

Podophyllotoxin. Podophyllotoxin is a natural compound isolated from the root of the May apple (*Podophyllum peltatum*) that competitively inhibits the binding of colchicine to tubulin, but does not share an identical binding site (Cortese *et al.*, 1977). Like colchicine, it blocks both *in vitro*

and *in vivo* MT assembly, inhibits cell division and contains the trimethoxyphenyl ring structure hypothesized to be significant in tubulin binding.
Podophyllotoxin reversibly binds tubulin at a rate 10 times faster than
colchicine and has a dissociation constant of 8.3×10^{-7} M. In addition to
the different binding kinetics, important structural differences exist
between these two molecules. The tropolone ring structure of colchicine
which serves as an attachment point for tubulin is lacking in podophyllotoxin. These data are confusing when considering the competitive
tubulin binding of these agents. However, evidence indicates that colchicine and podophyllotoxin each have two binding domains, one of which
they share (Cortese *et al.*, 1977). Podophyllotoxin-resistant mutants were
reported to exhibit an increased sensitivity to colchicine, strengthening the
hypothesis that the sites of interaction on tubulin of these two drugs do
interact with one another but are not identical (Gupta *et al.*, 1982).
Although podophyllotoxin has been evaluated as an anticancer agent, its
side effects were too toxic for clinical application in cancer treatment. This
led to the development of semisynthetic podophyllotoxin derivatives,
VP-16 (4′-demethylepipodophyllotoxin ethylidene β-D-glucoside) and
VM-26 (4′-demethylepipodophyllotoxin thenylidene β-D-glucoside) for
use as potential antitumour agents. In contrast to podophyllotoxin, these
derivatives block cells in the S or G2 (as opposed to M) phase of the cell
cycle and do not inhibit MT assembly (Krishan *et al.*, 1975). VP-16 is
currently used clinically as an anticancer agent and is believed to inhibit
cell growth by forming a cleavable complex of DNA with topoisomerase
II (Liu *et al.*, 1989).

Steganacin. Steganacin, a lignan lactone derived from the alcoholic extract
of *Steganataenia araliacea* inhibits MT assembly, causes a slow depolymerization of preformed MTs *in vitro*, exhibits antitumour activity *in vivo*,
and prevents formation of mitotic spindle apparatus in sea urchin eggs
(Wang *et al.*, 1977; Schiff *et al.*, 1978; Kupchan *et al.*, 1973). The drug
competitively inhibits colchicine binding to tubulin and has an apparent
K_i value of 3.1×10^{-6} M (Schiff *et al.*, 1978). The trimethoxybenzene ring
structure of steganacin which is shared with colchicine and podophyllotoxin is a likely determinant for its binding to tubulin.

MPTP and combretastatin. MPTP (2-methoxy-5-(2-′,3′,4′-trimethoxy-
phenyl) tropone, a structural analogue of colchicine differing only in the
B ring, and related compound, combretastatin, isolated from the South
African tree *Cambretum caffrum*, both inhibit tubulin polymerization,
have antimitotic activity, and stimulate tubulin-dependent GTP hydrolysis (Fitzgerald, 1976; Ray *et al.*, 1981; Hamel & Lin, 1983). Both agents
bind to tubulin almost instantaneously and reversibly at 4°C and 37°C and
inhibit the binding of colchicine to tubulin with apparent K_i values of

Nocodazole

Benzimidazole carbamates

Dihydropyrido pyrazine

16 μM and 1.1 μM, respectively. Studies with these drugs have helped elucidate the role of colchicine's B ring in tubulin binding. Findings indicate that although the B ring is not required for colchicine's interactions with tubulin, its substituents are important in determining the binding properties of the drug.

Thiocolchicine and derivatives. Alterations in the C ring of colchicine have resulted in compounds that are more powerful inhibitors of tubulin polymerization and cell growth. These include thiocolchicine with a sulphur atom replacing the oxygen atom at C-10 and 4-*N*-acetylcolchinol *O*-methyl ether (NCME) with a benzenoid ring conversion of the tropone C ring (Kang *et al.*, 1990). Both analogues are more effective than colchicine in L1210 murine leukaemia cells (IC$_{50}$ values of 10 nM and 70 nM, respectively) and are more potent inhibitors of tubulin polymerization (Muzaffar *et al.*, 1990). While both analogues bind more rapidly than colchicine, to tubulin only NCME exhibits a readily reversible, temperature-independent binding capacity. NCME and a related compound, allocolchicine, exhibit nearly identical *in vitro* effects including cytotoxicity, prevention of tubulin polymerization, inhibition of colchicine binding and a lack of guanosine triphosphatase (GTPase) effects and polymerization enhancement through drug preincubation (Brossi *et al.*, 1988). Similar to MPTP and allocolchicine, NCME exhibits a biphasic binding to the colchicine site of tubulin, which is hypothesized to be due to the drug binding to two separate species of tubulin (Kang *et al.*, 1990). A battery of thiocolchicine derivatives were demonstrated to be equally effective at binding tubulin as colchicine, but exhibited only weak antitumour activities (Kerekes *et al.*, 1985); indicating that tubulin binding is not solely responsible for biological activity.

Benzimidazole carbamate derivatives. Benzimidazole carbamates include a diverse class of synthetic antifungal and antihelminthic compounds that are known to inhibit the polymerization of tubulin and consequently block cell division (Friedman & Platzer, 1978; Lacey & Watson, 1985; Gupta, 1986). The single structural feature common to this heterogeneous class of antimitotics appears to be the carbamate group.

Nocodazole/oncodazole. Methyl[5-(2-thienylcarbonyl)-1H-benzimidazol-2-yl] carbamate and TN-16: 3-(1-anilinoethylidene)-5-benzylpyrrolidine-2,4-dione are synthetic anticancer agents that exhibit antimitotic activity *in vitro* through interactions with the colchicine binding-site of tubulin (De Brabander *et al.*, 1976). Nocodazole has antitumour activity *in vivo* (Atassi & Tagnon, 1975), stimulates the GTP hydrolysis of tubulin (Lin & Hamel, 1981) and inhibits *in vitro* polymerization of rat brain tubulin, however, it does not depolymerize preformed MTs (Hoebeke *et al.*, 1976). The drug binds tubulin in a mole to mole ratio, is able to bind both tubulin dimers and the polymeric form, and is a competitive inhibitor of colchicine binding to tubulin (apparent K_i value of 0.95×10^{-5}M). TN-16 binds to tubulin in the same manner and has almost equal affinity for the protein as nocodazole (Aria, 1983). Studies with nocodazole-resistant mutants suggest that the mechanism of action of nocodazole is distinct from those of colchicine, taxol, vinblastine, maytansine and griseofulvin, but similar to those of podophyllotoxin (Gupta, 1986). Studies indicate that the carbamate group of nocodazole and related drugs is critical in their interactions with tubulin. A second common structural feature of agents exhibiting nocodazole-like activity is two rings fused in the 3,4-β position; one being a six-membered ring, the other a five- or six-membered ring (Gupta, 1986). Lastly, the presence of a non-polar group in the R_3 position may act to stabilize nocodazole's binding to tubulin.

Tubulozole-C. *cis*-ethyl-4-[2-(2,4-dichlorophenyl)-2-(1H-imidazol-1-ylmethyl)-1,3-dioxolan-4-ylmethylthio]phenyl carbamate exhibits *in vitro* antimitotic effects in both interphase and mitotic tumour cells. Tubulozole-C treatment of cells results in cytoplasmic MT disassembly, arrest of subcellular organelle saltatory movements, dispersion of Golgi cisternae and lysosomes, and the accumulation of IFs into bundles. This agent demonstrates activities similar to other typical antimitotics such as colchicine and the vinca alkaloids including, prevention of MT spindle formation and division in mitotic cells, *in vitro* tubulin polymerization and malignant invasion. Interestingly, the *trans*-isomer, tubulozole-T, has no effect on *in vitro* tubulin polymerization or cellular MT-dependent processes. Such an agent which is both an active and inactive isomer provides a model system for distinguishing specific MT-related changes from non-specific side effects. Presently, the molecular mechanism by which tubulozole-C inhibits tubulin polymerization is not well-defined, but is hypothesized that the carbamate moiety may be required for its anti-MT activity (Geuens *et al.*, 1985).

1,2-dihydropyrido(3,4-b)pyrazines.   1,2-dihydropyrido(3,4-b)pyrazine(1-deaza-7,8-dihydropteridine) compounds cause antimitotic responses in both cultured and *in vivo* cells similar to those of other anticancer agents; however, they have a parent ring structure distinct from any known anticancer agent (Wheeler *et al.*, 1981; Temple *et al.*, 1982). Structurally, the presence of a 6-substituent containing an aryl group is required for antimitotic activity which can be augmented with a methyl group substitution at position 7 (Temple *et al.*, 1983). One of these compounds (NSC 370147) which has been selected for potential preclinical development, completely inhibits colchicine binding to purified tubulin (apparent K_i value of 0.62 μM) and when combined with vincristine, exhibits synergistic effects in prolonging the lives of P388 leukaemic bearing mice as well as killing cultured L1210 cells (Bowdon *et al.*, 1987).

Drugs interacting with the vinblastine binding-site on tubulin

Vinca alkaloids. Vinblastine and vincristine, isolated from the Madagascan periwinkle plant *Catharanthus rosea* are clinically the most important mitotic inhibitors and serve as major players in cancer chemotherapeutic regimens. These asymmetrical, dimeric compounds exhibit differential, concentration-dependent effects on MTs. Lower concentrations of vinblastine cause mammalian cells to arrest in mitosis, coinciding with a depolymerization of cellular MTs, while higher drug levels elicit the unique formation of paracrystalline arrays of tubulin associated with the cytoskeleton. The paracrystals formed are short, rod-like structures containing large macrotubules consisting of two intertwined helical tubulin aggregates, arranged in parallel along their axis (Fujiwara & Tilney, 1975). Paracrystals isolated from sea urchin eggs as well as those prepared from purified tubulin *in vitro* contain one molar equivalent of vinblastine and are capable of binding an additional molar equivalent of drug (Bryan, 1972; Na & Timasheff, 1982). Wilson *et al.* (1978) demonstrated that the two vinblastine binding-sites in the paracrystals had similar drug affinities and drug-binding properties were independent of temperature. Although colchicine and podophyllotoxin do not cause paracrystal formation, they are able to bind to vinblastine-induced paracrystals (Na & Timasheff, 1982). Immunofluorescent studies showed these paracrystals to be retained in the cytoskeleton of extracted cells and stable to polymerization by calcium. The fact that vinblastine does not cause MT depolymerization or tubulin paracrystal formation in extracted cells suggestes that vinca akaloids require tubulin dimers to produce antimitotic effects, rather than a direct interaction with MTs (Manfredi & Horwitz, 1984b). Vinblastine binds tubulin at two distinct sites in a rapid, reversible manner. However, values for the reported binding affinities and the number of these sites remains controversial (Wilson et al., 1975; Bhattacharyya & Wolff, 1976b; Mandelbaum-Shavit et al., 1976; Lacey et al., 1987). While numerous groups report one class of vinblastine binding-site (Owellen et al., 1972; Wilson et al., 1975; Conrad et al., 1979), others provide strong evidence for two distinct classes. Reports by Bhattacharyya and Wolff (1976) demonstrated both a high-affinity site, responsible for inhibition of MT assembly, and a low-affinity site, which when occupied causes paracrystal formation. These studies are supported by those of Safa et al. (1987) who also describe two classes of tubulin vinblastine binding-sites. In addition, others have found multiple low-affinity sites on tubulin, perhaps involved in tubulin precipitation (Lee et al., 1975; Na & Timasheff, 1986).

In addition to inhibiting MT assembly, the vinca alkaloids effect tubulin–GTP interactions. While vinblastine and vincristine augment GTP binding to tubulin at both 0 and 37°C (Tan & Lagnado, 1975), they either weakly inhibit or have no effect on nucleotide exchange in the tubulin–colchicine complex at 0 and 37°C; respectively (Tan & Lagnado, 1975). In addition, vinblastine binding to tubulin causes a marked inhibition of the protein's GTPase activity (David-Pfeuty et al., 1977, 1979).

The actions of the vincas are quite distinct in that they do not merely prevent tubulin polymerization. Lower concentrations of the drug disassemble steady-state MTs yielding oligomeric and polymeric rings (David-Pfeuty et al., 1977; Batra et al., 1986; Safa et al., 1987) and tightly coiled spirals which form from protofilaments peeling off MT ends (Warfield & Bouck, 1974; Himes et al., 1976; Parness & Horwitz, 1981). Formation of the spiral coils is strongly enhanced by the presence of tau proteins, and these coils are stable to cold, calcium-induced and colchicine-induced polymerization (Haskins et al., 1981; Luduena et al., 1981). Although controversy still exists, most of the reported observations indicate that the predominant effects of the vincas are due to their binding at a single site on tubulin.

Structural modification of the vincas has provided some insight into the portion of the molecule responsible for its biological activity. Although few analogues have been examined, studies indicate that modifications of the pentacyclic (vindoline) portion of vinblastine have little effect on activity (Owellen et al., 1976; Wilson et al., 1978); whereas alterations in the tetracyclic (catharanthine) moiety can alter biological responses. A single high-affinity vinca site on tubulin is believed to be responsible for the effects of a number of structurally diverse antimitotic natural products including maytansine, rhizoxin, phomopsin A and dolastatins (Mandelbaum & Shavit et al., 1976).

Maytansine. Maytansine is a novel ansa macrolide isolated from numerous *Maytenus* plant species that exhibits potent antimitotic effects (Remillard *et al.*, 1975), produces MT disassembly both *in vitro* (Luduena & Roach, 1981a) and *in vivo* (Schnaitman *et al.*, 1975), and inhibits tubulin-dependent GTP hydrolysis and nucleotide exchange (Lin & Hamel, 1981) and MAP-mediated MT assembly (York *et al.*, 1981; Huang *et al.*, 1985). Maytansine binding to tubulin is rapid, reversible and occurs with a higher affinity than the vinca alkaloids (Mandelbaum-Shavit *et al.*, 1976; York *et al.*, 1981). The presence of the 19-member macrolide ring is critical to anti-MT activity; however, antibiotics can differ in their R groups while possessing *in vitro* and *in vivo* activities similar to maytansine (Ootus *et al.*, 1980).

Rhizoxin. Rhizoxin, isolated from the fungus *Rhizopus chinensis*, is a 16-membered macrolide exhibiting both antifungal and antitumour activities (Iwasaki, 1985). The drug produces MT disassembly, interferes with *in vitro* tubulin polymerization and inhibits mitosis. Rhizoxin binds tubulin in a rapid, reversible manner with a K_D of 1.7×10^{-7} M (Takahashi *et al.*, 1987). Although rhizoxin's tubulin binding-site is distinct from vinblastine and colchicine, it is identical with maytansine and ansamitocin P-3. The structural feature hypothesized to be most critical for the drug's activity is its macrocyclic lactone ring (Takahashi *et al.*, 1987). However, the epoxide groups at positions 2, 3 and 11, 12 are critical, since their reduction causes significant loss in activity. This suggests a possible role for thiol reactivity at these sites. Of interest, rhizoxin produces strong effects in both plant and animal tissues, placing it in a select group of antimitotic agents.

Phomopsin A. Phomopsin A, a fungal toxin produced by *Phomopsis leptostromiformis*, is a hexapeptide mycotoxin containing a 13-membered ring formed by an ether bridge. It is the causative agent in the livestock disease lupinosis, characterized by mitotic arrest of hepatocytes (Van Warmelo *et al.*, 1970). The most active ingredient of the fungal extract is phomopsin A, which was found to be a potent inhibitor of tubulin polymerization with concentrations of less than 1 μM sufficient to block MT assembly. This drug inhibits the binding of vinblastine, while enhancing that of colchicine's to tubulin. Phomopsin's high levels of toxicity limits its therapeutic usefulness, however, its anti-MT activities warrant further study to elucidate structural requirements for such microtubule inhibitory effects.

Dolastatin. Dolastatin 10, a potent antimitotic peptide isolated from the marine shell-less mollusc *Dolabella auricularia*, is the first natural antimitotic product from an animal source (Bai *et al.*, 1990a). It is a linear

Taxol

Dolavaline | Valine | Dolaisoleuine | Dolaproine | Dolaphenine

Dolastatin 10

peptide containing four amino acid residues (three of these are unique: dolavaline, dolaisoleucine and dolaproline) linked to the primary amine dolaphenine. The drug inhibits *in vitro* MT assembly, mitosis in cultured cells, tubulin-dependent GTP hydrolysis and the binding of vinblastine and vincristine to tubulin (Bai *et al.*, 1990b). A comparative analysis of dolastatin with other antimitotics that effect the binding of vinca alkaloids to tubulin showed that maytansine, rhizoxin and vinblastine were competitive inhibitors of vincristine binding to tubulin while dolastatin 10 and phomopsin A demonstrated non-competitive inhibition. Dolastatin 10 and phomopsin are believed to bind the same peptide site of tubulin and share similar activites. These include the inhibition of tubulin polymerization, tubulin-dependent GTP hydrolysis and nucleotide exchange on tubulin, and the stabilization of colchicine binding activity of tubulin. Although there are numerous possible vinca alkaloid binding-sites on tubulin, the effects of the drugs studied appear to involve a high-affinity vinca site, located primarily on β-tubulin. Interestingly, these four compounds are highly diversified structurally and show no apparent common features with the vincas to explain their inhibition of vinca binding.

Taxol

Taxol, isolated from the plant *Taxus brevifolia*, was first reported to have antitumour effects by Wani *et al.* (1971). The drug's chemical structure, an ester containing a taxane derivative with an oxetan ring is unusual. Schiff *et al.* (1979) reported that taxol promotes *in vitro* calf brain MT assembly by reducing the critical concentration of tubulin and shifting the equilibrium between the tubulin dimer and polymer towards the polymer. The drug is a unique MT poison in being the only agent to promote MT assembly and stabilize MTs to depolymerization, even at low temperatures and in the presence of antimitotics such as colchicine (Manfredi & Horwitz, 1984a). MTs can form in the presence of taxol under conditions that normally would prevent their assembly, including the absence of MAPs and the presence of exogenously added GTP and organic buffers (Hamel *et al.*, 1981; Kumar, 1981). Taxol blocks cells in late $G2/M$ phase of the cell cycle and has no significant effect on DNA, RNA or protein synthesis in cells. An unusual structure anomaly in taxol-treated cells is the formation of prominent MT bundles, which are concentration-, time- and energy-dependent (Manfredi *et al.*, 1982). Evidence indicates that the intracellular binding-sites for taxol is the polymerized form of tubulin. This binding site is distinct from the exchangeable GTP site as well as the colchicine, vinblastine and podophyllotoxin sites (Kumar, 1981; Schiff & Horwitz, 1981). Taxol binds specifically and reversibly with maximal effects at a concentration stoichiometric with tubulin dimer concentration (Parness & Horwitz, 1981). In addition, MTs polymerized in the presence of $10 \mu M$ taxol are shorter than control MTs (average length $4.12 \mu m$ versus $1.49 \mu m$), suggesting that taxol increases the number of nucleation events prior to MT formation (Schiff & Horwitz, 1981). Furthermore, taxol changes the kinetics of tubulin assembly, practically eliminating the typical 3–4 min lag time prior to onset of polymerization.

Sulphhydryl-reacting compounds

Sulphhydryl groups are believed to play a role in mitosis. Thiol-containing molecules, such as glutathione, have been shown to be critical for optimal MT assembly in cells and for maintaining MT structure and organization of the mitotic spindle during cell division (Nathan & Rebhun, 1976; Tew *et al.*, 1986). In addition, alkylation of a small number of tubulin sulphhydryl groups results in a complete inhibition of *in vitro* MT assembly. Numerous agents are believed to inhibit MT assembly through their interactions with tubulin's sulphhydryl groups.

Included in this class are the chlorinated derivatives of benzyl thiocyanate. The initial compound in this series of antimitotic agents, 2,4-dichlorobenzyl thiocyanate (DCBT), was shown to induce mitotic arrest, irreversibly inhibit *in vitro* tubulin polymerization and disrupt intracellular

MTs (Abraham *et al.*, 1986). Although additional studies were not able to show a significant effect of DCBT on purified tubulin polymerization or assembly of MTs, they did reveal that tubulin was the intracellular target of DCBT (Bai *et al.*, 1989). DCBT was shown to be an alkylating agent forming a mixed disulphide with tubulin. β-tubulin is preferentially alkylated at low drug concentrations, while at higher DCBT concentrations, both α- and β-tubulin are alkylated.

Cis-dichlorodiammine-platinum (CDDP), a widely used anticancer agent, exhibits antitumour activity through interactions with DNA. Recent evidence indicates that CDDP is an *in vitro* inhibitor of MT polymerization (Peyrot *et al.*, 1986). CDDP binds covalently and irreversibly to tubulin thiol residue sites, and one blocked sulphhydryl group (approximately 20 sulphhydryl groups per tubulin dimer) is sufficient for polymerization inhibition. Evidence indicates that the binding sites for CDDP are distinct from those of colchicine or the vinca alkaloids.

Other compounds that have been shown to inhibit MT assembly through their interactions with tubulin's sulphhydryl groups include: (i) triethyl-lead ion (Et_3PB^+), which interacts with two of tubulin's 18 thiol groups leading to inhibition of *in vitro* tubulin polymerization and disassembly of preformed MTs (Faulstich *et al.*, 1984); (ii) 4-hydroxy-alkenals which are metabolic products of polyunsaturated fatty acids produced during lipid peroxidation that cause numerous damaging effects in cells. They interact with tubulin's sulphhydryl groups, resulting in a dose-dependent (0.1–1 mM) inhibition of tubulin polymerization, and an inhibition of colchicine binding to the protein (Gabriel *et al.*, 1985); and (iii) the organic sulphhydryl-blocking reagents, *p*-chloromercuribenzene sulphinic acid (PCMBS) and *N*-ethylmaleimide (NEM) are capable of inhibiting polymerization of tubulin (Kuriyama & Sakai, 1974; Abe *et al.*, 1975) as well as influencing MT-associated adenosine triphosphatase (ATPase) activity. At low concentrations (pH of 6.8), both agents stimulate Mg^{2+}– ATPase activity, while higher concentrations are inhibitory (Wallin *et al.*, 1979).

Estramustine

Estramustine was synthesized in the mid-1960s (Fex *et al.*, 1967), as a compound which could improve specificity for the treatment of breast cancer. Interestingly, it has turned out that the rationale for the drug design has resulted in a drug with considerable specificity and biological activity. Moreover, such characteristics arise for reasons unrelated to conceptual considerations in the drug's design. The molecule is oestradiol attached to nor-nitrogen mustard via a carbamate–ester linkage. In proprietary form, the drug has a phosphate at the 17β position of the steroid D ring in order to enhance its solubility in water. Treatment of animals or

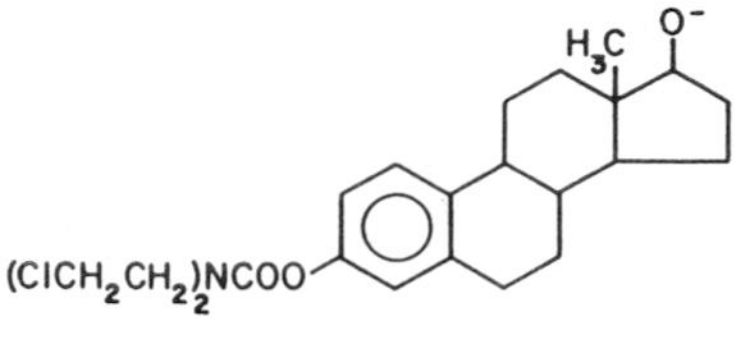

Estramustine

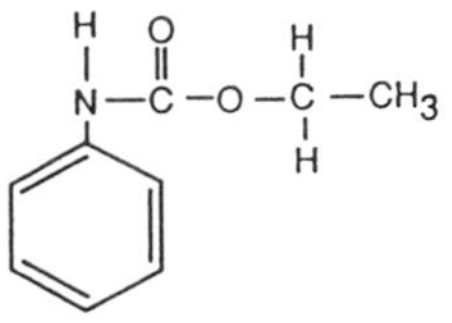

Isopropyl carbamate

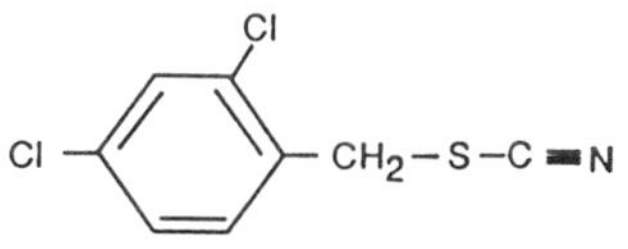

2,4-Dichlorobenzyl thiocyanate

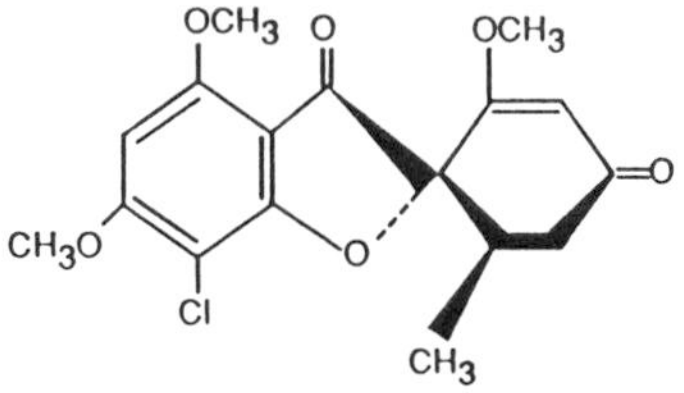

Griseofulvin

cells with the compound results in a rapid dephosphorylation and subsequent production of estramustine or its oxidized metabolite, estromustine (Gunnarsson et al., 1981).

The initial rationale dictated that the steroid moiety would facilitate selective uptake of estramustine in oestrogen receptor-positive tumours, producing elevated levels of drug in malignant tissue. Subsequently, the drug would undergo intracellular cleavage, via hydrolytic enzymes, to form oestradiol and nor-nitrogen mustard. The release of the nor-nitrogen mustard would then presumably result in covalent drug-induced damage to cellular nucleophilic sites contained in nucleic acids and proteins.

In earlier studies, several observations indicated that an unusual mechanism of action underlay the drug's pharmacological properties. In addition to showing activity in oestrogen receptor-negative cell lines, estramustine binding was not competitively inhibited by greater than 1000-fold excess concentrations of oestradiol (Tew, 1983). Further, the drug possessed no alkylating activity *in vitro* at concentrations which induced cytotoxicity (Tew et al., 1983). Accumulation of data from a large number of clinical experiences also was consistent with a lack of alkylating activity since toxicity to rapidly dividing tissues such as bone marrow and gastrointestinal epithelia was not apparent.

A clue to the possible mechanism of action of estramustine was revealed when the drug was shown to accumulate cells in metaphase (Hartley-Asp, 1984; Tew et al., 1986). Since that time it has become apparent that the pharmacological activity of estramustine is due to its effects on the cytoskeleton, specifically MAPs rather than via covalent interactions with proteins and/or nucleic acids (Kanje et al., 1985; Stearns & Tew, 1985). The drug was shown to effect rapid disassembly of MTs at concentrations between 30 and 120 μM. Interphase and mitotic MTs were

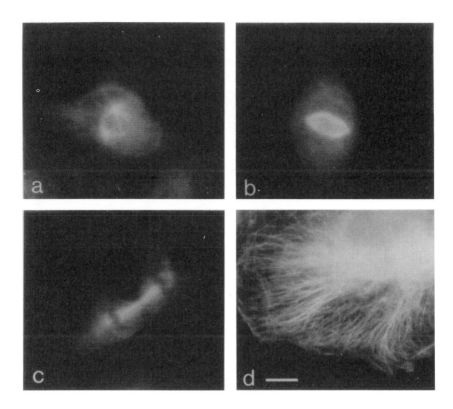

Fig. 3.2. Immunofluorescent micrographs of mitotic (a–c) and interphase DU 145 cells labelled with antibody raised against β-tubulin. (a) Prophase, (b) metaphase, (c) intercellular microtubules and midbody between daughter cells, and (d) interphase microtubules were not destroyed in 20 μM estramustine (bar = 10 μM).

both shown to be disrupted by estramustine. The only subset of MTs which appeared resistant to the drug were those composing the intra-cellular bridge between daughter cells during telophase and cytokinesis (Stearns & Tew, 1985). Experiments conducted *in vitro* showed that estramustine exerts a cytotoxic effect on cells via MT distribution through non-covalent binding to MAPs.

The precise mechanism(s) by which the drug induces cytolysis remain to be elucidated, Firstly, it is not yet known whether estramustine has a primary cytotoxic effect on one phase (e.g. mitosis) of the cell cycle or instead exerts a multiplicity of effects on several MT-regulated processes (Fig. 3.2). In fact, Mareel *et al.* (1988) have shown that the drug also inhibits the invasive activity of malignant mouse MO_4 cells and human DU 145 cells, suggesting that estramustine may inhibit cell motility and/or secretory processes, presumably by effecting the disassembly of interphase MTs. Secondly, the concentrations of estramustine utilized in the majority of studies to date range from 10 to 120 μM, which are relatively high for a compound with a target specificity. Such concentrations could possibly exert pleiotropic effects on metabolic processes and create an imbalance in the thiol–disulphide balance existent within cells. Indeed, estramustine affects both the level of intracellular glutathione as well as glutathione S-transferase activity (Tew *et al.*, 1986). Other antimitotic agents such as the vinca alkaloids have been shown to cause a shift in the thiol–disulphide balance in cells (Beck, 1980). It therefore seems critical to an understanding of estramustine's mechanism(s) of action to know whether the drug acts in a specific way in the cell cycle, and if so, then what concentration is necessary for this activity.

Griseofulvin

Initial reports suggested that relatively high concentrations of the antifungal drug griseofulvin (isolated from *Penicillium griseofulvin*) caused mitotic arrest in mammalian cells (Paget & Walpole, 1958; Grisham *et al.*, 1973). The anti-MT effects have been linked to drug binding to both tubulin (Sloboda *et al.*, 1982) and MAPs (Roobol *et al.*, 1977). Although there is presently no consensus upon the precise nature of the drug binding-site, drug-induced stimulation of tubulin-dependent GTP hydrolysis and enhancement of vinblastine-induced paracrystal formation in ova from sea urchins (Starling, 1976; David-Pfeuty *et al.*, 1979) suggest a more likely role for direct binding to tubulin.

Miscellaneous agents

DDP (5,6 diphenylpyriadazin-3-one) derivatives. DDP is an active herbicide that has significant antimitotic effects in intact animals as well as activity against murine P388 leukaemia. *In vitro* effects of these derivatives include stimulation of tubulin-dependent GTP hydrolysis and inhibition of MT assembly (10 μM results in complete inhibition of nucleation, elongation and polymerization of purified tubulin and MAPs). This new class of antimitotic agents is believed to bind tubulin at a site distinct from any previously described, as inferred from a lack of interference of tubulin's interactions with GTP, vinblastine, colchicine or maytansine. Structural requirements for antitubulin activity appear to include the two phenol rings which are capable of exhibiting some degree of mobility. In addition, the substituents at position 4 of the pyridazinone ring appear to be important factors in the antimitotic effects (Batra *et al.*, 1986).

2-styrylquinazolin-4(3H)-ones. Compounds in this series of novel antimitotic agents which exhibit significant *in vitro* tumour cell inhibitory activity in L1210 murine leukaemia cells contain a 2-styryl-quinazolin-4(3H)-one structure. Five of the 23 compounds tested *in vivo* prolong the life-spans of tumour-bearing animals. The mechanisms of action for most of the inhibitory compounds include inhibition of MAP-dependent MT assembly, inhibition of polymerization of purified tubulin and accumulation of cells in metaphase. Inhibition of tubulin polymerization is maximized when compounds contain an intact core 2-styrylquinazolin-4(3H)-one structure with position 6 having either a halide or methyl/methoxy substituent. This class of compounds shares structures and activities similar to combretastatin and derivatives. Both classes of drugs have quantitatively similar effects on tubulin polymerization inhibition and both have a two-carbon bridge separating two aromatic rings. Combretastatin is a powerful competitive inhibitor of colchicine binding to tubulin, however, the 2-styrylquinazolin-4(3H)-ones demonstrate weak effects on this interaction. Current studies hope to elucidate the characteristics of the interaction of this novel antimitotic agent with tubulin (Jiang *et al.*, 1990).

Chlorpromazine. Chlorpromazine (chlorpromazine hydrochloride,2-chloro-10-(3-dimethylaminopropyl)-phenothiazine: CPZ) is a tranquillizing drug which interacts reversibly with tubulin, causing MT disruption and the *in vitro* arrest of cells in mitosis (Boder *et al.*, 1983). Comparative studies of antitubulin activity of other phenothiazines demonstrated that while trifluoperazine is a more potent inhibitor of tubulin polymerization than CPZ, the non-tranquillizing agent, promethazine, causes a slight enhancement of assembly (Appu Rao & Cann, 1981).

Other agents which have been shown to exhibit anti-MT activity include: (i) rotenone, widely used as a respiratory inhibitor, is a potent, but reversible inhibitor of tubulin polymerization (Marshall & Himes, 1978); (ii) methylmercury (MeHg), a potent neurotoxic agent (Sager *et al.*, 1983); (iii) rifampicin, a semisynthetic antibiotic (Rajagopalan & Gurnani, 1983); (iv) the metahalone class of antimitotics which arrest cells in metaphase and are dependent on the presence of a halogen atom in the molecule (Gacek *et al.*, 1979) including 5-fluoropyrimidin-2-one (Oftebro *et al.*, 1972) and 1-propargyl-5-chloropyrimidin-2-one (Dornish *et al.*, 1984). Diethylstilboestrol (DES), the synthetic oestrogen, has colcemid-like effects on cells, causing mitotic spindle abnormalities and an increase in mitotic index (Parry *et al.*, 1982).

MF poisons

Cytochalasins and phalloidins

Cytochalasins and phalloidins have no apparent clinical utility. However, they have been of value in furthering studies of cytoskeletal proteins, as well as the fundamental processes of actin polymerization. An analogy may be drawn between the opposing mechanisms of action of these actin-binding drugs with those of the previously described MT inhibitors. While the cytochalasins' actions as 'capping proteins' are similar to those of the vinca alkaloids, phalloidin serves to stabilize actin filaments in a manner similar to taxol's effects on MTs.

The cytochalasins are a family of fungal metabolites which freely permeate cell membranes and bind to actin, leading to an inhibition of many types of cellular motility functions, including ruffling and translocating (Schliwa, 1982; Yahara *et al.*, 1982), phagocytosis and cytokinesis. Cytochalasins bind to the fast-growing end of actin filaments with a 1 : 1 stoichiometry, causing an inhibition both of association and dissociation of subunits at that end (Flanagan & Lin, 1980).

Phalloidin is a bicyclic heptapeptide derived from the poisonous mushroom *Amanite phalloides*. Its mechanism of action is the opposite of the cytochalasins, serving to stabilize actin filaments and thereby preventing depolymerization. Phalloidin lowers the critical concentration for polymerization by binding to actin filaments and shifting the equilibrium between monomers and filaments towards filaments (Faulstich *et al.*, 1977; Estes *et al.*, 1981). Because phalloidins do not freely permeate cell membranes, their usefulness in experiments with living cells is limited. However, their specific binding to actin filaments renders them useful for the fluorescent staining of actin filaments in fixed cells.

Structural determinants of anti-MT effects

Many agents which affect cytoskeletal structures in eukaryotic cells appear to have evolved as part of the continuing struggle of members of the less evolved phyla to protect themselves from predators. It is virtually certain that an abundant number of such toxins still exist in the natural environment waiting to be identified. Man's early experiences with anti-MT agents will have been with concentrated fractions of plants such as *Colchicum autumnale* or other members of the *Liliaceae* family. However, not until 1928 was an efficient extraction procedure for colchicine published (Chemnitius, 1928) and the elucidation of structure took a further 17 years (Dewar, 1945). Used by many authors of fiction as a convenient method of murdering unfortunate victims, the early therapeutic uses of colchicine were in the treatment of gout with considerably less focus on antineoplastic activity. Further evidence that plant alkaloids had potential in the treatment of cancer has more recently been provided by extracts from the *Vinca rosea* from which first vinblastine (Noble *et al.*, 1958) and then vincristine (Svoboda *et al.*, 1961) were isolated.

It is apparent even in comparing the chemical structures of the *Colchicum* and *Vinca* alkaloids that no simple master formula exists in the design of active anti-MT drugs. Indeed, other agents which cause similar effects are shown in Table 3.1. Any concordance or commonality of source or

Table 3.1. Drugs with reported antimicrotubule activities

Benzimidazole carbamate(s)	Estramustine
Chalcones	Griseofulvin
Chlorpromazine	Isopropyl-*N*-phenylcarbamate
Colchicine/colcemid (colchicum alkaloids)	Maytansine
	Nocodazole
Combretastatin	Podophyllotoxin derivatives
Cyclohexyl isocyanate and 2,4-dichlorobenzyl thiocyanate	Rhizoxin
	Rifampicin
Diethylstilboestrol	Rotenone
Dihydropyridopyrazine(s)	Steganacin
Diphenylpyridazine derivatives	Tubulozole
Dolastatin(s)/phomopsin A	Taxol
Ergot derivatives (ergocryptine/bromocryptine)	Vincristine/vinblastine (vinca alkaloids)

structure would be difficult to discern. Drugs such as taxol or the dolastatin family are relative newcomer natural products, the former an alkaloid extract from the bark of a yew tree, *Taxus baccata*, the latter an unusual series of pentapeptides from the sea hare *Dolabella auricularia*. Although each of the drugs or class of drugs shown in Table 3.1 cause a similar anti-MT end-point, they do not have the same pharmacological mechanism of action. For those agents that interact with tubulin, multiple and distinct binding sites are present. However, in overview, two generalities appear to distinguish most of these drug structures. The first is that all have ring structures of varying degrees of complexity. The second is the presence of simpler aliphatic residues which are connected to the rings through a linking group, which in many cases has the characteristics of a peptide bond. In fact, a structure–activity analysis with a series of dihydropyridopyrazines (Wheeler *et al.*, 1983) has suggested that while a great deal of flexibility exists in the ring substitutions, stepwise removal of the aminocarboalkoxy moiety essentially eliminates both the toxicity and the antimitotic activity of the drug. Ring substituents containing either oxygen or sulphur also reduced the efficacy, presumably through destabilization of these ring structures.

Perhaps the most detailed structure–activity analysis of the critical nature of the aminocarboalkoxy group in determining anti-MT effects was carried out in a series of benzimidazole carbamates (Gupta, 1986). In determining commonalities in both the cytotoxic and MT inhibitory activities of nocodazole and agents of similar chemical structure and biological activity (albendazole, benomyl, cambendazole, carbendazim, fenbendazole, mebendazole, oxibendazole and parbendazole), Gupta was able to make several inferences concerning critical groups. Each of the cytotoxic anti-MT derivatives bore the aminocarboalkoxy group, while inactive congeners did not. In addition, two other anti-MT agents TN-16 and NSC 181928 (Arai, 1983; Wheeler *et al.*, 1983) possessing similar pharmacological activity to the benzimidazole carbamates, also incorporate the aminocarboalkoxy group.

The importance of the ring structures to the anti-MT activity of the benzimidazole series was also addressed (Gupta, 1986). Two fused rings, either two six-membered rings (one of which may be heterocyclic), as represented by NSC 181928, or one six- and one five-membered ring (as in benzimidazole), appeared necessary for activity. TN-16 would, on first analysis, appear contrary to this prediction. However, the possibility of intramolecular hydrogen bonding between the –NH group and the carbonyl (C=O) on position 4 of the pyrrolidine ring would mimic a five-membered ring. Indeed, the overall importance of the carbamate motif may be in permitting internal hydrogen bonding in such a way as to modify or constrain the drug to allow stearic interaction with the protein target site. The alternative explanation of hydrogen bonding with target sites on the MT–peptide remains a possibility. Both hydrophobic and hydrogen bonding are relatively weak stabilizing forces, but in most cases would be sufficient to account for the drug binding constants to tubulin or other MAPs. Once again, for benzimidazole derivatives, the presence of a large non-polar group such as an aromatic or heterocyclic ring, or even an aliphatic chain, confers increased anti-MT properties. Similar non-polar substituents appear for TN-16 and NSC 181928, again emphasizing the significance of this common property.

For the MAP-binding drug estramustine, some observations similar to those for the benzimidazole carbamates can be made. Crystallographic studies (Punzi *et al.*, 1991) have shown that the hydrophobic ring structures of the steroid nucleus resemble the 'chair' configuration which would normally be associated with oestradiol. Although the nitrogen is not protonated the presence of the carbonyl group could facilitate hydrogen bonding. The chloroethyl moieties, as already discussed, do not act as leaving groups but tend to 'bend back' over the molecule serving to hinder the possible enzymatic catalysis of the carbamate or ester linkages. It should be noted that a major factor which distinguishes estramustine from the plethora of other steroid-alkylating agent drugs is the presence of the carbamate moiety. Drugs such as prednimustine do not possess antimitotic activity. This is because the linkage of predisolone to chlorambucil is via an ester group. The multipurpose and ubiquitous esterases in cells rapidly break this linkage liberating both the steroid and the alkylating mustard which enact commensurate pharmacological properties. This factor is true for all similar drugs which use an ester as the linking group. The antimitotic properties of diethylstilboesterol (Parry *et al.*, 1982) although certainly not the primary pharmacological property of this agent, also indicate the possible role of the planar, hydrophobic steroid nucleus in determining binding to MT.

An analysis of the structures of the antimitotic drugs confirms that the carbamate motif appears in many of them, including the simplest of the structures, isopropyl-*N*-phenylcarbamate. It may be of interest to consider compounds such as acetaminophen, acetanilide or acetazolamide for antimitotic activity, since next to isopropyl-*N*-phenylcarbamate, they represent some of the simplest compounds with moieties structurally similar. In this drug, nocodazole (and related analogues), colchicine and ergocryptine, the nitrogen is attached to the ring system. For estramustine, the ester links the alkyl side chain to the steroid A ring. This may be of some significance to the different cytoskeletal target of estramustine compared to standard tubulin binders, since to date griseofulvin and estramustine are the only two agents that have reported binding avidity for MAPs although the evidence for the former is limited.

The participation of each component of the drugs possessing ring structures and 'peptide-bond' like linking groups should be addressed. Many of the drugs which interact with cytoskeletal proteins do so in a non-covalent manner, with varying extents of reversibility. Effective, in many instances, at low concentrations, binding avidity is primarily determined by hydrophobic interactions and hydrogen bonding. The nature of both the ring structures and substituents vary widely, however, it is likely that they provide stearic properties consistent with hydrophobic binding domains within 'grooves' of target proteins such as tubulin or MAPs. Substituents that alter the planarity and/or hydrophobicity of the ring structures will influence the binding constant of the drug for the target protein.

For colchicine a number of structural modifications have suggested that the B ring is not the major determinant of binding stringency to tubulin (Ray *et al.*, 1981). Indeed, both the thimethoxyphenyl (A ring) and the tropolone (C ring) moieties appear critical to the stringent binding of the drug (Bhattacharyya & Wolff, 1974; Fitzgerald, 1976). For example, replacement of the tropolone ring with a phenyl ring (colchinol) produces an inactive drug (Zweig & Chugnell, 1973). In addition, changes in this ring such as interchanging the positions of the carbonyl and methoxy groups (isocolchicine) produce analogues which do not bind tubulin (Bhattacharyya & Wolff, 1974). Alterations in the B ring do not negate the tubulin-binding properties of this drug class. However, some changes may influence the binding mechanism and avidity. For example, colcemid binds tubulin fairly rapidly and reversibly, while colchicine is slower and less readily reversible (Borisy & Taylor, 1967). Generally, the smaller the substituents on the B ring the faster the binding and such analogues may bind tubulin at 4°C as opposed to 37°C for a more heavily substituted ring.

More recently, combretastatins, natural products isolated from a South African tree (Pettit *et al.*, 1982), have been shown to have significant antitubulin properties (Hamel & Lin, 1983). The trimethoxy A ring of combretatstatin is identical to colchicine, whereas the C ring is a substituted benzene ring. The absence of the seven-membered tropone B ring does not negate the tubulin-binding potential, however, it does alter the binding affinity (Hamel & Lin, 1981). With respect to the B ring substituent aminocarboalkoxy group, these findings would indicate that the ring structures are the initial determinant of drug tubulin interaction with the aminocarboalkoxy functioning to stabilize the binding, perhaps through inter- or intramolecular hydrogen bonding.

In drugs such as podophyllotoxin or ergot derivatives, the R group is represented by a complex of ring systems. Methoxy substituents are present in many of the ring systems, presumably contributing to the overall hydrophobicity of the rings. It is possible that stacking and/or intercalating of these drugs into protein hydrophobic domains may be influenced by such ring substituents and by other more complicated stearic considerations.

In most instances the nature of the alkyl and alkyl–halide R group is not a major determinant in the selectivity or avidity of binding for cytoskeletal proteins. However, in herbicidal analogues of the 5,6-diphenyl-pyridazin-3-one-series, the phenyl rings of the most potent anti-MT agents are either unsubstituted or bear fluorine atoms (Batra et al., 1986). By substituting chlorines into the ring systems, the herbicidal activity is lost, but the interactions with calf brain tubulin are enhanced. The electro-negativity of the halogen substitutions will be a consideration in the overall binding affinity. Their presence, either as a ring substituent, or as part of an alkyl–halide side chain will be of consequence in the design of new anti-MT drugs. Conversely, the relatively large number of antimitotic drugs which lack halogen atoms would argue against the mandatory requirement of such atoms.

An intriguing corollary to the halogen requirement is provided by estramustine. As discussed previously, the nor-nitrogen mustard moiety bears two chloroethyl groups designed to act as bifunctional alkylating species. Because of constraints enacted upon the molecules by the carbamate, the chlorines do not act as effective leaving groups and the formation of alkylating intermediate aziridinium species does not occur (Punzi et al., 1991). The cytotoxic effect of estramustine is not impaired by the replacement of the chlorines with hydroxyl groups substituents which are ineffective leaving groups and would be expected to have no alkylating potential. Indeed, the complete absence of covalent binding of estramustine with cellular targets confirms the unimportance of alkylation in inducing the antimitotic effect (Tew, 1983). A schematic representation of how the drug causes MT disassembly is shown in Fig. 3.3.

The importance of the peptide bond in stabilizing the polypeptide chain of a protein has been appreciated for some time. Functional hydrogen bonding between donor atoms, such as –NH groups, and recipi-

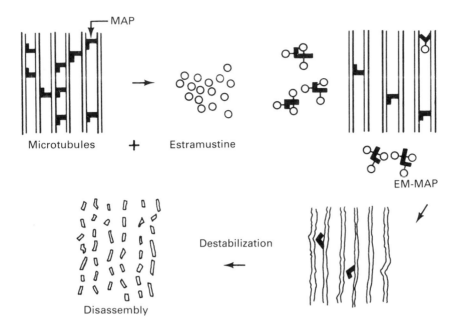

Fig. 3.3. Schematic of estramustine (EM) binding to microtubule-associated proteins (MAPs).

ents, such as C=O groups, stabilize both proteins and nucleic acids against external forces such as thermal motion and are critical in maintaining these molecules in a structurally and functionally viable state. As shown in Table 3.2, the proportion of antimitotic drugs which possess peptide bond-like moieties is quite high. Estramustine possesses a carbonyl residue which can act as an effective hydrogen bond recipient. For estramustine, it has been suggested that by intermolecular hydrogen bonding, multiple drug molecule lattices can form. Crystallization of estramustine (Punzi *et al.*, 1992) has predicted that such lattices may be feasible and B_{max} values (Stearns *et al.*, 1988) are consistent with the

Table 3.2. Antimitotic drugs which incorporate a carbamate/amide into their structure

Isopropyl-*N*-phenylcarbamate
Colchicine and analogues
Benzimidazole carbamates
Dihydropyridopyrazines
Ergocryptine (other ergot analogues)
Maytansine
Dolastatins
Styrylquinazolinones
Taxol
Cytochalasin B

binding of approximately 10–15 molecules of estramustine to each MAP target protein.

The analogy of the carbamoyl linker to a peptide bond is perhaps further emphasized by a novel group of antimitotic drugs, the dolastatins. The most potent of these is dolastatin 10. A tripeptide segment of dolastatin 10 was found to inhibit both tubulin polymerization and GTP hydrolysis but to have no effect upon nucleotide exchange (Bai *et al.*, 1990a). These authors also demonstrated that the tripeptide fragment failed to compete for vinca alkaloid binding sites on tubulin and propose that this site, purportedly on the β-tubulin subunit, is the same one recognized by another natural product polypeptide, phomoposin A (Lacey *et al.*, 1987). The presence of nine asymmetrical carbon atoms in the four amino acid–complex primary amine molecule is important to drug binding. Five of these are carried over into the tripeptide and the authors have determined that proper configuration at positions 18 and 19 are required for the most avid binding of the drug to tubulin (Bai *et al.*, 1990c). Whatever the chirality requirements, the similarity between dolastatins, other natural product polypeptides and the 'standard' anti-MT agents would not appear to be unreasonably related to ring structures of various degrees of hydrophobicity and the presence of simple or modified peptide bonds. In suggesting a schematic model for the binding of dolastatin to β-tubulin, Bai *et al.* (1990a) have theorized that the peptide backbone interacts with the three-dimensional groove on the tubulin monomer. The side chains may provide a stearic hindrance to the binding of other antimitotics such as vinca alkaloids, maytansine or rhizoxin. The extremely low concentrations of dolastatin 10 required to cause an anti-MT effect (10^{-13} M) predicate either a high-affinity binding to a critical site or effective intracellular localization of the drug. A summary of the relative efficacy of common anti-MT agents for inhibiting MT assembly is shown in Table 3.3.

The reversibility of drug-induced anti-MT activity also appears to be a commonality of effect for many drugs. This is presumably a function of the non-covalent binding properties of most of these agents. Many alkylating and carbamoylating agents have produced anti-MT effects in cell lines through covalent modifications of nucleophilic sites on tubulin. The isocyanate species produced through the decomposition of alkyl nitrosoureas has been found to produce mitotic dysfunction through carbamoylation, presumably of the thiol groups of tubulin (Tew *et al.*, 1983). Similarly, 2,4-dichlorobenzyl thiocyanate has been shown to alkylate tubulin with resultant mitotic arrest. These effects can be related to the high molar concentration of cysteine in tubulin (20/mol) conferring a degree of intracellular nucleophilic selectivity for the active alkylating species. Aberrant mitotic figures are frequently seen in those cells treated with such drugs. Although resultant incomplete or inadequate spindle

Table 3.3. Drug concentrations for IC$_{50}$ inhibition of mictotubule assembly*

Classification of tubulin binding-site	IC$_{50}$ (μM)
Colchicine	
Colchicine	0.2–0.5
Rhizoxin	0.2
Dihydropyrido pyrazine derivatives	0.3–3
Tubulozole	0.5
Rotenone	0.5
Podophyllotoxins	0.6–0.7
Nocodazole	1 (analogues 2–9)
Steganacin	2–4
TN16	2
Vinca	
Vinca alkaloids	1–2
Phomopsin A	0.4–0.6
Maytansine	1–5
Rhizoxin	5
Miscellaneous	
2,4-dichlorobenzyl thiocyanate	4
5,6-diphenyl-pyridazinone	10
Methylmercuric chloride	> 20
Estramustine	> 20
Griseofulvin	> 50

*Based upon values published values for standard *in vitro* assay conditions.
IC$_{50}$, inhibitory concentration 50% of maximum.

formation was found to result in chromosomal abnormalities such as polyploidy, chromosome decondensation and endoreduplication (Tew *et al.*, 1983), the block in metaphase and concomitant synchronization of cellular populations is not a standard effect of these drugs. Thus the relative non-selectivity of the alkylating/carbamoylating drugs confers anti-MT effects primarily on the basis of the high content of nucleophilic sulphhydryl residues in tubulin. These cysteines have critical intracellular functions, both in maintaining a normal redox (SH : SS) balance and in the stabilization of tubulin polymers through intra β-sulphhydryl crosslinks (Luduena *et al.*, 1985).

Tumour cell resistance and cytotoxicity

It is possible to learn much about the mechanism of action of a drug by studying the change(s) acquired by a cell to counteract the toxic effect. The development of resistance to a particular class of anticancer drug is frequently the underlying cause of failure in the successful eradication of a patient's cancer. Tumour cells possess a degree of genetic plasticity prerequisite for adaptation to treatment with toxins such as antimitotic drugs. Because anticytoskeletal drugs target the basic architecture of a cell, it could be argued that acquired resistance to a drug may involve a dramatic change in cell structure. However, one of the important properties of MTs is their flexibility, not in the sense of structural 'bendability', but in terms of their constant assembly and disassembly (Kirschner & Mitchison, 1986a). To allow normal structure and function of cytoskeletal events, a balance between the assembly/disassembly process is constantly required. Although in tumour cells this qualitative balance is likely to be extremely varied, specific threshold limits will presumably be inherent. For example, if a ratio of greater than 3:1 polymerized to depolymerized tubulin occurs, the cell may not be able to maintain normal MT arrays (or mitotic spindle) or to transport intracellular organelles in an ordered manner. Internal control mechanisms may include genetic regulation of tubulin production or alterations in its subsequent post-translational modification. In addition, MAP interactions could influence functionality, as could MT organization within the framework of actin domains and IF structures. Given the complexity and obvious flexibility of the cytoskeletal components, it is not unreasonable to assume that cells can survive drugs which affect the polymerization ratio, as long as certain threshold limits are not surpassed. For this reason, cell lines with resistance to vinca alkaloids which express mutant forms of either α- or β-tubulin (Cabral et al., 1980; Houghton et al., 1983), have only a limited proportion of the total protein as the mutant form. Because of this, only low levels of resistance occur and in hybrids, formed between resistant and wild-type cells, the resistance is frequently codominant. Thus, the 'diluting effect' of normal tubulin with the mutant serves as a controlling element in the expression of resistance.

Crossresistance patterns amongst and between antimitotic drugs also contribute to an understanding of drug mechanism and have been used in many instances to distinguish tubulin binding-sites for unrelated drugs. For example, the tubulin binding-site of vincristine or vinblastine is frequently used as the standard to which other tubulin binding agents are compared. As discussed, the natural product polypeptides such as dolastatins and phomopsin, although causing antimitotic events, have distinct, but overlapping tubulin binding-sites compared to vincas. Similarly, podophyllotoxin-resistant cells have been shown to have distinct cellular changes that do not confer resistance to all other antimitotics (Gupta et al., 1982). The precise nature of the binding to the MT domain has yet to be defined (see earlier discussion). However, obviously commonality of chemical structure will be a crucial determinant in the crossresistance profile. For example, nocodazole-resistant cells show crossresistance to benzimidazole urea. Compounds of similar structure but lacking a urea group were not part of the resistance profile.

The much studied multidrug resistant (MDR) phenotype encompasses some of the anticytoskeletal agents. This is not surprising, since the classic MDR cells overexpress a membrane P glycoprotein, the function of which is to efflux hydrophobic natural products, thereby protecting the cell from toxic insult. Since this glycoprotein has ubiquity throughout both pro-karyotes and eukaryotes, it is quite possible that its evolution paralleled that of the plant toxins themselves. The fact that so many chemically divergent drugs are affected by this phenotype would indicate a lack of specificity for anti-MT agents. Mechanistically, any efflux pump which can maintain the intracellular concentration of an anti-MT drug below the critical threshold value required for MT destabilization would be of obvious physiological advantage. Alterations in the target proteins, or in the propensity of the cell to detoxify antimitotic drugs, appear to occur at significantly lower, but nonetheless meaningful, rates. Interestingly, taxol may be a drug which fits into the MDR profile. However, its distinctive mechanism of action has resulted in a number of interesting resistant cell lines which will not grow in the absence of the drug (Schibler & Cabral, 1985). Presumably, this reflects the loss of an inherent ability to stabilize MT arrays, but the underlying mechanism remains obscure.

For MAP-binding drugs such as estramustine, an entirely different resistance profile is found. No crossresistance to vinca alkaloids or cyto-chalasin B is apparent and indeed the phenotype appears to be indepen-dent of MDR, since such cell lines show sensitivity to estramustine (Speicher et al., 1991). Because estramustine seems to circumvent MDR, there is a sound rationale for including the drug in clinical regimens which include other antimitotic agents. Indeed, this was a determinant factor in the formulation of the estramustine/vinblastine protocol for the treatment of prostate cancer (Seidman et al., 1991).

Although relevant to all anticancer drugs, the question of how tumour cell kill is specifically achieved by antimitotic drugs remains contentious. The enigma of programmed cell death has gained renewed momentum since initial descriptions of apoptosis (see Chapter 2). Antimitotic drugs generally cause a stathmokinetic effect, i.e. a block and subsequent build-up of cells in metaphase. This event presumably is the result of inadequate spindle functionality as a consequence of interference with tubulin or MAP cycling. However, cells blocked in mitosis may remain viable for long periods, resuming normal cell division upon removal of the drug. As mentioned, there is a good deal of flexibility in what constitutes normal stoichiometry of MT components and cell death and need not be a consequence of a temporary interference with the ratio of free to poly-merized MTs. The concept of unbalanced cell growth has been proposed to account for cell death resulting from anticancer drug treatment. Recent studies of vincristine-induced cell death have shown that protein synthesis is required for a cell to proceed to the lysis phase (Kung et al., 1990). Such data are interpreted to mean that the enactment of cell death requires continued active cellular processes involving protein synthesis. Concluding that death results from 'the dissociation of normally integrated cell cycle events (i.e. karyokinetic/nuclear reformation events), Kung *et al.* suggest that differential sensitivity of tumours to antimitotic agents may be a function of varying degrees of stringency in control of events leading to cell cycle progression. Such an idea would make anticytoskeletal agents indistinct from other drugs which interfere with either DNA synthesis or other events responsible for the fidelity of cycle progression.

Conclusion and perspectives

It is evident that toxins targetting the eukaryotic cytoskeleton have provided many plants and lower animals a selective advantage in deterring predacity. A large number of these natural products have been isolated and used in the treatment of human diseases as disparate as gout and cancer. It is equally plausible that many further natural products have yet to be identified and that these agents will have a use in medicinal therapy. Of the antimitotic agents most frequently used in cancer chemotherapy, those that affect the MT domain of a cell predominate over those which target MFs or IFs. The reasons for this are not at first obvious, however, it may be that molecules such as actin and vimentin are less critical to the formation of a mitotic spindle in dividing cells. Thus, interference with the regulation and/or turnover of these proteins has more limited cytotoxic consequences in rapidly dividing tumours. Of the existent anti-MT drugs, colchicine and vinca alkaloids are perhaps the most studied and best understood. It is unlikely that significant increases in the therapeutic value of these classes of agents will be forthcoming by synthesis of novel analogues. This does not mean that improvements in drug delivery or targetting to tumours may not be achieved, but the basic underlying inhibitory effects upon tubulin equilibrium will probably only be mildly influenced by minor improvements in the drug binding constants. Circumvention of resistance to vinca alkaloids may be achieved with novel congeners, but this will most likely result from overcoming or bypassing efflux pump changes as exemplified by the MDR phenotype. Thus, while a rationale for continued synthesis of novel vinca alkaloids has merit, significant increases in therapeutic index through altered mechanism of action remain less likely.

The significant list of antimitotic drugs includes mainline development of lead compounds which have tubulin binding-sites either overlapping with, or distinct from, those characterized for vinca alkaloids. Continued study of these drugs may well lead to their inclusion into clinical regimens. This may be especially valuable in circumventing resistance, or in some cases, achieving synergistic cell kill in combination. If overlapping normal tissue toxicities are avoided, such an approach may be warranted. Indeed, recent information on combinations of vinblastine and estramustine may provide a precedent for this approach. Estramustine is perhaps one of the more unusual antimitotic agents. Because of a natural predilection to base conclusions on the mechanism of action upon the synthetic rationale and chemical structural properties, acceptance of the drug as a MAP-binding agent has been slow to achieve. However, preclinical studies of a vinblastine/estramustine combination (Mareel *et al.*, 1988) and subsequent clinical utility in the treatment of human prostate cancer (Seidman *et al.*, 1991) suggest that sequential and additive targetting of tubulin and MAPs may be a novel and worthwhile approach to the management of cancer patients. It would be valuable to screen for other agents which may target MAPs, especially since there is some indication that tumour cells may vary in their MAP components from other normal tissues. It is also of interest that tumour cells developing resistance to tubulin-binding drugs, such as podophyllotoxins, have been shown to overexpress a protein of mol. wt 66 kDa suggested to be a MAP (Gupta *et al.*, 1982). The somewhat limited information presently available on the tumour-specific MAPs and the possibility that differential expression exists between tumour and normal tissues suggests that this may be a fruitful arena for future research.

A further encouraging aspect of the utility of MT-targetted chemotherapy has been the recent success of taxol in the treatment of refractory ovarian cancer. As a single agent, at dose ranges from 110 to 250 mg/m^2, taxol induced remissions lasting from 3 to 15 months. Dose-limiting toxicity was myelosuppression with leucocytes more sensitive than thrombocytes or reticulocytes. Conclusions from this non-randomized, prospective, phase II trial were that taxol studies should be extended to combination therapies (McGuire *et al.*, 1989). Unfortunately, the supply of this natural product is limited by the paucity and geographic distribution of the yew tree source. Consequently, extensive trials must await the elucidation and implementation of large scale chemical synthesis. Such approaches are the focus of much present attention.

The overall approach of targetting cellular structural proteins has provided a reasonably successful mechanism for chemotherapeutic control of cancer cells. As is always the case, selectivity remains a major obstacle in the improvement of therapeutic index. Although tubulin *per se* has, to this time, been a primary target, some novelty has been invoked by the use of taxol to stabilize MTs and this may be the forerunner of other stabilizing agents. In addition, the expanding knowledge of MAPs and these drugs which bind to these proteins may provide a fertile area for future drug development. Each of these approaches gains credibility from the seemingly endless source of natural products from plants and invertebrates, many of which have yet to be classified, let alone analysed.

References

Abe, T., Haga, T. & Kurokawa, M. (1975). Blockage of axoplasmic-transport and depolymerization of reassembled microtubules by methyl mercury. *Brain Research* **86**, 504–508.

Abraham, I., Dion, R.L., Duanmu, C., Gottesman, M.M. & Hamel, E. (1986) 2,4-dichlorobenzyl thiocyanate, an antimitotic agent that alters microtubule morphology. *Proceedings of the National Academy of Sciences, USA* **83**, 6839–6843.

Aizawa, H., Kawasaki, H., Murofush, H., Koten, S., Suzuki, K. & Sakai, H. (1989). A common amino acid sequence in 190-kDa microtubule-associated protein and tau for the promotion of microtubule assembly. *Journal of Biological Chemistry* **264**, 5885–5890.

Albrecht-Buehler, G. (1977). Daughter 3T3 cells. Are the mirror images of each other? *Journal of Cell Biology* **72**, 595–603.

Appu Rao, A.G. & Cann, J.R. (1980). A comparative study of the interaction of chlorpromazine, trifluoperazine, and promethazine with mouse brain tubulin. *Molecular Pharmacology* **19**, 295–301.

Arai, T. (1983). Inhibition of microtubule assembly *in vitro* by TN-16, a synthetic antitumour drug. *FEBS Letters* **155**, 273–276.

Atassi, G. & Tagnon, H.J. (1975). R17934-NSC 238159: a new antitumor drug—I. Effect on experimental tumors and factors influencing effectiveness. *European Journal of Cancer* **11**, 599–607.

Aubin, J.E., Osborn, M., Franke, W.W. & Weber, K. (1980). Intermediate filaments of the vimentin type and the cytokeratin type are distributed differently during mitosis. *Experimental Cell Research* **129**, 149–165.

Avila, J. (1990). Microtubule dynamics. *FASEB Journal* **4**, 3284–3290.

Bai, R., Duanmu, C. & Hamel, E. (1989). Mechanism of action of the antimitotic drug 2,4-dichlorobenzyl thiocyanate: alkylation of sulfhydryl group(s) of β-tubulin. *Biochimica et Biophysica Acta* **994**, 12–20.

Bai, R., Pettit, G.R. & Hamel, E. (1990a). Binding of dolastatin 10 to tubulin at a distinct site for peptide antimitotic agents near the exchangeable nucleotide and vinca alkaloid sites. *Journal of Biological Chemistry* **265**, 17141–17149.

Bai, R., Pettit, G.R. & Hamel, E. (1990b). Dolastatin 10, a powerful cytostatic peptide derived from a marine animal. *Biochemical Pharmacology* **39**, 1941–1949.

Bai, R., Pettit, G.R. & Hamel, E. (1990c). Structure–activity studies chiral isomers and with segments of the antimitotic marine peptide dolastatin 10. *Biochemical Pharmacology* **40**(8), 1859–1864.

Banerjee, A.C. & Bhattacharyya, B. (1979). Colcemid and colchicine binding to tubulin. Similarity and dissimilarity. *FEBS Letters* **99**, 333–336.

Batra, J.K., Jurd, L. & Hamel, E. (1985). Structure–function studies with derivatives of 6-benzyl-1,3-benzodioxole, a new class of synthetic compounds which inhibit tubulin polymerization and mitosis. *Molecular Pharmacology* **27**, 94–102.

Batra, J.K., Powers, L.J., Hess, F.D. & Hamel, E. (1986). Derivatives of 5,6-diphenylpyridazin-3-one: synthetic antimitotic agents which interact with plant and mammalian tubulin at a new drug-binding site. *Cancer Research* **46**, 1889–1893.

Beck, W.T. (1980). Increase by vinblastine of oxidized glutathione in cultured mammalian cell. *Biochemical Pharmacology* **29**, 2333–2337.

Bhattacharyya, B. & Wolff, J. (1974). Promotion of fluorescence upon binding of colchicine to tubulin. *Proceedings of the National Academy of Sciences USA* **71**, 2627–2632.

Bhattacharyya, B. & Wolff, J. (1976a). Anion-induced increases in the rate of colchicine binding to tubulin. *Biochemistry* **15**, 2283–2288.

Bhattacharyya, B. & Wolff, J. (1976b). Tubulin aggregation and disaggregation: mediation by two distinct vinblastine-binding sites. *Proceedings of the National Academy
  of Sciences USA* **73**, 2375–2381.
Bignami, A., Dahl, D. & Rueger, D.C. (1980). Glial fibrillary acidic protein (GFA) in
  normal neural cells and in pathological conditions. *Advances in Cellular Neurobiology*
  7, 285–310.
Bloom, G.S., Luca, F.C. & Vallee, R.B. (1984). Widespread cellular distribution of
  MAP 1A (microtubule-associated protein 1A) in the mitotic spindle and on interphase microtubules. *Journal of Cell Biology* **98**, 331–340.
Bloom, G.S., Luca, F.C. & Vallee, R.B. (1985). Microtubule-associated protein 1B:
  identification of a major component of the neuronal cytoskeleton. *Proceedings of the
  National Academy of Sciences USA* **82**, 5404–5408.
Boder, G.H., Paul, D.C. & Williams, D.C. (1983). Chlorpromazine inhibits mitosis of
  mammalian cells. *European Journal of Cell Biology* **31**, 349–353.
Bonder, E.M., Fishkind, D.J. & Mooseker, M.S. (1983). Direct measurement of critical
  concentrations and assembly rate constants at the two ends of an actin filament. *Cell*
  34, 491–501.
Borisy, G.G. & Taylor, E.W. (1967). The mechanism of action of colchicine: binding
  of colchicine-^{3}H to cellular protein. *Journal of Cell Biology* **34**, 525–531.
Bowdon, B.J., Waud, W.R., Wheeler, G.P., Hain, R., Dansby, L. & Temple, C. Jr
  (1987). Comparison of 1,2-dihydropyridol[3,4-b]pyrazines(1-deaza-7,8-dihydrop-
  teridines) with several other inhibitors of mitosis. *Cancer Research* **47**, 1621–1626.
Bray, D., Heath, J. & Moss, D. (1986). The membrane-associated cortex of animal cells:
  its structure and mechanical properties. *Journal of Cell Science* **4** (Suppl.), 71–88.
Brinkley, B.R., Fuller, G.M. & Highfield, D.P (1975). Cytoplasmic microtubules in
  normal and transformed cells in culture: analysis by tubulin antibody immuno-
  fluorescence. *Proceedings of the National Academy of Sciences USA* **72**, 4981–4985.
Brossi, A., Yeh, H.J.C., Chrzanowska, M., Wolff, J., Hamel, E., Lin, C.M., Quinn, F.,
  Suffness, M. & Silverton, J. (1988). Colchicine and its analogs—recent findings.
  Medical Research Reviews **8**, 77–94.
Bryan, J. (1972). Definition of three classes of binding sites in isolated microtubule
  crystals. *Biochemistry* **11**, 2611–2616.
Buckley, I.K. & Porter, K.R. (1967). Cytoplasmic fibrils in living cultured cells. A light
  and electron microscope study. *Protoplasma* **64**, 349–380.
Bulinski, J. & Borisy, G.G. (1979). Self-assembly of microtubules in extracts of cultured
  HeLa cells and the identification of HeLa microtubule-associated proteins. *Proceed-
  ings of the National Academy of Sciences USA* **76**, 293–297.
Cabral, F., Sobel, M. & Gottesman, M. (1980). CHO mutants resistant to colchicine,
  colcemid or griseofulvin have an altered β-tubulin. *Cell* **20**, 29–36.
Carley, W.W., Barak, L.S. & Webb, W.W. (1981). F-actin aggregates in transformed
  cells. *Journal of Cell Biology* **90**, 797–802.
Carlier, M.F., Melki, R., Pantaloni, D., Hill, T. & Chen. Y. (1987). Oscillations in
  microtubule polymerization. *Proceedings of the National Academy of Sciences USA*
  84, 5257–5261.
Carlier, M.F. & Pantaloni, D. (1981). Kinetics analysis of guanosine 5′-triphosphate
  hydrolysis associated with tubulin polymerization. *Biochemistry* **20**, 1918–1924.
Cassimeris, L.U., Walker, R.A., Pryer, N.K. & Salmon, E.D. (1988). Dynamic instability of microtubules. *Bioessays* **7**, 149–154.
Chemnitius, F. (1928). Preparation of colchicine. *Journal of Praktische Chemie* **118**, 29.
Conrad, R.A., Cullinan, G.J, Gerzon, K. & Poore, G.A. (1979). Structure–activity
  relationships of dimeric *Catharanthus* alkaloids. II. Experimental antitumour activi-

ties of *n*-substituted deacetyl vinblastine amide (vindesine) sulfates. *Journal of Medicinal Chemistry* **22**, 391–398.

Cortese, F., Bhattacharyya, B. & Wolff, J. (1977). Podopyllotoxin as a probe for the colchicine binding site of tubulin. *Journal of Biological Chemistry* **252**, 1134–1140.

David-Pfeuty, T., Erickson, H.P. & Pantalini, D. (1977). Guanosine triphosphatase activity of tubulin associated with microtubule assembly. *Proceedings of the National Academy of Sciences USA* **74**, 5372–5376.

David-Pfeuty, T., Simon, C. & Pantaloni, D. (1979). Effect of antimitotic drugs on tubulin GTPase activity and self-assembly. *Journal of Biological Chemistry* **254**, 11696–11702.

De Brabander, I.J., Van de Veire, R.M.L., Aerts, F.E.M., Borgers, M. & Janssen, P.A.J. (1976). The effects of methyl [5-(2-thienylcarbonyl)-1H-benzimidazol-2-yl]carbamate, (R 17934; NSC 238159), a new synthetic antitumoral drug interfering with microtubules on mammalian cells cultured *in vitro*. *Cancer Research* **36**, 905–916.

Dewar, J. (1945). Structure of colchicine. *Nature* **155**, 141.

Dornish, J.M., Pettersen, E.O. & Oftebro, R. (1984). Interaction of 1-propargyl-5-chloropyrimidin-2-one (a methalone) with rat brain tubulin. *Biochimica et Biophysica Acta* **797**, 156–162.

Dustin, P. (1984). *Microtubules*, 2nd edn. Springer-Verlag, New York.

Edelman, G.M. & Yahara, I. (1976) Temperature-sensitive changes in surface modulating assemblies of fibroblasts transformed by mutants of Rous sarcoma virus. *Proceedings of the National Academy of Sciences USA* **73**, 2047–2051.

Edwards, M.L., Stemerick, D.M. & Sunkara, P.S. (1990). Chalcones: a new class of antimitotic agents. *Journal of Medicinal Chemistry* **33**, 1948–1954.

Engelborghs, Y. (1990). Dynamic aspects of microtubule assembly. In Avila, J. (ed.) *Microtubule Proteins*, pp. 1–36. CRC Press, Florida.

Erickson, H.P. & Voter, W. (1986). Nucleation of microtubule assembly. *Annals of the New York Academy of Science* **466**, 552–565.

Estes, J.E., Selden, L.A. & Gershman, L.C. (1981). Mechanism of action of phalloidin on the polymerization of muscle actin. *Biochemistry* **20**, 708–712.

Faulstich, H.A., Schafer, A.J. & Weckauf, M. (1977). The dissociation of the phalloidin–actin complex. *Hoppe–Seyler's Zeitschrift für Physiological Chemistry* **358**, 181–184.

Faulstich, H.A., Stournaras, C., Doenges, K.H. & Zimmermann, H.-P. (1984). The molecular mechanism of interaction of Et_3Pb^+ with tubulin. *FEBS Letters* **174**, 128–131.

Feit, H., Neudeck, U. & Baskin, F. (1977). Comparison of the isoelectric and molecular weight of properties of tubulin subunits. *Journal of Neurochemistry* **28**, 697–702.

Fex, H.J., Hogberg, K.B., Konyves, I. & Kneip, Ph.O.J. (1967). Certain steroid *N-bis*-(halo-ethyl)-carbamates. US Patent No. 3 229 104, 17.1.

Fitzgerald, T.J. (1976). Molecular features of colchicine associated with antimitotic activity and inhibition of tubulin polymerization. *Biochemical Pharmacology* **25**, 1383–1387.

Flanagan, M.D. & Lin, S. (1980). Cytochalasins block actin filament elongation by binding to high affinity sites associated with F-actin. *Journal of Biological Chemistry* **255**, 835–838.

Folkman, J. & Moscona, A. (1978). Role of cell shape in growth control. *Nature* **273**, 345–349.

Fonte, V. & Porter, K.R. (1974). In *Electron Microscopy*, pp. 334–335. Proceedings of the Eight International Congress on Electron Microscopy, Australian Academy of Sciences, Canberra.

Friedman, P.A. & Platzer, E.G. (1978). Interaction of anthelmintic benzimidazoles and benzimidazole derivatives with bovine brain tubulin. *Biochimica et Biophysica Acta* **544**, 604–614.

Fujiwara, K. & Tilney, L.G. (1975). Substructures analysis of the microtubule and its polymorphic forms. *Annals of the New York Academy of Sciences* **253**, 27–50.

Fuller, G.M., Brinkley, B.K. & Boughter, M.J. (1975). Immunofluorescence of mitotic spindles by using monospecific antibody against bovine brain tubulin. *Science* **187**, 948–950.

Gabriel, L., Miglietta, A. & Dianzani, M.U. (1985). 4-hydroxy-alkenals interactions with purified microtubular protein. *Chemical–Biological Interactions* **56**, 201–212.

Gacek, M., Undheim, K., Oftebro, R. & Laland, S.G. (1979). Metahalones, a new class of metaphase inhibitors. *FEBS Letters* **98**, 355–358.

Garland, D.L. (1978). Kinetics and mechanism of colchicine binding to tubulin: evidence for ligand-induced conformation change. *Biochemistry* **17**, 4266–4272.

Geiger, B. (1987). Intermediate filaments: looking for a function. *Nature* **329**, 392–393.

Geuens, G.M.A., Nuydens, R.M., Willebrords, R.E., Van de Veire, R.M.L., Goossens, F., Dragonetti, C.H., Mareel, M.M.K. & De Brabander, M.J. (1985). Effects of tubulozole on the microtubule system of cells in culture nd *in vivo*. *Cancer Research* **45**, 733–742.

Goldman, R.D. (1985). Intermediate filaments: passive functions as cytoskeletal connecting links between nixlous and the cell surface. *Annals of the New York Academy of Sciences USA* **455**, 1–17.

Grisham, L.M., Wilson, L. & Bensch, K.G. (1973). Antimitotic action of griseofulvin does not involve disruption of microtubules. *Nature* **244**, 294–296.

Gundersen, G.G., Kalnoski, M.H. & Bulinski, J.C. (1984). Distinct populations of microtubules: tyrosinated and nontyrosinated alpha tubulin are distributed differently *in vivo*. *Cell* **38**, 779–789.

Gunnarsson, P.O., Forshell, G.P., Fritjofson, A. & Norlen, B.J. (1981). Plasma concentrations of estramustine phosphate and its major metabolites in patients with prostatic carcinoma treated with different doses of estramustine phosphate (Estracyt). *Scandinavian Journal of Urology and Nephrology* **15**, 201–205.

Gupta, R.S. (1986). Cross-resistance of nocodazole-resistant mutants of CHO cells toward other microtubule inhibitors: similar mode of action of benzimidazole carbamate derivatives and NSC 181928 and TN-16. *Molecular Pharmacology* **30**, 142–148.

Gupta, R.S., Ho, T.K.W., Moffat, M.R.K. & Gupta, R. (1982). Podophyllotoxin-resistant mutants of Chinese hamster ovary cells. *Journal of Biological Chemistry* **257**, 1071–1078.

Hamel, E. & Lin, C.M. (1981). Glutamate-induced polymerization of tubulin: characteristics of the reaction and application to the large-scale purification of tubulin. *Archives of Biochemistry and Biophysics* **209**, 29–40.

Hamel, E. & Lin, C.M. (1983). Interactions of combretastatin, a new plant-derived antimitotic agent, with tubulin. *Biochemical Pharmacology* **32**, 3864–3867.

Hamel, E., del Campo, A.A., Lowe, M.C. & Lin, C.M. (1981). Interactions of taxol, microtubule-associated proteins and guanine nucleotides in tubulin polymerization. *Journal of Biological Chemistry* **256**, 11887–11894.

Hamel, E., del Campo, A.A., Lustbader, J. & Lin, C.M. (1983). Modulation of tubulin–nucleotide interactions by microtubule associated proteins. *Biochemistry* **22**, 1271–1279.

Hargreaves, A.J., Wandosell, F. & Wandosell, F. & Avila, J. (1986). Phosphorylation of tubulin enhances its interaction with membranes. *Nature* **323**, 827–828.

Hartley-Asp, B. (1984). Estramustine-induced mitotic arrest in two human prostatic carcinoma cell lines, DU 145 and PC-3. *The Prostate* **5**, 93–100.

Hartung, E.F. (1954). History of the use of colchicum and related medicaments in gout. *Annals of Rheumatoid Disease* **13**, 190–200.

Haskins, K.M., Donoso, J.A. & Himes, R.H. (1981). Spirals and paracrystals induced by vinca alkaloids: evidence that microtubule-associated proteins act as polycations. *Journal of Cell Science* **47**, 237–247.

Hill, T.L. & Chen, Y.D. (1984). Phase changes at the end of a microtubule with a GTP cap. *Proceedings of the National Academy of Sciences USA* **81**, 5772–5776.

Hiller, G. & Weber, K. (1978). Radioimmunoassay for tubulin: a quantitative comparison of the tubulin content of different established tissue culture cells and tissues. *Cell* **14**, 795–804.

Himes, R.H., Kersey, R.N., Heller-Bettinger, I. & Samson, F.E. (1976). Action of the vinca alkaloids vincristine, vinblastine, and desacetylvinblastine amide on microtubules *in vitro*. *Cancer Research* **36**, 3798–3802.

Himmler, A., Dreschsel, D., Kirscher, M.W. & Martin, D.W. (1989). Tau consists of a set of proteins with repeated C-terminal microtubule-binding domains and variable N-terminal domains. *Molecular and Cellular Biology* **9**, 1381–1388.

Hoebeke, J., Van Nijen, G. & De Brabander, M. (1976). Interaction of oncodazole (R17934), a new anti-tumoral drug, with rat brain tubulin. *Biochemical and Biophysical Research Communications* **69**, 319–324.

Horio, T. & Hotani, H. (1986). Visualization of the dynamic instability of individual microtubules by dark-field microscopy. *Nature* **321**, 605–607.

Houghton, J.A., Houghton, P.J., Hazelton, B.J. & Douglass, E.C. (1985). *In situ* selection of a human rhabdomyosarcoma resistant to vincristine with altered β-tubulins. *Cancer Research* **45**, 2706–2713.

Huang, A.B., Lin, C.M. & Hamel, E. (1985). Mayansine inhibits nucleotide binding at the exchangeable site of tubulin. *Biochemical and Biophysical Research Communications* **128**, 1239–1246.

Iwasaki, S., Kobayashi, J., Furukawa, J., Namikoshi, M., Okuda, S., Sato, Z., Matsuda, I. & Noda, T. (1985). Studies on macrocyclic lactone antibiotics. *Journal of Antibiotics* **37**, 354–362.

Jiang, J.B., Hesson, D.P., Dusak, B.A., Dexter, D.L., Kang, G.J. Hamel, E. (1990). Synthesis and biological evaluation of 2-styrylquinazolin-4(3H)-ones, a new class of antimitotic anticancer agents which inhibit tubulin polymerization. *Journal of Medicinal Chemistry* **33**, 1721–1728.

Kahn, P. & Shin, S. (1979). Cellular tumorigenicity in nude mice. *Journal of Cell Biology* **82**, 1–16.

Kang, G.-J., Getahung, Z., Muzaffar, A., Brossi, A. & Hamel, H. (1990). N-acetylcolchinol O-methyl ether and thiocolchicine, potent analogs of colchicine modified in the C ring. *Journal of Biological Chemistry* **265**, 10355–10259.

Kanje, M., Deinum, J., Wallin, M., Ekstrom, P., Edstrom, A. & Hartley-Asp, B. (1985). Effect of estramustine phosphate on the assembly of isolated bovine brain microtubules and fast axonal transport in the frog sciatica nerve. *Cancer Research* **45**, 2234–2239.

Kerekes, P., Sharma, P.N., Brossi, A., Chignell, C.F. & Quinn, F.R. (1985). Synthesis and biological effects of novel thiocolchicines. 3. Evaluation of N-acyldeacetylthiocolchicines, N-(alkoxycarbonyl)deacetylthiocolchicines, and O-ethyldemethylthiocolchicines. New synthesis of thiodemecolcine and antileukemic effects of 2-demethyl- and 3-demethylthiocolchicine. *Journal of Medicinal Chemistry* **28**, 1204–1208.

Kimura, I. (1973). Further evidence of the similarity of microtubule protein from mitotic apparatus and sperm tail of the sea urchin as a substrate in thiol:disulfide exchange reaction. *Experimental Cell Research* **79**, 445–448.

Kirschner, M.W. & Mitchison, T. (1986a). Beyond self assembly: from microtubules to morphogenesis. *Cell* **45**, 329–342.

Kirschner, M.W. & Mitchison, T. (1986b). Scientific correspondence: microtubule dynamics. *Nature* **324**, 621.

Korn, E.D. (1982). Actin polymerization and its regulation by proteins from nonmuscle cells. *Physiology Reviews* **6**, 672–737.

Korn, E.D., Carlier, M.-F. & Pantaloni, D. (1987). Actin polymerization and ATP hydrolysis. *Science* **238**, 638–644.

Koska, C., Leichtfried, F.E. & Wiche, G. (1985). Identification and spatial arrangement of high molecular weight proteins (M_r 300,000–330,000) co-assembling with microtubules from a cultured cell line (rat glioma C6) *European Journal of Cell Biology* **38**, 149–156.

Krishan, A., Paika, K. & Frei, E. III (1975). Cytofluorometric studies on the action of podophyllotoxin and epipodophyllotoxins (VM-26 and VP-16-213) on the cell cycle traverse of human lymphoblasts. *Journal of Cell Biology* **66**, 521–530.

Kumar, N. (1981). Taxol-induced polymerization of purified tubulin: mechanism of action. *Journal of Biological Chemistry* **256**, 10435–10441.

Kung, A.L., Zetterberg, A., Sherwood, S.W. & Schimke, R.T. (1990). Cytotoxic effects of cell cycle phase specific agents: result of cell cycle perturbation. *Cancer Research* **50**, 7307–7317.

Kupchan, S.M., Britton, R.W., Ziegler, M.F., Gilmore, C.J., Restivo, R.J. & Bryan, R.F. (1973). Steganacin, novel antileukemic lignan lactone from *Steganataenia araliacea. Journal of the American Chemical Society* **95**, 1335–1336.

Kuriyama, R. & Sakai, H. (1974). Role of tubulin–SH groups in polymerization to microtubules. *Journal of Biochemistry* **76**, 651–654.

Lacey, E., Edgar, J.A. & Culvenor, C.C.J. (1987). Interaction of phomopsin A and related compounds with purified sheep brain tubulin. *Biochemical Pharmacology* **36**, 2133–2138.

Lacey, E. & Watson, T.R. (1985). Activity of benzimidazole carbamates against L1210 mouse leukaemia cells: correlation with *in vitro* tubulin polymerization assay. *Biochemical Pharmacology* **34**, 3603–3605.

Lazarides, E. (1980). Intermediate filaments as mechanical integrators of cellular space. *Nature* **283**, 249–256.

Lee, G., Cowan, N. & Kirscher, M. (1988). The primary structure and heterogeneity of tau protein from mouse brain. *Science* **239**, 285–288.

Lee, J.C., Harrison, D. & Timasheff, S.N. (1975). Interaction of vinblastine with calf brain microtubule protein. *Journal of Biological Chemistry* **250**, 9276–9282.

Lewis, S.A., Ivanov, I.E., Lee, G.-H. & Cowan, N.J. (1989). Organization of microtubules in dendrites and exons is determined by a short hydrophobic zipper in microtubule-associated proteins MAP 2 and tau. *Nature* **342**, 498–505.

Lewis, S.A., Wang, D. & Cowan, N.J. (1988). Microtubule associated MAP 2 shares a microtubule binding motif with tau protein. *Science* **242**, 936–939.

Lin, C.M. & Hamel, E. (1981). Effects of inhibitors of tubulin polymerization on GTP hydrolysis. *Journal of Biological Chemistry* **256**, 9242–9248.

Liu, S.-Y., Hwang, B.-D., Haruna, M., Imakura, Y., Lee, K.-H. & Cheng, Y.-C. (1989). Podophyllotoxin analogs: effects on DNA topoisomerase II, tubulin polymerization, human tumour KB cells and their VP-16-resistant variants. *Molecular Pharmacology* **36**, 78 82.

Luduena, R.F. & Roach, M.C. (1981a). Contrasting effects of maytansine and vinblastine on the alkylation of tubulin sulfhydryls. *Archives of Biochemistry and Biophysics* **210**, 498–504.

Luduena, R.F., & Roach, M.C. (1981b). Interaction of tubulin with drugs and alkylating agents. Effects of colchicine, podophyllotoxin and vinblastine on the alkylation of tubulin. *Biochemistry* **20**, 4444–4450.

Luduena, R.F., Fellous, A., Francon, J., Nunez, J. & McManus, L. (1981). Effect of tau on the vinblastine-induced aggregation of tubulin. *Journal of Cell Biology* **89**, 680–683.

Luduena, R.F., Roach, M.C., Jordan, M.A. & Murphy, D.B. (1985). Different reactivites of brain and erythrocyte tubulins toward a sulfhydryl group-directed reagent that inhibits microtubule assembly. *Journal of Biological Chemistry* **260**, 1257–1264.

McGuire, W.P., Rowinsky, E.K., Rosenshein, N.R., Grumbine, F.C., Ettinger, D.S., Armstrong, D.K. & Donehower, R.C. (1989). Taxol: a unique antineoplastic agent with significant activity in advanced ovarian epithelial neoplasms. *Annals of Internal Medicine* **111**, 273–279.

Magendantz, M. & Solomon, F. (1985). Analyzing the components of microtubules: antibodies against chartins, associated proteins from cultured cells. *Proceedings of the National Academy of Sciences USA* **82**, 6581–6585.

Mandelbaum-Shavit, F., Wolpert-DeFilippes, M.K. & Johns, D.G. (1976). Binding of maytansine to rat brain tubulin. *Biochemical Biophysical Research Communications* **72**, 47–54.

Manfredi, J.J. & Horwitz, S.B. (1984a). Taxol: an antimitotic agent with a new mechanism of action. *Pharmacology and Therapeutics* **25**, 83–125.

Manfredi, J.J. & Horwitz, S.B. (1984b). Vinblastine paracrystals from cultured cells are calcium stable. *Experimental Cell Research* **150**, 205–217.

Manfredi, J.J., Parness, J. & Horwitz, S.B. (1982). Taxol binds to cellular microtubules. *Journal of Cell Biology* **94**, 688–696.

Mareel, M.M., Storme, G.A., Dragonetti, C.H., De Bruyne, G.K., Hartley-Asp, B., Segers, J.L. & Rabaey, M.L. (1988). Antiinvasive activity of estramustine on malignant MO$_4$ mouse cells and on DU-145 human prostate carcinoma cells *in vitro*. *Cancer Research* **48**, 1842–1849.

Margolis, R.L. & Wilson, L. (1977). Addition of colchicine–tubulin complex to microtubule ends: the mechanism of substoichiometric colchicine poisoning. *Proceedings of the National Academy of Sciences USA* **74**, 3466–3470.

Margolis, R.L. & Wilson, L. (1978). Opposite end assembly and disassembly of microtubules at steady state *in vitro*. *Cell* **13**, 1–8.

Margolis, R.L. & Wilson, L. (1981). Microtubule treadmilling—possible molecular machinery. *Nature* **293**, 705–711.

Margolis, R.L., Rauch, C.T. & Wilson, L. (1980). Mechanism of colchicine-dimer addition to microtubule end: implications for the microtubule polymerization mechanism. *Biochemistry* **19**, 5550–5557.

Marshall, L.E. & Himes, R.H. (1978). Rotenone inhibition of tubulin self-assembly. *Biochimica et Biophysica Acta* **543**, 590–594.

Matus, A., Huber, G. & Bernhardt, R. (1983). Neuronal microdifferentiation. *Cold Spring Harbor Symposium on Quantitative Biology* **48**, 775–782.

Mautner, V. & Hynes, R.O. (1977). Surface distribution of LETS protein in relation to the cytoskeleton of normal and transformed cells. *Journal of Cell Biology* **75**, 743–768.

Mitchison, T.J. & Kirschner, M.W. (1984). Dynamic instability of microtubule growth. *Nature* **312**, 237–242.

Mitchison, T.J. & Kirschner, M.W. (1987). Some thoughts on the partitioning of tubulin between monomer and polymer under conditions of dynamic instability. *Cell Biophysics* **11**, 35–55.

Muzaffar, A., Brossi, A., Lin, C.M. & Hamel, E. (1990). Antitubulin effects of derivatives of 3-demethylthiocolchicine, methylthio ethers of colchicinoids, and thioketones derived from thiocolchicine. Comparison with colchicinoids. *Journal of Medicinal Chemistry* **33**, 567–571.

Na, G.C. & Timasheff, S.N. (1982). *In vitro* vinblastine-induced tubulin paracrystals. *Journal of Biological Chemistry* **257**, 10387–10391.

Na, G.C. & Timasheff, S.N. (1986). Interaction of vinblastine with calf brain tubulin: multiple equilibria. *Biochemistry* **25**, 6214–6222.

Nathan, J. & Rebhun, L.I. (1976). Effects of caffeine and other methylxanthines on the development and metabolism of sea urchin eggs: involvement of NADP$^+$ and glutathione. *Journal of Cell Biology* **68**, 440–451.

Noble, M., Lewis, S.A. & Cowan, N.J. (1989). The microtubule binding domain of MAP 1B contains a repeated sequence motif unrelated to that of MAP 2 and tau. *Journal of Cell Biology* **109**, 3367–3376.

Noble, R.L., Beer, C.T. & Cutts, J.H. (1958). Role of chance observations in chemotherapy: vinca rosea. *Annals of the New York Academy of Sciences USA* **76**, 882–894.

Oftebro, O., Grimmer, O., Owen, T.B. & Laland, S.G. (1972) 5-fluoropyrimidin-2-one, a new metaphase arresting agent. *Biochemical Pharmacology* **21**, 2451–2456.

Olmsted, J.B. (1986). Microtubule-associated proteins. *Annual Review of Cell Biology* **2**, 421–457.

Olmsted, J.B. & Borisy, G.G. (1973). Characterization of microtubule assembly in porcine brain extracts by viscometry. *Biochemistry* **12**, 4282–4289.

Olmsted, J.B. & Lyon, H.D. (1981). A microtubule-associated protein specific to differentiated neuroblastoma cells. *Journal of Biological Chemistry* **256**, 3507–3511.

Olmsted, J.B., Asnes, C.F., Parysek, L.M., Lyon, H.D. & Kidder, G.M. (1986). Distribution of MAP 4 in cells and in adult and developing mouse tissues. *Annals of the New York Academy of Science USA* **466**, 292–305.

Oosawa, R. & Asakura, S. (1975). *Thermodynamics of the Polymerization of Protein.* Academic Press, New York.

Ootsu, K., Kozai, Y., Takeuchi, M., Ikeyama, S., Igarashi, K., Tsukamoto, K., Sugino, Y., Tashiro, T., Tsukagoshi, S. & Sakurai, Y. (1980). Effects of new antimitotic antibiotics, ansamitocins, on the growth of murine tumors *in vivo* and on the assembly of microtubules *in vitro*. *Cancer Research* **40**, 1707–1717.

Osborn, M. & Weber, K. (1983). Tumor diagnosis by intermediate filament typing: a novel tool for surgical pathology. *Laboratory Investigation* **48**, 372–394.

Ostlund, R. & Pastan, I. (1975). Fibroblast tubulin. *Biochemistry* **14**, 4064–4068.

Owellen, R.J., Hartke, C.A., Dickerson, R.M. & Hains, F.O. (1976). Inhibition of tubulin–microtubule polymerization by drugs of the vinca alkaloid class. *Cancer Research* **36**, 1499–1507.

Owellen, R.J., Owens, A.H. Jr & Donigian, D.W. (1972). The binding of vincristine, vinblastine and colchicine to tubulin. *Biochemical and Biophysical Research Communications* **47**, 685–691.

Pabion, M., Job, D. & Margolis, R.L. (1984). Sliding of STOP proteins on microtubules. *Biochemistry* **23**, 6642–6648.

Paget, G.E. & Walpole, A.L. (1958). Some cytological effects of griseofulvin. *Nature* **182**, 1320–1321.

Parness, J. & Horwitz, S.B. (1981). Taxol binds to polymerized tubulin *in vitro*. *Journal of Cell Biology* **91**, 479–487.

Parry, E.M., Danford, N. & Parry, J.M. (1982). Differential staining of chromosomes and spindle and its use as an assay for determining the effect of diethylstilbestrol on cultured mammalian cells. *Mutation Research* **105**, 243–252.

Paschal, B.M. & Vallee, R.B. (1987). Retrograde transport by the microtubule-associated protein MAP 1C. *Nature* **330**, 181–183.

Penningroth, S.M. & Kirschner, M.W. (1977). Nucleotide binding and phosphoryla-tion in microtubule assembly *in vitro*. *Journal of Molecular Biology* **115**, 643–673.

Pettit, G.R., Gragg, G.M., Herald, D.L., Schmidt, J.M. & Lohavanijaya, P. (1982). Isolation and structure of combretastatin. *Canadian Journal of Chemistry* **60**, 1374–1381.

Peyrot, V., Briand, C., Momburg, R. & Sari, J.C. (1986). *In vitro* mechanism study of microtubule assembly inhibition by *cis*-dichlorodiammine-platimum (II). *Biochemical Pharmacology* **35**, 371–375.

Pollard, T.D. (1986). Actin and actin-binding proteins. A critical evaluation of mechanisms and functions. *Annual Review of Biochemistry* **55**, 987–1035.

Puck, T.T. (1977). Cyclic AMP, the microtubule–microfilament system, and cancer. *Proceedings of the National Academy of Sciences USA* **74**, 4491–4495.

Punzi, J.S., Duax, W.L., Strong, P., Griffin, J.F., Flocco, M., Zacharias, D., Tew, K.D. & Glusker, J.P. (1992). Molecular conformation of estramustine and two analogues. *Molecular Pharmacology* **41**, 569–576.

Rajagopalan, R. & Gurnani, S. (1985). Effect of rifampicin on the biological activity of tubulin. *Biochemical Pharmacology* **34**, 3515–3419.

Ray, K., Bhattacharyya, B. & Biswas, B.B. (1981). Role of B-ring colchicine in its binding to tubulin. *Journal of Biological Chemistry* **256**, 6241–6244.

Raz, A. & Ben-Ze'ev, A. (1983). Modulation of the metastatic capability in B16 melanoma by cell shape. *Science* **221**, 1307–1310.

Remillard, S., Rebhun, L.I., Howie, G.A. & Kupchan, M. (1975). Antimitotic activity of the potent tumor inhibitor maytansine. *Science* **189**, 1002–1005.

Rohrschneider, L.R. & Najita, L. (1984). Detection of the v-abl gene product of cell-substratum contact sites in Abelson murine leukemia virus-transformed fibro-blasts. *Journal of Virology* **51**, 547–552.

Roobol, A., Gull, K. & Pogson, C.I. (1977). Evidence that griseofulvin binds to a microtubule-associated protein. *FEBS Letters* **75**, 149–152.

Safa, A.R., Hamel, E. & Felsted, R.L. (1987). Photoaffinity labeling of tubulin subunits with a photoactive analogue of vinblastine. *Biochemistry* **26**, 97–102.

Sager, P.R., Doherty, R.A. & Olmsted, J.B. (1983). Interaction of methylmercury with microtubules in cultured cells and *in vitro*. *Experimental Cell Research* **146**, 127–137.

Salmon, E.D., Leslie, R.J., Saxton, W.M., Kasow, M.L. & McIntosh, J.R. (1984). Spindle microtubule dynamics in sea urchin. *Journal of Cell Biology* **99**, 2165–2174.

Schibler, M.J. & Cabral, F. (1985). In Gottesman, M.M. (ed.) *Microtubule Mutants in Molecular Cell Genetics*. John Wiley, New York.

Schiff, P.B. & Horwitz, S.B. (1981). Taxol assembles tubulin in the absence of exoge-nous guanosine 5'-triphosphate or microtubule-associated proteins. *Biochemistry* **20**, 3247–3252.

Schiff, P.B., Fant, J. & Horwitz, S.B. (1979). Promotion of microtubule assembly *in vitro* by taxol. *Nature* **277**, 665–667.

Schiff, P.B., Kende, A.S. & Horwitz, S.B. (1978). Stegnanacin: an inhibitor of HeLa cell growth and microtubule assembly *in vitro*. *Biochemical and Biophysical Research Communications* **85**, 737–746.

Schliwa, M. (1982). Action of cytochalasin D on cytoskeletal networks. *Journal of Cell Biology* **92**, 79–91.

Schnaitman, T., Rebhun, L.I. & Kupchan, S.M. (1975). Antimitotic activity of the antitumour agent, maytansine. *Journal of Cell Biology* **67**, 388a.

Seidman, A., Scher, H., Petrylak, D., Tew K., Krigel, R., Comis, R. & Hudes, G. (1991). Estramustine and vinblastine: effects on serum prostate specific antigen in hormone-refractory prostate cancer. *Proceedings of the American Association for Cancer Research* **32**, 1991.

Serpinskaya, A.S., Gelfand, V.T. & Koprin, B.P. (1981). Comparison of mitostatic effect, cell uptake and tubulin-activity of colchicine and colcemid. *Biochimica et Biophysica Acta* **673**, 86–92.

Shaw, G., Osborn, M. & Weber, K. (1981). An immunofluorescence microscopical study of the neurofilament triplet proteins, vimentin and glial fibrillary acidic protein within the adult rat brain. *European Journal of Cell Biology* **26**, 68–82.

Shelanski, M.L. & Taylor, E.W. (1967). Isolation of a protein subunit from microtubules. *Journal of Cell Biology* **34**, 549–554.

Sheptner, H.S. & Vallee, R.B. (1989). Identification of dynamin, a novel mechano-chemical enzyme that mediates interactions between microtubules. *Cell* **59**, 421–432.

Shin, S., Freedman, V.H., Risser, R. & Pollack, R. (1975). Tumorigenicity of virus-transformed cells in nude mice is correlated specifically with anchorage independent growth *in vitro*. *Proceedings of the National Academy of Sciences USA* **72**, 4435–4439.

Sloboda, R.D., Van Blaricom, G., Creasey, W.A., Rosenbaum, J.L. & Malawista, S.E. (1982). Griseofulvin: association with tubulin and inhibition of *in vitro* microtubule assembly. *Biochemical and Biophysical Research Communications* **105**, 882–88.

Small, J.V. & Sobieszek, A. (1977). Studies of the function and composition of the 10-NM (100-A) filaments of vertebrate smooth muscle. *Journal of Cell Science* **23**, 243–268.

Speicher, L.A., Sheridan, V.R., Godwin, A.K. & Tew, K.D. (1991). Resistance to the antimitotic drug estramustine is distinct from the multidrug resistant phenotype. *British Journal of Cancer* **64**, 267–273.

Starling, D. (1976). The effects of mitotic inhibitors on the structure of vinblastine-induced tubulin paracrystals from sea-urchin eggs. *Journal of Cell Science* **20**, 91–98.

Stearns, M.E. & Tew, K.D. (1985). Antimicrotubule effects of estramustine, an anti-prostatic tumour drug. *Cancer Research* **45**, 3891–3897.

Stearns, M.E., Wang, M., Tew, K.D. & Binder, L.I. (1988). Estramustine binds a MAP-1-like protein to inhibit microtubule assembly *in vitro* and disrupt microtubule organization in Du 145 cells. *Journal of Cell Biology* **107**, 2647–2656.

Steinert, P.M. & Roop, D.R. (1988). Molecular and cellular biology of intermediate filaments. *Annual Review of Biochemistry* **57**, 593–626.

Steinert, P.M., Jones, J.C. & Goldman, R.D. (1984). Intermediate filaments. *Journal of Cell Biology* **99**(1), 225–275.

Stossel, T.D., Chaponries, C., Ezzell, R.M., Hartwig, J.H. (1985). Non-muscle actin binding proteins. *Annual Review of Cell Biology* **1**, 353–402.

Suck, D., Kabasch, W. & Mannherz, H.G. (1981). Three-dimensional structure of the complex skeletal muscle actin and bovine pancreatic DNAse I at 6-Å resolution. *Proceedings of the National Academy of Sciences USA* **78**, 4319–4323.

Sunkara, P.S., Lachman, P.J., Stemerick, D.M. & Edwards, M.L. (1987). MDL 27,048: a novel and potent inhibitor of microtubule assembly. *Journal of Cell Biology* **105**, 2020–2026.

Svoboda, F.H., Gorman, M., Neuss, N. & Barnes, A.L. (1961). Alkaloids of *Vinca rosea Linn*. Preparation and characterization of minor alkaloids. *Journal of Pharmacological Sciences* **50**, 407–413.

Takahashi, M., Iwasaki, S., Kobayashi, H., Okuda, S., Murai, T. & Sato, Y. (1987). Rhizoxin binding to tubulin at the maytansine-binding site. *Biochimica et Biophysica Acta* **926**, 215–223.

Tan, P.T. & Lagnado, J.R. (1975). Effects of indole alkaloids and related compounds on the properties of brain microtubular protein. *Biochemical Society Transactions* **3**, 121–124.

Taylor, E.W. (1965). The mechanism of colchicine inhibition of mitosis. *Journal of Cell Biology* **25**, 145–160.

Temple, C. Jr, Wheeler, G.P., Elliott, R.D., Rose, J.D., Comber, R.N. & Montgomery, J.A. (1983). 1,2-dihydropyrido(3,4-b)pyrazines: structure–activity relationships. *Journal of Medicinal Chemistry* **26**, 91–95.

Temple, C. Jr, Wheeler, G.P., Elliott, R.D., Rose, J.D., Kussner, C.L., Comber, R.N. & Montgomery, J.A. (1982). *Journal of Medicinal Chemistry* **25**, 1045–1050.

Teng, M., Bartholomew, J.C. & Bissell, M.J. (1977). Synergism between anti-microtubule agents and growth stimulants in enhancement of cell cycle traverse. *Nature* **268**, 739–741.

Tew, K.D. (1983). The mechanism of action of estramustine. *Seminars in Oncology* **10**, 21–26.

Tew, K.D., Erickson, L.C., White, G., Wang, A.L., Schein, P.S. & Hartley-Asp, B. (1983). Cytotoxicity of estramustine, a steroid-nitrogen mustard derivative, through non-DNA targets. *Molecular Pharmacology* **24**, 324–328.

Tew, K.D., Woodworth, A. & Stearns, M.E. (1986). Antimitotic properties of estra-mustine are accomplished by a depletion in intracellular glutathione and an inhibition in glutathione S-transferase. *Cancer Treatment Reports* **70**, 715–720.

Vallee, R.B., Wall, J.S., Paschal, B.M. & Schpetner, H.S. (1988). Microtubule associat-ed protein IC from brain is a two-headed cytosolic dynein. *Nature* **332**, 561–563.

Van Warmelo, K.T., Marasas, W.F.O., Adelaar, T.F., Kellerman, T.S., Van Rensbrug, I.B.J. & Minne, J.A. (1970). Experimental evidence that lupinosis of sheep is a mycotoxicosis caused by the fungus *Phomopsis leptostromiformis*. *Journal of the South African Medical Association* **41**, 235–241.

Vandekerckhove, J. & Weber, K. (1978). The amino acid sequence of physarum actin. *Nature* **276**, 720–721.

Wallin, M., Larsson, H. & Edstrom, A. (1979). Effects of sulfhydryl reagents on brain microtubule-associated ATPase activity *in vitro*. *Journal of Neurochemistry* **33**, 1095–1099.

Wang, R.W.-J., Rebhun, L.I. & Kupchan, S.M. (1977). Antimitotic and antitubulin activity of the tumour inhibitor steganacin. *Cancer Research* **37**, 3071–3079.

Wani, M.C., Taylor, H.L., Wall, M.E., Coggon, P. & McPhail, A.T. (1971). Plant antitumor agents. VI. The isolation and structure of taxol, a novel antileukemic and antitumor agent from *Taxus brevifolia*. *Journal of the American Chemical Society* **93**, 2325–2327.

Warfield, R.K.N. & Bouck, G.B. (1974). Microtubule–macrotubule transitions: inter-mediates after exposure to the mitotic inhibitor vinblastine. *Science* **186**: 1219–1221.

Way, M. & Weeds, A. (1990). Cytoskeletal ups and downs. *Nature* **344**, 292–294.

Weatherbee, J.A., Sherline, P., Mascardo, R.N., Izant, J.G., Luftig, R.B. & Weihing, R.R. (1982). Microtubule-associated proteins of HeLa cells: heat stability of the 200,000 mol. wt HeLa MAPs and detection of the presence of MAP 2 in HeLa cell extracts and cycled microtubules. *Journal of Cell Biology* **92**, 155–163.

Weisenberg, R.C. & Deery, W.J. (1976) Role of nucleotide hydrolysis in microtubule assembly. *Nature (London)* **263**, 792–793.

Weisenberg, R.C., Derry, W.J. & Dickinson, P.J. (1976). Tubulin–nucleotide interac-tions during polymerization of microtubules. *Biochemistry* **15**, 4248–4254.

Wheeler, G.P., Bowdon, B.J., Temple, C. Jr, Adamson, D.J. & Webster, J. (1983). Biological effects and structure–activity relationships of 1,2-dihydropyrido[3,4-b]pyrazines. *Cancer Research* **43**, 3567–3575.

Wheeler, G.P., Bowdon, B.J., Werline, J.A. & Temple, C. Jr (1981). 1-deaza-7,8-di-hydropteridines, a new class of mitotic inhibitors with anticancer activity. *Biochemi-cal Pharmacology* **30**, 2381–2384.

Wiche, G., Briones, E., Koszka, C., Artlich, U. & Krepler, R. (1984). Widespread occurrence of polypeptides related to neurotubule-associated proteins (MAP 1 and MAP 2) in nonneuronal cells and tissues. *EMBO Journal* **3**, 991–998.

Willingham, M.C., Jay, G. & Pastan, I. (1979). Localization of the ASV *src* gene product to the plasma membrane of transformed cells by electron microscopic immunocytochemistry. *Cell* **18**, 125–134.

Wilson, L. (1975). Microtubules as drug receptors: pharmacological properties of microtubule protein. *Annals of the New York Academy of Sciences USA* **253**, 213–231.

Wilson, L., Creswell, K.M. & Chin, D. (1975). The mechanism of action of vinblastine. Binding of [acetyl-^{3}H]vinblastine to embryonic chick brain tubulin and tubulin from sea urchin sperm tail outer doublet microtubules. *Biochemistry* **14**, 5586–5592.

Wilson, L., Morse, A.N.C. & Bryan, J. (1978). Characterization of acetyl-^{3}H-labeled vinblastine binding to vinblastine–tubulin crystals. *Journal of Molecular Biology* **121**, 255–268.

Wittelsberger, S.C., Kleene, K. & Penman, S. (1981). Progressive loss of shape-responsive metabolic controls in cells with increasing transformed phenotype. *Cell* **24**, 859–866.

Wright, T.C., Ukena, T.E., Campbell, R. & Karnovsky, M.J. (1977). Rates of aggregation, loss of anchorage dependency and tumorigenicity of cultured cells. *Proceedings of the National Academy of Sciences USA* **74**, 258–262.

Wyllie, A.H. (1980). Glucorcorticoid-induced thymocyte apoptosis is associated with endogenous nuclease activation. *Nature* **284**, 555–556.

Yahara, I., Harada, F., Sekita, S., Yoshihira, K. & Natori, S. (1982). Correlation between effects of 24 different cytochalasins on cellular structures and events and those on actin *in vitro*. *Journal of Cell Biology* **92**, 69–78.

Yang, J.T., Laymon, R.A. & Goldstein, L.S.B. (1989). A three domain structure of kinesin heavy chain revealed by DNA sequence and microtubule binding analysis. *Cell* **56**, 879–889.

York, J., Wolpert-DeFilippes, M.K., Johns, D.G. & Sethi, V.S. (1981). Binding of maytansinoids to tubulin. *Biochemical Pharmacology* **30**, 3239–3243.

Zweig, M.H. & Chignell, C.F. (1973). Interaction of some colchicine analogs, vinblastine and podophyllotoxin with rat brain microtubule protein. *Biochemical Pharmacology* **22**, 2141–2149.

Chapter 4
Tyrphostins—a novel concept for antiproliferative drugs
Alexander Levitzki and Chaim Gilon

Introduction

Cell proliferation is governed by cell division/cycle proteins, by the gene products of the proto-oncogene family and by the products of tumour-suppressor genes. Proto-oncoproteins can be classified according to their cellular localization as well as according to their biochemical activity. Proto-oncoproteins when mutated or amplified become highly active or even constitutively active thus generating sustained proliferative signals (Bishop, 1987). Since proto-oncoproteins and oncoproteins are directly involved in regulating cell proliferation, they are excellent targets for antiproliferative agents (see Chapter 1). Such agents should be less cytotoxic, since they are targetted to antagonize a selective set of proteins specifically involved in cell proliferation. This is in contrast to conventional chemotherapeutic agents used in cancer therapy which employ chemical agents that interfere with DNA, RNA and protein synthesis or are cytoskeleton-disrupting agents (Calabresi & Parks, 1985) (but see Chapter 3, this volume). These agents potentially interfere with all cellular functions and therefore are toxic also to non-proliferating cells. From examination of oncogene targets, it is apparent that a number of approaches can be adopted for generating antiproliferative agents. The most successful approach in medical practice so far has been the development of synthetic compounds which selectively block the action of a target protein. Thus, it is likely that the so-called chemical approach to combat proliferative diseases stands to gain momentum. This is also true for

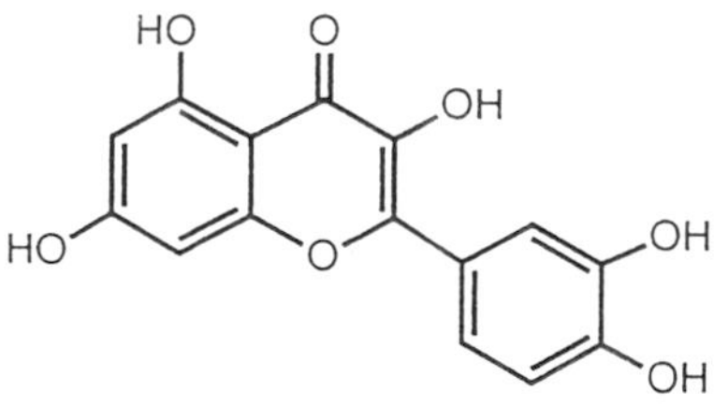

Quercetin
($K_i \simeq 10 \, \mu\text{M}$)

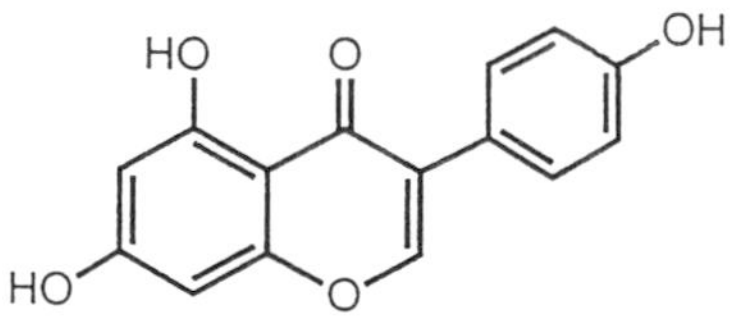

Genistein
($K_i \simeq 2.6 \, \mu\text{M}$)

Fig. 4.1. Tyrosine kinase inhibitors that compete with the adenosine triphosphate (ATP) subsite.

non-neoplastic proliferative diseases such as psoriasis, atherosclerosis and myofibrosis. There is no doubt that other valid approaches to combat proliferative diseases are likely to develop. For example, the employment of cytokines, growth factors, antibodies and hormones, as detailed in this book. The combination of synthetic antineoplastic agents and a biological reagent is definitely a realistic possibility, as we have demonstrated for inhibitors of protein tyrosine kinase (PTK) inhibitors (tyrphostins) and anti-epidermal growth factor (EGF) receptor antibodies (see below). Among the targets for future drugs, PTKs stand out. It is by now clear that enhanced PTK activity is associated with abnormal cell proliferation and malignancies (Bishop, 1987; Ullrich & Schlessinger, 1990).

Protein tyrosine kinase inhibitors

Naturally occurring PTK inhibitors

Soon after the PTK reaction was discovered and their unique role in transforming cells was established, the search for inhibitors of such reactions began. The first inhibitor discovered was the natural product quercetin (Glossman *et al.*, 1981; Graziani *et al.*, 1983) and a related compound genistein (Akiyama *et al.*, 1987) was discovered later (Fig. 4.1).

Quercetin, as well as some of its synthetic analogues, were found also to inhibit various serine/threonine kinases such as cyclic adenosine monophosphate (cAMP)-dependent kinase, protein kinase C and $Ca^{2+}/$ calmodulin-dependent kinase. This feature rendered these compounds highly cytotoxic and therefore of little or no potential to us as candidates for antiproliferative drugs. Recently, however, certain synthetic derivatives of quercetin have been synthesized and demonstrated to be more selective towards PTKs (Cushman *et al.*, 1991). Genistein is much more selective towards PTK as compared to serine/threonine kinases (Akiyama *et al.*, 1987).

Other naturally occurring compounds such as erbstatin (Umezawa

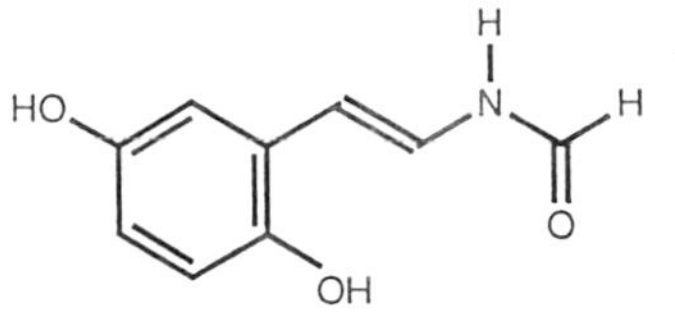

Erbstatin
($IC_{50} \simeq 0.63\ \mu M$)

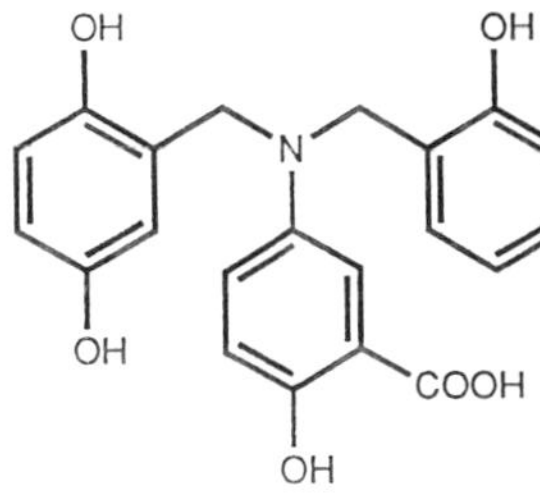

Lavendustin A
($IC_{50} \simeq 50\ nM$)

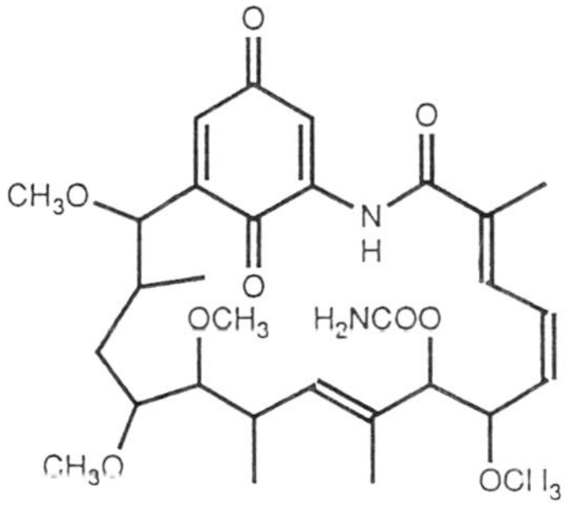

Herbimycin A
($IC_{50} \simeq 1\ \mu M$)

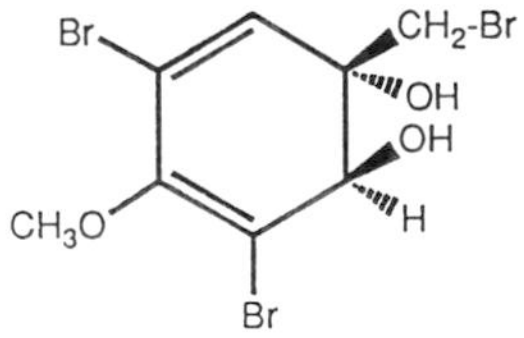

(+) Aeroplysinin-1
($IC_{50} = 0.2\ \mu M$)

Fig. 4.2. Some naturally occurring protein tyrosine kinase (PTK) inhibitors.

et al., 1986), herbimycin A (Murakami *et al.*, 1988), lavendustin (Onoda *et al.*, 1989) and aeroplysinin-1 (Kreuter *et al.*, 1990) have also been identified as PTK blockers (Fig. 4.2). These compounds, in contrast to quercetin, are highly selective inhibitors of PTKs and therefore are potential leads for the design of novel and more selective antiproliferative agents.

Design of tyrphostins

We have also recognized the potential of PTK inhibitors as antiproliferative drugs and therefore have embarked on a systematic synthetic programme to develop non-peptidic inhibitors of PTKs. The lack of unambiguous structural information of PTKs such as X-ray crystallographic data or conformation analysis by two-dimensional nuclear magnetic resonance (NMR) (Wutrich 1989a,b) led us to base our design on the structure of the substrate or the structure of known natural products which inhibit PTKs and on the knowledge of the reaction mechanism. Since the exact mechanism of the PTK catalysed reaction is unknown, we based our design on the mechanism of other adenosine triphosphate (ATP)-dependent kinases. Kinetic studies and the use of ATP-analogous bearing chiral P_{γ} groups have indicated that the phosphorylation reaction of many ATP-dependent kinases proceeds via a 'direct displacement' mechanism rather than a 'double displacement' type (Knowles, 1980). According to this mechanism the nucleophile, which is activated by a basic side chain of the kinase attacks the P_γ of ATP by a direct nucleophilic attack to give phosphorylated substrate and ADP (see Fig. 4.6, and section on bisubstrate tyrphostins, below). Our systematic programme to generate potent selective PTK inhibitors is guided by the following principles (Yaish *et al.*, 1988; Gazit *et al.*, 1989, 1991):

1   To use simple straightforward synthetic procedures in order to facilitate structure–activity relationship (SAR) studies, and allow synthetic scale up of successful compounds.

2   To prepare small molecules which by initial design considerations should compete with the substrate subsite rather than with the ATP subsite on the PTK.

3   To prepare selective compounds for key PTKs. Towards this end, we have established *in vitro* biochemical assays as well as cell bioassays for various PTKs such as EGF-receptor kinase (EGFRK) (HER1), InsRK, neu/erbB2(HER2) kinase and *abl* kinases.

4   To control pharmacokinetic properties of the inhibitors such as appropriate solubility properties that will allow them to traverse the cell membrane and therefore be tested on intact cells and later in experimental animals.

We have ruled out the use of small synthetic peptides containing tyrosine as potential inhibitors mainly for two reasons. Firstly, small linear peptides composed of natural amino acids suffer from several drawbacks that prevent them from becoming effective drugs. These include metabolic instability due to fast degradation by peptidases, lack of selectivity due to their conformational instability (Gilon *et al.*, 1991) and inferior pharmacokinetic properties such as poor permeation through cell membranes and poor absorption into the intestinal tract. Secondly, tyrosine-containing peptides are rather poor substrates for PTKs with high K_m values, close to the millimolar range. The best peptide substrates, with K_m values in the 50 to 100 μM range, are too long and therefore poor 'guideline' molecules.

In view of these considerations, we decided to design small molecules (called tyrphostins) that will complement spatially and electronically the PTK substrate subsite based on structural elements of tyrosine and erbstatin (Fig. 4.3) We felt that the *p*-hydroxyphenyl moiety of tyrosyl residue of a PTK substrate and the conjugated doubled bond of erbstatin were excellent guidelines for the initial PTK blockers we made. This was especially true since it was claimed that erbstatin is a competitive inhibitor with the substrate tyrosine subsite and not with the ATP subsite although Posner *et al.* (1993) and others (Bishop *et al.*, 1990) have recently shown

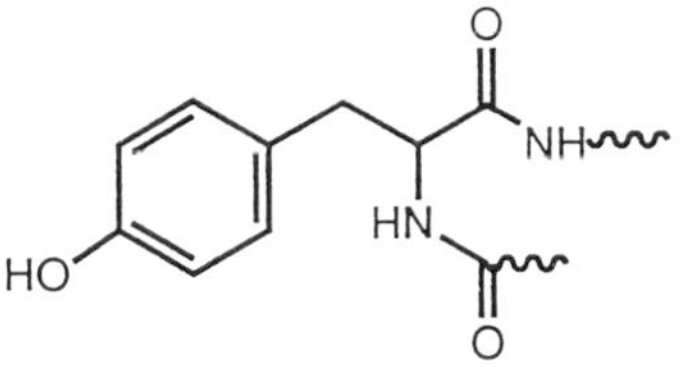

Tyrosine residue in a PTK substrate

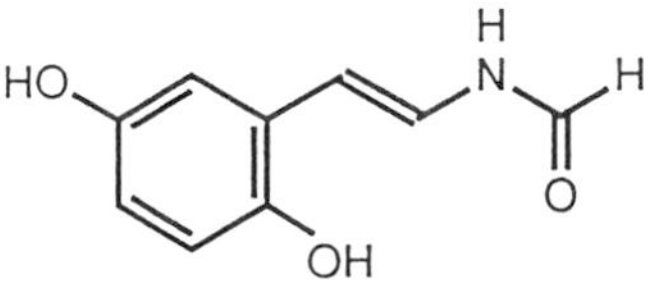

Erbstatin (IC$_{50}$ ≃ 0.63 μM)

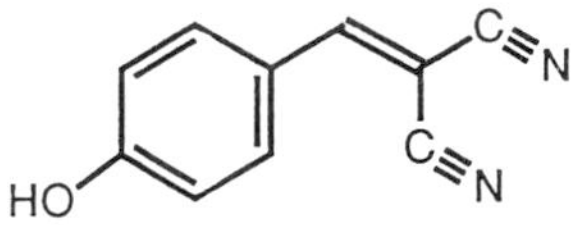

Tyrphostin AG10
(IC$_{50}$ = 560 μM)

Fig. 4.3. Structural leads for tyrphostins.

that erbstatin is actually a 'mixed type' competitive inhibitor which also affects the affinity of EGFRK towards both substrate and ATP.

Synthesis of tyrphostins

Erbstatin is an unstable compound due to the presence of the trans eneformamido group and its synthesis is complicated. Moreover, erbstatin is limited in structural elements that permit modifications intended to improve selectivity, potency and pharmacokinetic properties. We, therefore, chose to incorporate the phenolic residue of tyrosine into a benzylidenemalononitrile framework which permitted greater synthetic flexibility. From a synthetic point of view most benzylidenemalononitriles can be easily prepared by a straightforward Knoevenagel condensation of benzaldhydes or acetophenones with malononitriles and their derivatives (Fig. 4.4). The synthetic scheme presented in Fig. 4.4 allows for modification on the aromatic nucleus (R′) and the double bond (α and β). These modifications are necessary for SAR studies.

Studies of structure activity relationships

Benzylidenemalononitrile-based tyrphostins

One of the first compounds synthesized by Gazit et al. (1989) was 4-hydroxybenzylidenemalononitrile (compound 1, Table 4.1 and Fig. 4.3). As can be seen from the structures in Fig. 4.3, this compound contains structural elements which resemble both erbstatin and a tyrosyl residue in a PTK substrate. Tyrphostin 1 (as we called the benzylidenemalononitrile-

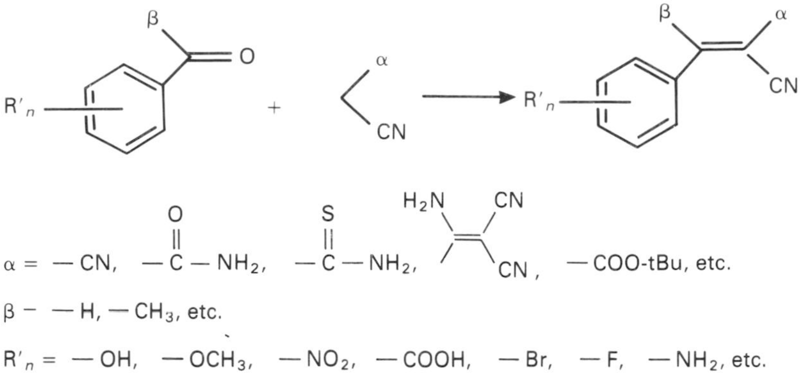

$$\alpha = -CN, \quad \overset{O}{\underset{\parallel}{-C}} - NH_2, \quad \overset{S}{\underset{\parallel}{-C}} - NH_2, \quad \overset{H_2N}{\diagdown}\overset{CN}{\diagup}_{CN}, \quad -COO\text{-}tBu, \text{ etc.}$$

$\beta - -H, -CH_3$, etc.

$R'_n = -OH, \quad -OCH_3, \quad -NO_2, \quad -COOH, \quad -Br, \quad -F, \quad -NH_2$, etc.

Fig. 4.4. Synthesis of tyrphostins.

derived PTK inhibitors) has a 4-hydroxybenzene moiety like tyrosine and a conjugated double bond-like erbstatin. Tyrphostin 1 has two cyano groups that resemble both the formamido group of erbstatin and the two flanking amide bonds of a tyrosyl residue.

The low inhibitory activity ($IC_{50} = 560 \,\mu M$) of tyrphostin 1 prompted Yaish et al. (1988) and Gazit et al. (1989) to incorporate other structural elements aimed to improve its inhibitory activity. First, more hydroxyls were introduced on the aromatic ring to enhance similarity to erbstatin. Indeed, two hydroxyls in positions 3 and 4 on the aromatic ring, increased potency 20-fold (compound 2, Table 4.1). The relative positions of the two hydroxyls, in positions 2 and 5, like in erbstatin, led to a cyclic compound (compound 3, Table 4.1) which was much less active (Fig. 4.5).

Introduction of a third hydroxyl or a methoxy group on the aromatic ring further improved activity (compounds 4 and 5, Table 4.1). Compound 4, however, was unstable and underwent fast oxidation. Substituents other than hydroxyls or addition of electron withdrawing groups on the aromatic ring (such as NO_2, F, Cl, Br, I, etc.) have some effects on the potency of compound 2 (not shown). Replacement of the dihydroxyphenyl ring by other aromatic or heteroaromatic rings (e.g. compound 6, Table 4.1) yielded inactive compounds towards EGFRK. These and other inactive compounds towards EGFRK were routinely checked as potential leads for selective inhibitors for other PTKs. Indeed, compound 6, which was found to be inactive as an inhibitor of EGFRK ($IC_{50} = 2200 \,\mu M$) (Gazit et al., 1991), is a potent inhibitor of platelet-derived growth factor (PDGF) receptor kinase activity and PDGF-induced mitogenesis ($IC_{50} = 15 \,\mu M$) (Bryckaert et al., 1992). The authors have indeed recognized that indole tyrphostins are potent and selective blockers of the PDGF-receptor system.

Further SAR studies (Gazit et al., 1991) have demonstrated the importance of the cis cyano group for biological activity of tyrphostins

Table 4.1. Structure and biological activity of tyrphostins

Chemical data		Biochemical data	Biological data*
		PolyGAT phosphorylation	EGF-dependent proliferation
Compound No.	Structure	IC$_{50}$ (μM)	IC$_{50}$ (μM)
1 (AG10)		560	ND
2 (AG18)		35	30 (>30)
3 (AG111)		75	ND
4 (AG82)		3	20 (>60)
5 (AG34)		6	20 (>10)
6 (AG361)		2200	ND
7 (AG30)		70	53
8 (AG114)		2.5	ND
9 (AG99)		10	15(60)
10 (AG213)		2.4	50
11 (AG473)		1.3	15(120)
12 (AG336)		2.5	≫16 (unstable)
13 (AG308)		0.5	30 (>150)
14 (AG538)		0.37	8 (>50)

Table 4.1. Continued

		Biochemical data	Biological data[*]
Chemical data		PolyGAT phosphorylation	EGF-dependent proliferation
Compound No.	Structure	IC_{50} (μM)	IC_{50} (μM)
15 (AG455)	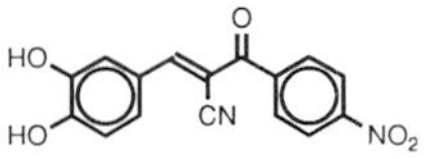	2.3	20 (>20)
16 (AG527)[†]	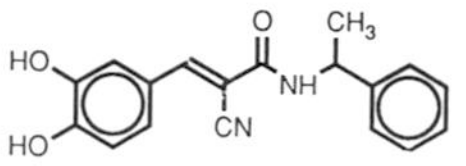	0.4	3.5 (10)
17 (AG555)	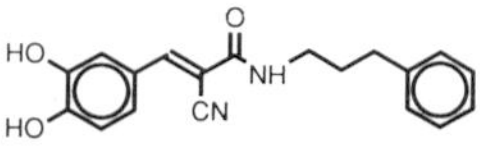	0.7	2.5 (25)

*Numbers in brackets refer to the concentration required to inhibit serum-dependent cell growth.
†The (-) enantiomer.
ND, not determined; PolyGAT, random co-polymer $Glu_6Ala_3Tyr_1$ (sigma).
Data for compounds 1-5, 7, 8 from Gazit et al. (1989); and for compounds 6, 9-17 from Gazit et al. (1991).

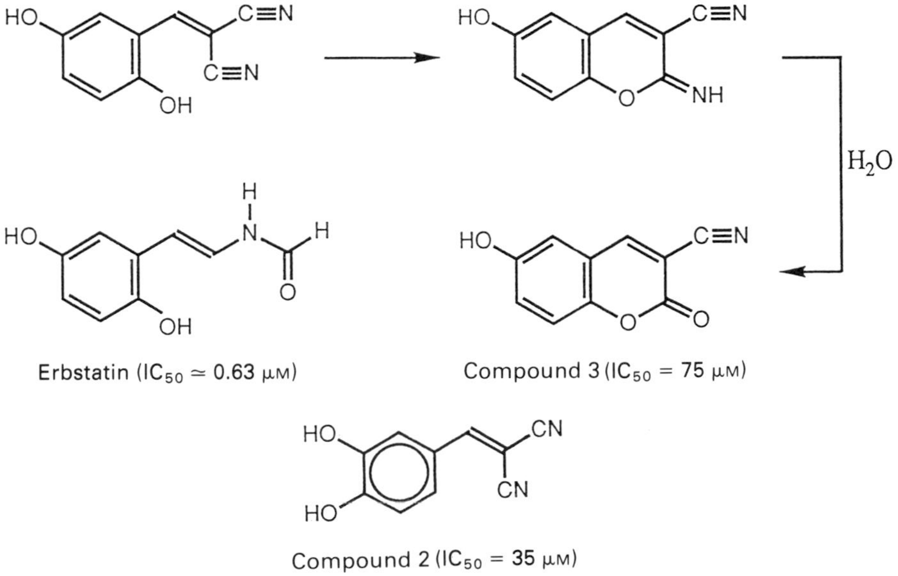

Erbstatin ($IC_{50} \simeq 0.63\ \mu M$)   Compound 3 ($IC_{50} = 75\ \mu M$)

Compound 2 ($IC_{50} = 35\ \mu M$)

Fig. 4.5. Cyclization of 2,5-dihydoxy benzylidenemalononitride.

(not shown). It was then decided to further explore the possibility of replacing the *trans* cyano group of compound 2 (position α in Fig. 4.4) to determine the degree of flexibility of this position. We decided to perform these modifications on the 3,4-dihydroxy benzylidene nucleus because of its relatively high potency and chemical stability.

Compounds 7–11 (Table 4.1) present modifications of 3,4-dihydroxy *cis*-cinnamonitrile at the α position. Introduction of a carboxyl group decreased the inhibitory activity on the EGFRK (compare compounds 2 and 7, Table 4.1) two-fold, but was found to be active ($IC_{50} = 4.5\,\mu M$) in inhibiting a yet unidentified tyrosine kinase from human colon carcinoma (Schwartz *et al.*, 1990). Other substituents at the α position, especially amido (compound 9), thioamido (compound 10) and keto (compound 11) exhibit at least 10-fold increase in inhibitory activity compared to the α-cyano group (compound 2). These compounds demonstrate the importance of a carbonyl group, be it a keto, amido or thioamido at the α position for improved activity. Moreover, these compounds enabled us to further modify the α position by the introduction of substituted amides and ketones (see below).

Conformationally constrained 3,4-dihydroxy cinnamonitriles

The authors prepared a series of analogues which have the dicyanoethylene moiety fixed *exo* to a dihydroxy phenyl-containing bicyclic structure (Gazit *et al.*, 1991). These rigid analogues were prepared in order to probe the conformational requirements of tyrphostins as PTK inhibitors. Compounds 1–11 (Table 4.1) are conformationally flexible due to the single bond character of the bond *exo* to the dihydroxy aromatic ring. In the conformationally restricted analogues, this bond is incorporated into another ring. The authors have prepared two classes of bicyclic compounds based on the 3,4-dihydroxy cinnamonitrile nucleus. The first group of compounds has the dicyano ethylene moiety *exo* to a dihydroxy isatin ring (compound 12). This compound and other isatin-containing analogues showed improved inhibitory activity, but were unstable in solution in an *in vitro* assay and especially in the whole cell (tissue culture) assays. The improved activity of the isatin series prompted preparation of their carbocyclic analogues based on an indane nucleus. Compound 13, which is a 3,4-dihydroxy–indanylidene malononitrile, has the dicyanoethylene moiety fixed *exo* coplanar to the catechol ring. Further studies, including enlargement of the five-membered indane ring to a more flexible six-membered ring led to the conclusion that the preferred orientation for inhibitory activity of the conformationally constrained dihydroxcinnamonitrile analogues is where the malononitrile moiety and the catechol ring are fixed in a coplanar *cis-'syn'* conformation (Gazit *et al.*, 1991).

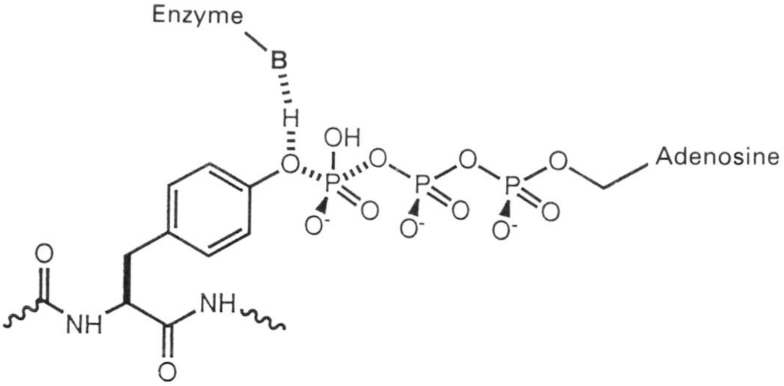

Fig. 4.6. Tentative transition state of tyrosine phosphorylation by protein tyrosine kinases (PTKs).

α-keto tyrphostins

The improved inhibitory and antiproliferative activity of α-keto tyrphostins (see compound 11, Table 4.1) prompted the authors to prepare a series of compounds which have various substituents on the α-keto aromatic ring. These substituents had little effect on the potency. The best inhibitor of this series was compound 14 with an IC_{50} of 0.37 μM. One of the α-keto tyrphostins showed enhanced efficiency towards the erbB2/neu PTK (e.g. compound 15 has an IC_{50} of 3 μM on the erbB2/neu PTK).

α-amido tyrphostins

The authors have found that substituted amides at the α-position, and especially those which contain aromatic rings, are more potent inhibitors than the parent unsubstituted amide (compound 9, Table 4.1). The authors have prepared a large number of aromatic and alicyclic amido tyrphostins with varied size, chemical nature and chirality of the spacer connecting the ring with the α-amido group. The best compound in the series was compound 16 with an IC_{50} of 0.4 μM. Compound 17 showed the best antiproliferative activity with an IC_{50} of 2.5 μM. Few of the α-amido tyrphostins, like some of the keto tyrphostins, could discriminate between the EGFRK and the erbB2/neu(HER2) kinase. For example, compound 17 is 50 times less potent on the erbB2/neu(HER2) kinase than on the EGFR(HER1) kinase (Gazit *et al.*, 1991). Other amide derivatives were shown to be more selective for erbB2/neu kinase (unpublished data).

Bisubstrate tyrphostins

Based on the mechanism presented in our discussion of the design of tyrphostins (above), it was assumed that the transition state of tyrosyl phosphorylation by PTK has a tyrosyl residue attached through its phenolic hydroxyl to an ATP as can be seen in Fig. 4.6. On theoretical

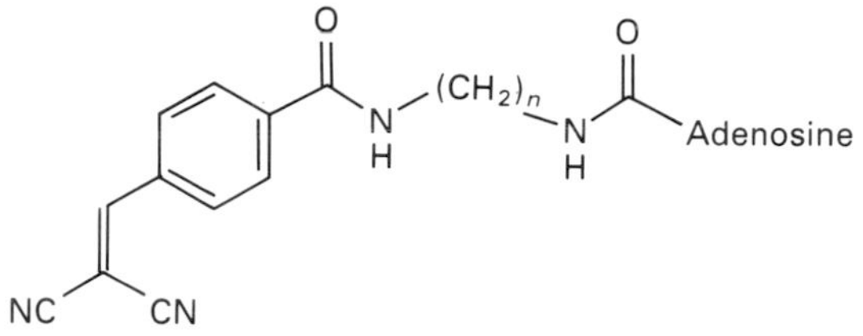

Fig. 4.7. Bisubstrate tyrphostin inhibitors.

grounds it can be argued that a single compound which possesses two structural elements, one of which would occupy the ATP subsite and the other the tyrosyl subsite, is expected to be a very potent bisubstrate inhibitor. Such an inhibitor is shown in Fig. 4.7 (unpublished).

This would be expected to bind to the active site with an affinity constant which is the product of the two affinity constants for the two separate moieties. This concept has been tested experimentally and was proven to be valid (Byers, 1978; Broom, 1989). Based on the tentative transitional state shown in Fig. 4.6, and on the assumption that tyrphostins such as compound 2 (Table 4.1) block the substrate subsite, the authors have designed and synthesized a series of bisubstrate inhibitors having an adenosine or an isoquinoline moiety attached through a spacer to the para position of a benzylidene malononitrile (Fig. 4.7). The length of the spacer linking the two moieties was varied to achieve maximal inhibitory activity (unpublished).

These, and other bisubstrate analogues, in which the spacers were connected through the para position of benzylidenemalononitrile tyrphostins, were found to be more potent than the monosubstrate inhibitors composing them but much less potent than most of the tyrphostins presented hitherto (Ataja *et al.*, in press).

Dimeric tyrphostins

One model of signal transduction in EGF and related growth factors assumes receptor dimerization induced by EGF binding which promotes the internal tyrosine kinase domains to phosphorylate each other (Ullrich & Schlessinger, 1990). This finding prompted the authors to prepare dimeric analogues in which two tyrphostins are linked through an appropriate spacer. The choice to connect the two tyrphostin moieties through their α positions had two reasons. Firstly, as can be seen from Table 4.1, various substitutions at the α position did not reduce inhibition and in many cases even improved it. Secondly, based on our study of α-amido tyrphostins described above, the authors found that the preparation of dimers with the general structure shown in Fig. 4.8 is synthetically facile (A. Gazit *et al.*, unpublished data).

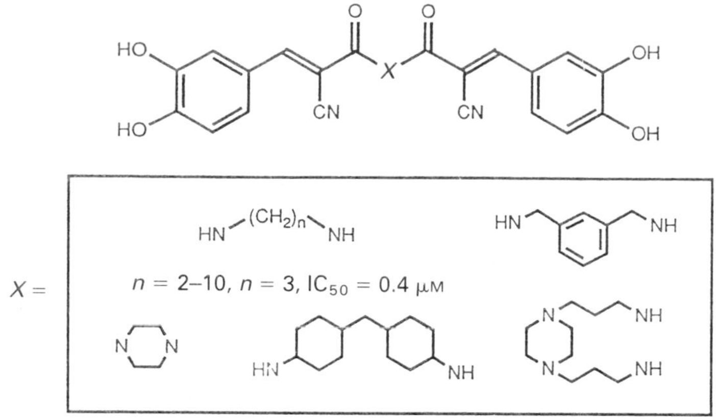

Fig. 4.8. Dimeric tyrphostins.

The authors have probed the chemical nature and optimal distance between the two dihydroxy cinnamonitrile moieties by changing the spacer. An optimal activity was obtained with the α, ω-diaminoalkylidene spacer (Fig. 4.8) where $n = 4$ (IC_{50} of $0.5\,\mu M$). An analogue where $n = 3$ was found by detailed kinetic studies to be a pure competitive inhibitor of EGFRK with an $IC_{50} = 0.4\,\mu M$, and $K_i = 0.06\,\mu M$ (Posner *et al.*, 1993).

Specificity of tyrphostins

Tyrphostins are either highly specific or possess rather 'relaxed' specificity. It seems that some of the tyrphostins interact with residues within the tyrosine kinase domain which may be common among many PTKs, thus probing similar structural elements. On the other hand, and strikingly, some tyrphostins even discriminate between the closely related EGF receptor (HER1) and the neu/erbB2(HER2) gene product which are 80% homologous in the kinase domain (Gazit *et al.*, 1991). The most striking results is our recent finding that some tyrphostins discriminate between p140^{c-abl}, p185$^{bcr-abl}$ and p210$^{bcr-abl}$, all of which possess identical catalytic domains, but differ in the N-terminal sequences. This result suggests that *abl* proteins may possess different substrate specificities and/or affinities towards intracellular target substrates. The authors have, therefore, examined the K_m values of the three human *abl* kinases towards ATP and tyrosine-containing substrates. Indeed the three *abl* proteins possess different affinities towards substrates and moreover towards ATP. Furthermore, certain tyrphostins discriminate rather sharply between *abl* and EGFRK (Anafi *et al.*, 1992).

Such findings are quite encouraging, since they strengthen the hypothesis that in spite of the belief that numerous PTKs have identical intracellular target substrates, like guanosine triphosphatase (GTPase)

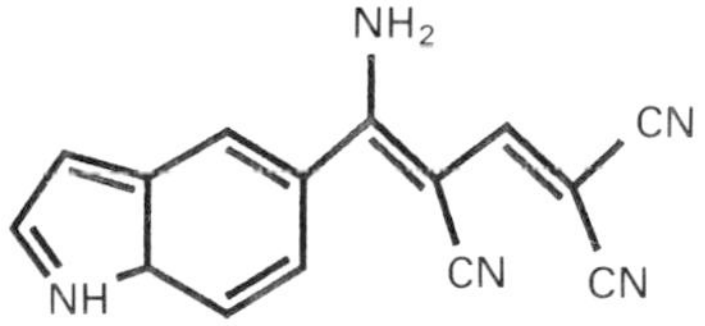

Fig. 4.9. AG370 blocker of platelet-derived growth factor (PDGF) signalling.

activating protein (GAP) or PLC$_\gamma$, they may differ from each other not only in their affinities towards identical putative substrates, but may have more specialized substrates. Thus selective tyrphostins may discriminate between even related PTKs and block selectively the action of a particular tyrosine kinase.

A related finding is the observation that a few tyrphostins, in contrast to many, are much more efficacious on EGF dependent cell proliferation as compared to their effect on EGFRK (A. Levitzki et al., unpublished data). This effect could be due to the accumulation of these tyrphostins in the cell or to their inhibitory action on an unknown PTK which is downstream in the EGF signalling pathway.

However, one would not always wish to use a highly selective tyrphostin, since in many proliferative processes a number of PTKs cooperate in generating the mitogenic process. For example, it has been known for a long time that PDGF-receptor activation by PDGF induces the activation of the intracellular pp $60^{c\text{-}src}$. Thus if one wishes to inhibit PDGF action, blocking of pp $60^{c\text{-}src}$ action concomitant to the inhibition of PDGFRK may be beneficial, if one wishes to block the action of PDGF. Indeed, in human bone marrow fibroblasts tyrphostin 6 (AG 361) or tyrphostin AG370 (Fig. 4.9) inhibit the PDGF-induced tyrosine phosphorylation and therefore the activation of pp $60^{c\text{-}src}$ (Bryckaert et al., 1992). The authors have not yet fully determined what is the relative contributions of the inhibition of PDGF-receptor kinase vis á vis the inhibition of the action of the PTK activity of pp $60^{c\text{-}src}$ by tyrphostin AG370 or AG361.

Similarly, we have recently demonstrated that a number of tyrphostins inhibit the EGF-dependent proliferation of human and guinea pig keratinocytes grown in culture and correspondingly the EGF-dependent growth of skin organ cultures (Dvir et al., 1991). Cells are arrested in the S phase of the cell cycle (H. Ben Bassat & A. Levitzki, unpublished data). We still, however, do not know whether these tyrphostins also affect the keratinocyte growth factor (KGF) receptor kinase (KGFRK) as well as other PTKs and whether the arrest of keratinocyte growth is due to the combined effects of tyrphostins on a number of PTKs.

Type of inhibition

Initially, the authors designed tyrphostins to compete with the substrate subsite and not with the ATP subsite. However, it was quickly discovered that tyrphostins can be effective tyrosine kinase blockers by competing with ATP and still not affect cAMP-dependent protein kinase or other threonine/serine kinases. In this respect, this family of tyrphostins behaves like the totally unrelated PTK blocker lavendustin A (Onada *et al.*, 1989) and its derivatives (A. Gazit *et al.*, unpublished data). This rather surprising finding strongly suggests that the ATP-binding domain in PTKs differs remarkably from that in other protein kinases. Although one can achieve selectivity of tyrphostins as ATP competitors, the authors consider this feature undesirable. The main reason being that the high intracellular concentration of ATP renders competition against ATP rather ineffective in intact cells or *in vivo*. Examination of highly potent tyrphostins which compete against ATP indeed show that they inhibit EGF-dependent cell growth at $IC_{50} = 2–15\,\mu M$ compared to K_i values of 40–100 nM as measured *in vitro* (Posner *et al.*, 1993 and unpublished data). Some of the tyrphostins which behave as ATP competitors have no effect at all on the affinity of *abl* kinases towards ATP and are strictly competitive with the substrate subsite (Anafi *et al.*, 1992). This difference in behaviour of the same tyrphostin towards two different PTKs is not only a manifestation of the selectivity of tyrphostins, but also demonstrates a fundamental difference between the kinase domains of EGFR and *abl* kinase.

This assertion is strengthened by the finding that AG537 (Fig. 4.8, $n = 4$) which has K_i of 60 nM as a competitive inhibitor of EGFRK *in vitro* (Gazit *et al.*, 1991; Posner *et al.*, 1993) is extremely specific for EGFRK, and is a poor inhibitor of *abl* kinase (Anafi *et al.*, 1992). Our synthetic approach, therefore, is directed toward tyrphostins which minimally affect the affinity towards ATP. It seems that PTKs differ in the structure of the kinase domain, specifically in the distance between the substrate site and the ATP site. As we make progress in our work, comparing the interaction between different PTKs and tyrphostins, more information on these relationships emerge.

Biological activity

A large number of tyrphostins have already been tested in a large variety of biological systems. Tyrphostins are proven to be successful experimental antiproliferative agents with low non-specific toxicity. The antiproliferative activity of these compounds is at present in the range of 0.1–50 μM. Most of the compounds become toxic at IC_{50}, a concentration which is 100-fold higher than that required to block 50% of the proliferative signal. Table 4.2 summarizes the experimental systems used and the tyrphostins used in those systems.

In one study, the authors have recently shown for the first time the antiproliferative effects of tyrphostins *in vivo*. Tyrphostins inhibit the growth of a human tumour which overexpresses EGF receptors, when implanted into nude mice. Tyrphostins, by intraperitoneal injection, prolong the survival of the mice and cause shrinking in the size of the tumours. One of the most exciting aspects of this study is the finding that the tyrphostin synergizes with a monoclonal antibody against the external EGF-binding domain of the EGF receptor, in blocking tumour growth (Yoneda *et al.*, 1991). The authors therefore anticipate that tyrphostins in combination with antibodies against cancer antigens or in combination with immunotoxins targetted to cancer cells can provide an effective antineoplastic chemotherapy.

Because of the success of tyrphostins in blocking EGF-dependent proliferation of keratinocytes (Dvir *et al.*, 1991), the authors have begun to test the potency of these as inhibitors of psoriatic keratinocytes. Initial findings demonstrate that a large number of EGFR-directed tyrphostins arrest the growth of psoriatic keratinocytes in culture (unpublished data).

This finding correlates with the assertion that the psoriatic condition is associated with the overexpression of the TGF-α gene (Elder *et al.*, 1989; Vassar & Fuchs, 1991 and references therein) and therefore sustained autocrine stimulation of keratinocytes. The persistent autocrine activation of the EGF receptor by TGF-α on keratinocytes seems to play a major role in the development and/or maintenance of the psoriatic condition. Indeed recently, Rhone Poulenc Rorer in collaboration with the authors, have begun clinical trials using tyrphostins as antipsoriatic ointments.

The antiproliferative activity of tyrphostins on the PDGF-dependent proliferation of vascular smooth muscles (Bilder *et al.*, 1991) suggests that tyrphostins can be considered as agents to combat restenosis following angioplasty and atherosclerosis. It is believed by many that PDGF plays a pivotal role in the development of the atherosclerotic plaque, especially in the initial stages of development (Ross, 1989).

PDGF also plays a role in other hyperproliferative conditions such as pulmonary fibrosis (Antoniades *et al.*, 1991) and myelofibrosis (Katoh *et al.*, 1990). The authors have recently identified tyrphostins which seem to be selective in the PDGFβ signalling system. These indole tyrphostins (AG361, Table 4.1) and another indole tyrphostin (AG370, Fig. 4.9) were found to be extremely effective in inhibiting PDGF-dependent proliferation of human bone marrow fibroblasts (Bryckaert *et al.*, 1992). In this study, it is also shown that the PDGF-dependent tyrosine phosphorylation of GAP, pp 60^{c-src} as well as PDGFR autophosphorylation itself are inhibited by tyrphostin AG370 (Fig. 4.9) with an $IC_{50} \sim 20\,\mu$M. The inhibitory dose response for PDGF-dependent phosphorylation is similar to the inhibitory dose response of PDGF-dependent cell proliferation. Recent analogs of AG370 were found to be more potent and more selective against PDGFR kinase and PDGF-dependent cell proliferation (unpublished).

Table 4.2. The biological activity of tyrphostins

Biological system	Type of biochemical activity inhibited by the tyrphostins	Class of tyrphostins used	References
EGF responsive system:			
NH3T3 cell expressing EGF receptors	EGF-dependent cell proliferation	Simple hydroxylated benzenemalononitriles	Yaish *et al.*, 1988
Human and guinea pigs keratinocytes	Inhibition of human tumour overexpressing EGF receptors grown in nude mice	Highly modified benzenemalononitriles	Gazit *et al.*, 1989
	PLC$_\gamma$ and other intracellular substrates		Lyall *et al.*, 1989
	EGF-induced production of phosphoinositides		Dvir *et al.*, 1991
			Gazit *et al.*, 1991
			Yoneda *et al.*, 1991
			Posner *et al.*, 1989
			Margolis *et al.*, 1989
PDGF responsive systems:			
Rabbit vascular smooth muscle cells grown in culture	Inhibition of cell proliferation	Indole malononitriles and some simple hydroxylated benzenemalononitriles	Bilder *et al.*, 1991
Human bone marrow fibroblasts grown in culture	Inhibition of PDGF-dependent phosphorylation of pp60[c-sr] other		Bryckaert *et al.*, 1992
Reversal of the pp60[c-src]:			
Transformed state in chicken lens cells	PTK activity of pp60[c-src] induced transformation	Simple hydroxylated benzene malononitriles	Vollberg *et al.*, 1992
Maturation of sea star oocytes	Inhibition of maturation	Hydroxylated benzene malonoitriles, erbstatin some which are different from EGFRK blockers	Daya-Makin *et al.*, 1991
	Inhibition of p34[cdc2] tyrosine phosphorylation		
	Inhibition of p44[mbp] tyrosine phosphorylation		

Inhibition of thrombin:			
Induced platelet aggregation	Inhibition of PtdIns$(4,5)$P$_2$ biosynthesis Inhibition of thrombin-induced tyrosine phosphorylation of pp60$^{c\text{-}src}$ and other intracellular substrates	Hydroxylated benzene malononitriles	Rendu *et al.*, 1991
Inhibition of proliferation of B and T lymphocytes	Inhibition of PLC$_\gamma$, inhibition of and Ca^{2+} mobilization Inhibition of tyrosine phosphorylation of proteins	Hydroxylated benzene malononitriles different from EGFRK blockers	Padeh *et al.*, 1991 Roifman *et al.*, 1991
Inhibition of bFGF-induced synaptic development	Not known	Hydroxylated benzene malononitriles	Peng *et al.*, 1991

EGF, epidermal growth factor; PDGF, platelet-derived growth factor; bFGF, basic fibroblast growth factor; PLC, phospholipase C; PTK, protein tyrosine kinase; PtdIns(4,5)P$_2$, phosphatidylinositol 4,5-bisphosphate; EGFRK, EGF-receptor kinase.

Tyrphostins as molecular tools

We have used tyrphostins to demonstrate that tyrosine phosphorylation is involved in thrombin-induced platelet aggregation and release of serotonin (Rendu *et al.*, 1991). Thrombin induces pp 60^{c-src} tyrosine phosphorylation as well as that of other intracellular target proteins. The inhibitory effect of tyrphostins on the thrombin-induced tyrosine phosphorylation correlates quantitatively with their inhibitory effect on platelet aggregation and serotonin release (Rendu *et al.*, 1992). This is an interesting case which may be the first example of many: that G proteins signal to protein tyrosine kinases. Thrombin interacts with a β-adrenoreceptor/rhodopsin-type receptor which is coupled to a G protein.

Similarly, tyrphostins were instrumental in demonstrating the involvement of protein tyrosine phosporylation on the signalling pathway of B-lymphocyte activation (Padeh *et al.*, 1991; Roifman *et al.*, 1991) as well as T-lymphocyte activation (Stanley *et al.*, 1990). In both the platelet system and the B-lymphocyte system, it was also shown that tyrphostins do not affect the signalling pathways elicited by the direct activation of protein kinase C using a phorbol ester. Independently, the authors have shown that cAMP-mediated pathways are not affected by tyrphostins (Schechter *et al.*, 1989) and that protein kinase A is inhibited *in vitro* by tyrphostin concentrations 100- to 10 000-fold higher than those required to block PTK activities of various tyrosine kinases (I. Posner & A. Levitzki, unpublished data).

Tyrphostins were instrumental in the elucidation of the signalling pathway leading from EGF-receptor activation to the mobilization of intracellular stores of Ca^{2+}. It was shown that tyrphostins block EGFR-induced phosphorylation of phospholipase C_γ (PLC$_\gamma$) (Margolis *et al.*, 1989) and therefore IP$_3$ formation (Posner *et al.*, 1989) and Ca^{2+} mobilization (Margolis *et al.*, 1989). Tyrphostins have no effect on IP$_3$ formation and Ca^{2+} mobilization induced by bradykinin and bombesin which most probably activate phospholipase $C\beta$ (PLCβ) which is not a substrate for PTK. These results also demonstrate the selectivity of tyrphostins and their relative non-toxicity.

The involvement of protein tyrosine phosphorylation in the maturation pathway of sea star oocytes was also clearly demonstrated by using tyrphostins and erbstatin (Daya-Makin *et al.*, 1991). In this system, we have shown that tyrosine phosphorylation of p44^{mbp} and the activation of p34^{cdc2} kinase are inhibited by tyrphostins, thus inhibiting oocyte maturation.

Conclusion

In the past 4 years, the authors have demonstrated that tyrphostins effectively block various PTKs and exhibit either narrow or broad specificities. These inhibitors have been demonstrated to be effective antiproliferative agents where their antiproliferative activity correlates with their PTK-blocking activity. Furthermore, tyrphostins act as antineoplastic agents *in vitro* and can synergize with antibodies which interact with cancer cells. These results demonstrate the potential of tyrphostins as antineoplastic agents. The arresting effects of EGFRK-directed tyrphostins on normal and psoriatic keratinocytes identifies tyrphostins as novel potential treatment of psoriasis. Also, the inhibition of PDGF-dependent proliferation of vascular smooth cells and bone marrow fibroblasts by PDGF-receptor directed tyrphostins suggest that tyrphostins can be considered as potential anti-atherosclerotic agents and as antiproliferative drugs on other conditions in which PDGF plays a major role.

Our studies also demonstrate that tyrphostins can be employed as molecular tools to dissect PTK signal transduction. Thus, for example, tyrphostins block PTK-induced PLC_γ activation and therefore inositol 1,4,5-trisphosphate $(Ins(1,4,5)P_3)$ formation and Ca^{2+} mobilization without interference of signalling to other PLC isozymes.

References

Akiyama, T., Ishida, J., Nakagawara, S., Ogawara, H., Watanabe, S., Itoh, N., Shibuya, M. & Fukami, Y. (1987). Genistein, a specific inhibitor of tyrosine specific protein kinases. *Journal of Biological Chemistry* **262**, 5592–5595.

Anafi, M., Gazit, A., Gilon, C., Ben-Neriah, Y. & Levitzki, A. (1992). Selective interactions of transforming and normal *abl* proteins with ATP, tyrosine copolymer substrates and tyrophostins. *Journal of Biological Chemistry* **267**, 4518–4523.

Antoniades, H.N., Bravo, M.A., Avila, R.E., Galanopulos, T., Neville-Godden, J., Maxwell, M. & Selman, M. (1991). Platelet-derived growth factor in idiopathic pulmonary fibrosis. *Journal of Clinical Investigation* **86**(4), 1055–1064.

Bilder A., Krawiec, J.A., Gazit, A., Gilon, C., McVety, K., Lyall, R., Zilberstein, A., Levitzki, A., Perrone, M. & Schreiber, A.B. (1991). Tyrphostins inhibit PDGF induced DNA synthesis, tyrosine specific protein kinase activity and c-*fos* mRNA expression in vascular smooth muscle cells. *American Journal of Physiology* **260**, c721–c730.

Bishop, J.M. (1987). The molecular genetics of cancer. *Science* **235**, 305–311.

Bishop, W.R., Petrin, J., Wang, L., Ramesh, U. & Doll, R.J. (1990). Inhibition of protein kinase C by the tyrosine kinase inhibitor erbstatin. *Biochemical Pharmacology* **40**(9), 2129–2135.

Broom, J. (1989). Rational design of enzyme inhibitors: multisubstrate analogue inhibitors. *Journal of Medical Chemistry* **32**, 2–7.

Bryckaert, M.C., Eldor, A., Gazit, A., Osherov, N., Gilon, C., Fontenay, M., Levitzki, A. & Tobelem, G. (1992). Inhibition of platelet derived growth factor (PDGF) induced mitogenic activity by PDGF receptor tyrosine kinase tyrphostin inhibitors. *Experimental Cell Research* **199**, 255–261.

Byers, L.D. (1978). Binding of reactic intermediate analogs to enzymes, *Journal of Theoretical Biology* **74**, 501–512.

Calabresi, P. & Parks, R.E. Jr. (1985). Chemotherpay of neoplastic diseases. In Gilman, A.G., Goodman, L.S., Rall, L.W. & Murad, F. (eds) *Goodman's and Gilman's: The Pharmacological Basis of Therapeutics*, pp. 1247–1306. Macmillan, New York.

Cushman, M., Nagarthnam, D., Burg, D.L. & Geahlen, R.L. (1991). Synthesis and protein-tyrosine kinase inhibitory activities of flavonoid analogues. *Journal of Medicinal Chemistry* **34**, 798–806.

Daya-Makin, M., Pelech, S., Levitzki, A. & Hudson, P.T. (1991). Erbstatin and tyrphostins block protein serine kinase activation and meiotic maturation of sea star oocytes. *Biochemica et Biophysica Acta* **1093**, 87–94.

Dvir, A., Milner, Y., Chomsky, O., Gilon, C. & Levitzki, A. (1991). The inhibition of EGF-dependent proliferation of keratinocytes by tyrosine kinase blockers. *Journal of Cell Biology* **113**, 857–865.

Elder, J.T., Fisher, G.J., Lindquist, P.S., Bennet, G.L., Pittelkow, M.R., Coffey, R.J., Ellingsworth, L., Derynck, R. & Voorhees, J.J. (1989). Overexpression of transforming growth factor a in psoriatic epidermis. *Science* **243**, 811–814.

Gazit, A., Osherov, N., Posner I., Yaish, R., Poradosu, E., Gilon, C. & Levitzki, A. (1991). Tyrphostins II: heterocyclic and α-substituted benzonemalononitrile tyrphostins as potent inhibitors of EGF receptor and erbB2/neu tyrosine kinases. *Journal of Medicinal Chemistry* **34**, 1897–1907.

Gazit, A., Yaish, P., Gilon, C. & Levitzki, A. (1989). Tyrphostins I: synthesis and biological activity of protein tyrosine kinase inhibitors. *Journal of Medical Chemistry* **32**, 2344–2352.

Gilon, C., Halle, D., Chorev, M., Selinger, Z. & Byk, G. (1991). Backbone cyclization: a new method for conferring conformational constraint on peptides. *Biopolymers* **31**, 745–750.

Glossman, H., Presek, P. & Eizenbrodt, E. (1981). Quercetin inhibits tyrosine phosphorylation of cyclic nucleotide independent transforming protein kinase pp 60^{src}. *Naunyn-Schmiedebergs Archives of Pharmacology* **317**, 100–102.

Graziani, Y., Erikson, E. & Erikson, R.L. (1983). The effect of quercetin on the phosphorylation activity of Rous sarcoma virus transforming gene product *in vitro* and *in vivo*. *European Journal of Biochemistry* **135**, 583–589.

Katoh, O., Kirmura, A., Itoh, T. & Kuramoto, A. (1990). PDGF messenger RNA is increased in bone marrow megacaryocytes with myeloproliferative disorders. *American Journal of Hematology* **35**, 145–150.

Knowles, J.R. (1980). Enzyme-catalyzed phosphoryl transfer reactions. *Annual Review of Biochemistry* **49**, 877–919.

Kreuter, M.-H., Leake, R.E., Rinaldi, F., Müller-Klieser, W., Maidhof, A., Müller, W.E.G. & Schröder, H.C. (1990). Inhibition of intrinsic protein tyrosine kinase activity of EGF receptor kinase complex from human breast cancer cells by the marine spone metabolite (+) Aeroplysinin-1. *Comparative Biochemistry and Physiology* **97B**(1), 151–158.

Lyall, R.M., Zilberstein, A., Gazit, A., Gilon, C., Levitzki, A. & Schlessinger, J. (1989). Tyrphostins inhibit EGF receptor tyrosine kinase activity in living cells and EGF-stimulated cell proliferation. *Journal of Biological Chemistry* **264**, 14503–14509.

Margolis, B., Phee, S-G., Felder, S., Lyall, R., Levitzki, A., Ullrich, A., Zilberstein, A. & Schlessinger, J. (1989). EGF induces tyrosine phosphorylation of phospholipase CII: a potential mechanism for EGF-receptor signalling. *Cell* **57**, 1101–1107.

Murakami, Y., Mizuno, S., Hori, M. & Uehara, Y. (1988). Reversal of transformed phenotype by herbimycin A in *src* oncogene expressed rat fibroblasts. *Cancer Research* **48**, 1587–1590.

Onoda, T., Iinuma, H., Sasaki, Y., Hamada, M., Isshibi, K., Naganawa, H., Tokeuchi, T., Tatsuta, K. & Umezawa, K. (1989). Isolation of a novel tyrosine kinase inhibitor lavendustin A from *Streptomyces griseolavendus*. *Journal of Natural Products* **52**, 1252–1257.

Padeh, S., Levitzki, A., Gazit, A., Mills, G.B. & Roifman, C.M. (1991). Activation of phospholipase C in human B cells is dependent on tyrosine phosphorylation. *Journal of Clinical Investigation* **87**, 1114–1118.

Peng, H.B., Baker, L.P. & Chen, Q. (1991). Inhibition of synaptic development in cultured muscle cells by basic fibroblast growth factor. *Neuron* **6**, 237–246.

Posner, I., Engel, M., Gazit, A. & Levitzki, A. (1993). Kinetics of inhibition of the tyrosine kinase activity of the epidermal growth factor receptor by tyrphostins. *Journal of Biological Chemistry*, in press.

Posner I., Gazit, A., Gilon, C. & Levitzki, A., (1989). Tyrphostins inhibit the epidermal growth factor receptor mediated breakdown of phosphoinositides, *FEBS Letters* **257**, 287–291.

Rendu, F., Eldor, A., Grelac, F., Gazit, A., Gilon, C., Levy-Toledano, S. & Levitzki, A. (1991). Tyrosine kinase blockers: new platelet activation inhibitors. Blood Coagulation and Fibrinolysis **1**, 713–716.

Rendu, F., Eldor, A., Gerlac, F., Gazit, A., Gilon, C., Levy-Toledano, S. & Levitzki, A. (1992). Inhibition of platelet activation by tyrosine kinase inhibitors. *Biochemical Pharmacology*, in press.

Roifman, C., Mills, G.B., Chin, K., Gazit, A., Gilon, C. & Levitzki, A. (1991). Tyrosine phosphorylation is an essential event in the stimulation of B lymphocytes by *Staphylococcus aureus* Cowen I. *Journal of Immunology* **146**, 2965–2971.

Ross, R. (1989). Platelet-derived growth factor. *Lancet* **ii**, 1179–1182.

Schechter, Y., Yaish, P., Chorev, M., Gilon, C., Braun, S. & Levitzki, A. (1989). Inhibition of insulin dependent lipogenesis and antilipolysis by protein tyrosine kinase inhibitors. *EMBO Journal* **8**(6), 1671–1676.

Schwartz, B., Cagnano, E., Braun, S. & Lamprecht, S.A. (1990). Characterization of tyrosine kinase associated with subcellular components of human colonic epithelium. *Anticancer Research* **10**, 1747–1754.

Stanley, J.B., Gorczynski, R., Huang, C-K., Love, J. & Mills, G.B. (1990). Tyrosine phosphorylation is an obligatory event in IL-2 secretion. *Journal of Immunology* **145**, 2189–2198.

Ullrich, A. & Schlessinger, J. (1990). Signal transduction by receptors with tyrosine kinase activity. *Cell* **61**, 203–212.

Umezawa, H., Imoto, M., Sawa, T., Isshikij, K., Matsuda, N., Uchida, T., Iinuma, H., Hamada, M. & Takeuchi, T. (1986). Studies on a new epidermal growth factor receptor kinase inhibitor, erbstatin, produced by MH435-hF3. *Journal of Antibiotics* **39**, 170–173.

Vassar, R. & Fuchs, F. (1991). Transgenic mice provide new insights into the role of TGFα during epidermal development and differentiation. *Genes and Development* **5**, 714–727.

Vollberg, T., Zik, Y., Dron, R., Sabanay, I., Gilon, C., Levitzki, A. & Geiger, B. (1992). The effect of tyrosine specific protein phosphorylation on the assembly of adherins type junctions. *EMBO Journal* **11**, 1733–1742.

Wutrich, K. (1989a). The development of nuclear magnetic resonance spectroscopy as a technique for protein structure determination. *Account Chemical Research* **22**, 36–44.

Wutrich, K. (1989b). Protein structure determination in solution by nuclear magnetic resonance spectroscopy. *Science* **243**, 45–50.

Yaish, P., Gazit, A., Gilon, C., Chorev, M., Braun, S. & Levitzki, A. (1988). Blocking of EGF-dependent cell proliferation by EGF receptor kinase inhibitors. *Science* **242**, 933–935.

Yoneda, T., Lyall, R., Alsine, M.M., Pearsons, P.E., Spada, A.P., Levitzki, A., Zilberstein, A. & Mundy, G.R. (1991). The antiproliferative effects of tyrosine kinase inhibitor tyrphostin on a human squamous cell carcinoma *in vitro* and in nude mice. *Cancer Research.* **51**, 4430–4435.

Chapter 5
Neuropeptide growth factors and antagonists

Penella J. Woll, Tariq Sethi and Enrique Rozengurt

Introduction

Cancer cells are characterized by unrestrained growth. Until recently pharmacologists have concentrated on disrupting cell division to kill cancer cells. The cytotoxic drugs developed have been extremely effective in the minority of rapidly growing tumours, but their effects on normal dividing tissues have led to dose-limiting toxicities. Attention has now moved to the biology of cancer, in the expectation that elucidation of the factors stimulating tumour growth and their modes of action will permit rational development of novel and specific antitumour agents, with activity in a wider range of solid tumours.

In recent years it has become evident that neoplastic cells acquire complete or partial independence of growth control through different mechanisms (Rozengurt, 1983; Sporn & Roberts, 1985; Goustin et al., 1986; Cross & Dexter, 1991). These include production of autocrine or paracrine growth factors, alterations in the number or structure of cellular receptors and changes in the activity of postreceptor signalling pathways (Sager, 1989; Bishop, 1991). Cancers are thought to result from the accumulation of multiple genetic changes, causing activation of oncogenes and deletion of tumour-suppressor genes. The discovery that many onco-genes code for growth factors, their receptors or for proteins involved in intracellular signalling has been central to this thesis.

Because of the complex interactions between growth factors *in vivo*, direct evidence for their effects has depended upon the development of homogeneous cell lines *in vitro*. The non-tumorigenic murine Swiss 3T3 fibroblast line has proved useful for identifying both the extracellular factors that modulate cell growth and the early signals and molecular events that lead to mitogenesis. These cells cease to proliferate when the medium is depleted of its growth-promoting activity and can be stimulated to reinitiate DNA synthesis and cell division either by replenishing the medium with fresh serum, or by the addition of purified growth factors, pharmacological agents or a variety of neuropeptides (Rozengurt, 1985). Studies performed using such quiescent cells and defined combinations of growth factors have revealed the existence of potent and specific synergistically acting signal transduction pathways initiated almost immediately after mitogen addition (Rozengurt, 1986; Rozengurt et al., 1988).

Neuropeptide growth factors may act on the secreting cell (autocrine) or nearby tumour or stromal cells (paracrine). These actions are increasingly implicated in a variety of important biological processes including wound healing, embryogenesis and oncogenesis (Zachary et al., 1987; Woll, 1991a). The evidence for neuropeptide growth factor action in tumours of the lung will now be briefly considered, and their modes of action outlined before discussing the development of drugs directed against them.

Lung cancer

Lung cancer is the commonest cause of cancer deaths in the developed world. It comprises small cell lung cancer (SCLC, 25%) and non-small cell lung cancer (NSCLC, 75%) including squamous cell, large cell and adeno-carcinoma. Epidermal growth factor (EGF) and transforming growth factor-α (TGF-α) are secreted by some NSCLC. These both bind to EGF receptors, which have been demonstrated on NSCLC cells, suggesting autocrine growth stimulation (Söderdahl et al., 1988; Veale et al., 1989; Tateishi et al., 1990). In contrast, SCLC does not express EGF receptors.

SCLC typically secretes a variety of hormones and growth factors including numerous neuropeptides. Many of these are now known to be mitogenic in diverse cell types, but their precise role in SCLC remains to be defined (Woll, 1991b). Of these, bombesin and its homologue gastrin-releasing peptide (GRP) have attracted most interest. This gut peptide was found to be secreted by SCLC 10 years ago (Moody et al., 1981; Wood et al., 1981; Erisman et al., 1982). The finding that it could also act as a growth factor for Swiss 3T3 cells focused attention on neuropeptides as possible mediators of cancer growth (Rozengurt & Sinnett-Smith, 1983). The mRNA for GRP has been demonstrated in SCLC (Suzuki et al., 1987) and GRP has been shown to stimulate SCLC growth in vitro and in vivo (Carney et al., 1987; Alexander et al., 1988). Cuttitta et al. (1985) used a monoclonal antibody to bombesin to inhibit the clonal growth of two SCLC cell lines in vitro and the growth of one as a xenograft in nude mice. Thus, there is persuasive evidence that bombesin/GRP can act as an autocrine growth factor in at least some SCLC. A detailed understanding

of the receptors and signal transduction pathways that mediate the mitogenic action of bombesin and GRP may identify novel targets for therapeutic intervention.

Early signalling events in bombesin action

The early cellular and molecular responses elicited by bombesin and
structurally related peptides have been elucidated in detail (Rozengurt &
Sinnett-Smith, 1990). The cause–effect relationships and temporal organization of these early signals and molecular events provide a paradigm
for the study of other growth factors and mitogenic neuropeptides and
illustrate the activation and interaction of a variety of signalling pathways
(Rozengurt, 1991).

Bombesin/GRP binds to a single class of high-affinity receptors in
Swiss 3T3 cells (Zachary & Rozengurt, 1985). The receptors are glycoproteins of M_r 75 000–85 000 with a core of M_r 43 000 (Kris et al., 1987;
Zachary & Rozengurt, 1987; Sinnett-Smith et al., 1988). The receptor is
coupled to one or more guanine nucleotide binding proteins (G proteins)
as judged by the modulation of ligand binding in membrane preparations
(Sinnett-Smith et al., 1990) and in receptor solubilized preparations
(Coffer et al., 1990a). The bombesin/GRP receptor has recently been
cloned and sequenced (Battey et al., 1990) and shown to be a member of
the G protein coupled receptor family. These receptors have seven predicted transmembrane domains which cluster to form a ligand-binding
pocket (Lefkowitz & Caron, 1988). Other neuropeptide mitogens with
receptors of this type include angiotensin, bradykinin, endothelin,
serotonin, substance K, substance P and vasopressin (Arai et al., 1990;
McEachern et al., 1991: Birnbaumer et al., 1992).

Binding of bombesin/GRP to its receptor initiates a cascade of intracellular signals culminating in DNA synthesis 10–15 h later (Rozengurt,
1986). One of the earliest events to occur after the binding of bombesin to
its specific receptor is a rapid mobilization of Ca^{2+} from intracellular
stores, which leads to a transient increase in the concentration of cytosolic
Ca^{2+} and subsequently to a decrease in the Ca^{2+} content of the cells. The
mobilization of Ca^{2+} by bombesin is mediated by inositol 1,4,5-trisphos-
phate ($Ins(1,4,5)P_3$), which acts as a second messenger in the action of
many ligands that stimulate inositol lipid turnover and Ca^{2+} efflux.
Bombesin causes a rapid increase in $Ins(1,4,5)P_3$, which coincides with the
increase in cytosolic Ca^{2+}. $Ins(1,4,5)P_3$ is formed as a result of phospholipase C catalysed hydrolysis of phosphatidyl inositol 4,5-bisphosphate in
the plasma membrane, a process that also generates 1,2-diacylglycerol
(DAG). DAG can also be generated from other sources, such as phosphatidylcholine hydrolysis, and acts as a second messenger in the activation of protein kinase C (PKC) by bombesin. In accord with this,

bombesin strikingly increases the phosphorylation of the acidic 80 kDa protein (Zachary *et al.*, 1986; Erusalimsky *et al.*, 1988), a major substrate of PKC which has been recently purified and molecularly cloned (Brooks *et al.*, 1990, 1991; Erusalimsky *et al.*, 1991). Bombesin/GRP also stimulates a rapid exchange of Na^+, H^+ and K^+ ions across the cell membrane, leading to cytoplasmic alkalinization and an increase in intracellular $[K^+]$ concentration.

Recently, bombesin, vasopressin and endothelin have been shown to induce a rapid and potent stimulation of tyrosine phosphorylation of several substrates in quiescent 3T3 cells (Zachary *et al.*, 1991). In addition, bombesin induces release of arachidonic acid and its cyclooxygenase metabolite prostaglandin E_2 (PGE_2) into the medium (Millar & Rozengurt, 1988, 1990a). Considerable evidence indicates that the liberation of arachidonic acid is an early signal that contributes to bombesin-mediated mitogenesis (Millar & Rozengurt, 1990a; Gil *et al.*, 1991). In common with many other growth factors, bombesin/GRP stimulates transient expression of the nuclear oncogenes c-*fos* and c-*myc* (Rozengurt & Sinnett-Smith, 1988). This complex network of signals (Fig. 5.1; see Rozengurt, 1991 for review) involves a degree of redundancy, suggesting the importance of the mitogenic pathway and ensuring the amplification of the stimulus. Strategies to block growth factor action must embrace this complexity. Importantly, studies with SCLC have demonstrated a similar set of early events. GRP stimulates mobilization of intracellular Ca^{2+} and inositol phosphate turnover in SCLC cells (Heikkila *et al.*, 1987; Moody *et al.*, 1987; Trepel *et al.*, 1988b).

The role of other neuropeptides

In addition to bombesin, several other regulatory peptides have been characterized as mitogens for Swiss 3T3 cells including vasopressin, bradykinin and endothelin-related peptides, and their signalling pathways have also been defined in detail (Issandou & Rozengurt, 1990; Millar & Rozengurt, 1990a; Rozengurt, 1991). It is central to our thesis that bradykinin, cholecystokinin, galanin, neurotensin, tachykinins and vasopressin have been shown to induce a rapid and transient increase in $[Ca^{2+}]_i$ in SCLC cell lines (Staley *et al.*, 1989a, b; Woll & Rozengurt, 1989a; Bunn *et al.*, 1990; Takuwa *et al.*, 1990). However, the precise relationship between these Ca^{2+}-mobilizing receptors and the long-term proliferation of SCLC remains unclear (e.g. see Takuwa *et al.*, 1990). In this respect, recent observations with galanin, a 29 amino acid neuropeptide, are relevant.

In pancreatic cells galanin activates an adenosine triphosphate (ATP)-sensitive K^+ channel, hyperpolarizes the plasma membrane and inhibits the activity of voltage-dependent Ca^{2+} channels (Dunne *et al.*, 1989). In this manner it reduces Ca^{2+} influx and blocks the activity of various agents

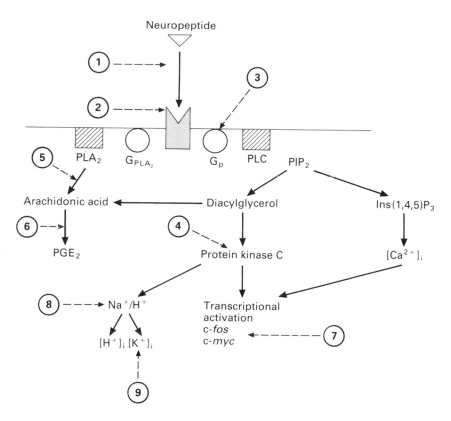

Fig. 5.1. Bombesin-mediated mitogenesis can be blocked at receptor and post-receptor levels. Growth factor-initiated cell proliferation in 3T3 cells is mediated by multiple signal transduction pathways that act in a synergistic fashion. The interactions have been well defined in these cells. The actions of the neuropeptide growth factors are demonstrated here and means of blocking the various pathways are indicated by broken lines as follows. (1) Specific and broad-spectrum neuropeptide antagonists; antibodies to the growth factors or receptors. (2) Down-regulation of the receptor. (3) GDPβS, a G protein antagonist that blocks signal transduction. (4) Phorbol dibutyrate down-regulation of protein kinase C. (5) Heterologous desensitization of arachidonic acid release. (6) Cyclo-oxygenase inhibitors, e.g. indomethacin. (7) Selective transcriptional block by antisense RNA. (8) Na^+/K^+ pump inhibitors, e.g. ouabain. (9) Blockers of N^+/H^+ antiport. $[Ca^{2+}]_i$, intracellular $[Ca^{2+}]$; G, guanine nucleotide binding protein; $Ins(1,4,5)P_3$, inositol 1,4,5-trisphosphate; PGE_2, prostaglandin E_2; PIP_2, phosphatidylinositol 4,5-bisphosphate; PLA_2, phospholipase A_2; PLC, phospholipase C. All other details are explained in the text.

that increase the intracellular concentration of Ca^{2+} in pancreatic cells. Surprisingly, in SCLC cell lines galanin caused a rapid and transient increase in $[Ca^{2+}]_i$ (Woll & Rozengurt, 1989a). Further studies showed that galanin induced rapid mobilization of Ca^{2+} from internal stores and stimulated early production of inositol phosphates, particularly $Ins(1,4,5)P_3$ (Sethi & Rozengurt, 1991). Thus, in contrast to the pancreatic cells, galanin receptors in SCLC are coupled to Ca^{2+} mobilization rather than to the control of membrane potential and indirectly, to the reduction of Ca^{2+} influx. Crucially, galanin has been shown to act as a growth factor for some SCLC cell lines, promoting clonal growth in semi-solid medium (Sethi & Rozengurt, 1991a). Consequently, we determined the effects of multiple Ca^{2+}-mobilizing neuropeptides to promote clonal growth in semisolid medium in different SCLC cell lines. We showed that at optimal concentrations, bradykinin, neurotensin, vasopressin, cholecystokinin, galanin and GRP induce comparable increases of SCLC clonal growth in responsive cell lines (Sethi & Rozengurt, 1991b). Opioid peptides have also been reported to stimulate SCLC growth *in vitro* (Davis *et al.*, 1989). Thus, the emerging picture is that of a heterogeneous SCLC tumour cell population secreting diverse neuropeptides, which act as autocrine and paracrine growth factors.

Blocking growth factor action

As understanding of the effects of growth factors in cancer increases, it has become possible to plan rational therapeutic interventions. If an autocrine growth loop is considered, in which cells synthesize, secrete, bind and respond to the same growth factor, it is evident that interruption of this cycle at any point will block mitogenesis. Paracrine growth could be blocked in the same way. As discussed in the preceding section, SCLC constitutes a special case in which unrestrained proliferation appears driven, as least in part, by multiple autocrine and paracrine circuits involving Ca^{2+}-mobilizing neuropeptides.

Secreted factors can be cleared by antibodies, such as the bombesin monoclonal antibody 2A11 used to retard the growth of SCLC xenografts in nude mice (Cuttitta *et al.*, 1985). This antibody has entered phase I clinical trials, but the use of antibodies continues to be hampered by the problems of immune reactions with repeated dosing. We have directed our efforts to develop peptide antagonists which are not antigenic and should have higher tissue penetration than antibody proteins. We have characterized two classes of neuropeptide antagonist in the model Swiss 3T3 fibroblast system and tested their effects on SCLC *in vitro*. These results are summarized as an example of growth factor antagonist development.

The first bombesin antagonist to be described was an analogue of substance P, [DArg[1], DPro[2], DTrp[7,9], Leu[11]]substance P (antagonist A, Table 5.1). Substance P is structurally unrelated to the bombesin-like peptides but antagonist A, which is a substance P antagonist, was found to block the secretory effects of bombesin on a pancreatic preparation (Jensen *et al.*, 1984). It was subsequently found to block ^{125}I-GRP binding and bombesin-stimulated mitogenesis in Swiss 3T3 cells with half-

Table 5.1. Broad-spectrum and specific antagonists of bombesin/GRP

Broad-spectrum antagonists (substance P analogues)
  Substance P: Arg-Pro-Lys-Pro-Gln-Gln-Phe-Phe-Gly-Leu-Met-NH$_2$
  Antagonist A: [DArg^1, DPro^2, DTrp^{7,9}, Leu^{11}]substance P
  Antagonist D: [DArg^1, DPhe^5, DTrp^{7,9}, Leu^{11}]substance P
  Antagonist G: [Arg^6, DTrp^{7,9}, MePhe^8]substance P(6–11)

Specific antagonists (bombesin analogues)
  Bombesin: pGlu-Gln-Arg-Leu-Gly-Asn-Gln-Trp-Ala-Val-Gly-His-Leu-Met-NH$_2$
  Antagonist L: [Leu^{13}-psi(CH$_2$NH)Leu^{14}]bombesin
  Antagonist N: *N*-acetyl-GRP(20–26)

---

maximal effect at 118 μM (Zachary & Rozengurt, 1985). It did not affect mitogenesis stimulated by polypeptide growth factors, such as EGF and platelet-derived growth factor (PDGF), but was found to block vasopressin-stimulated mitogenesis (Zachary & Rozengurt, 1986). Further substance P analogues were therefore studied in order to identify more potent bombesin antagonists that could be tested in SCLC (Woll & Rozengurt, 1988a, 1990).

Two interesting compounds were identified in this study. They were [DArg^1, DPhe^5, DTrp^{7,9}, Leu^{11}]substance P (antagonist D, Table 5.1) and [Arg^6, DTrp^{7,9}, MePhe^8]substance P(6–11) (antagonist G, Table 5.1). Both antagonists reversibly inhibited GRP-stimulated mitogenesis in Swiss 3T3 cells, and antagonist D was five-fold more potent than antagonist A, although antagonist G was less potent than A (half-maximal inhibitory concentrations with 3.6 nM GRP and 1 μg/ml insulin: 118 μM A, 22 μM D, 85 μM G). In contrast, when tested as competitive inhibitors of vasopressin-stimulated mitogenesis, antagonists D and G were equipotent, with half-maximal effect at 1 μM in the presence of 14 nM vasopressin and 1 μg/ml insulin. In addition, the antagonists were found to block mitogenesis stimulated by the neuropeptides bradykinin and endothelin (Woll & Rozengurt, 1988c; Fabregat & Rozengurt, 1990), but not that stimulated by the polypeptide growth factors EGF and PDGF, phorbol esters, prostaglandins or the cyclic adenosine monophosphate (cAMP) activators 8-bromo-cAMP and vasoactive intestinal peptide. Thus, the substance P analogue antagonists showed broad-spectrum specificity against several neuropeptide mitogens: bombesin/GRP, vasopressin, bradykinin and endothelin.

These findings prompted the question: is this growth inhibition receptor-mediated? Binding of radioisotope-labelled ligand to receptors provides evidence for receptor-mediated action. Consequently, ^{125}I-GRP, ^{3}H-vasopressin and ^{125}I-endothelin binding has been measured in Swiss 3T3 cells. Antagonists D and G competed with these radiolabelled ligands for binding in a dose-dependent fashion (Woll & Rozengurt, 1988c, 1990;

Fabregat & Rozengurt, 1990). Further evidence that these neuropeptides untilize independent receptors, which are all recognized by this class of antagonists was obtained using specific antagonists for bombesin, vasopressin and bradykinin. These had no crossreactivity against the other ligands (Woll & Rozengurt, 1988c).

The neuropeptide mitogens bombesin/GRP, vasopressin, bradykinin and endothelin thus act through distinct receptors in Swiss 3T3 cells, but a common feature in their signal transduction pathways is the rapid and transient mobilization of intracellular Ca^{2+}. Antagonists D and G inhibited Ca^{2+} mobilization stimulated by each of these peptides, in addition to other early intracellular signals triggered by them (Woll & Rozengurt, 1988a, 1990; Fabregat & Rozengurt, 1990). This has led us to speculate that the antagonists recognize a common domain on these neuropeptide receptors, each of which is a member of the G protein linked, Ca^{2+}-mobilizing receptor family, with seven helical transmembrane domains (Arai et al., 1990; Battey et al., 1990; McEachern et al., 1991; Birnbaumer et al., 1992).

Alternatively, the antagonists might bind to a separate protein that interacts with the receptor and regulates its activity. This would be analogous to the negative heterotropic effect of an allosteric ligand in an oligomeric protein. An obvious candidate would be the G proteins themselves, which are capable of binding basic and hydrophobic peptides (e.g. Gil et al., 1991). To distinguish between these models, it will be necessary to determine whether the broad-spectrum antagonists inhibit ligand binding to purified receptors. The availability of purified preparations of the bombesin receptor from Swiss 3T3 cells (Coffer et al., 1990b; Feldman et al., 1990) should make it possible to distinguish between these different molecular models.

Specific bombesin antagonists

The study of substance P analogues yielded several broad-spectrum antagonists more potent than antagonist A, but none more specific. [Leu^{13}-psi(CH_2NH)Leu^{14}]bombesin (antagonist L, Table 5.1) is a pseudopeptide bombesin analogue that was shown to inhibit bombesin-stimulated amylase release from guinea pig pancreatic acinar cells (Coy et al., 1988). We characterized its actions in Swiss 3T3 cells and found it to be a potent and specific, competitive antagonist of bombesin-stimulated mitogenesis (Woll & Rozengurt, 1988b). Half-maximal effect was obtained with 240 nM antagonist L in the presence of 2.7 nM GRP and 1 μg/ml insulin. It had no effect on mitogenesis stimulated by vasopressin, bradykinin, EGF, PDGF, phorbol 12,13-dibutyrate, cholera toxin, 8-bromo-cAMP, prostaglandins or vasoactive intestinal peptide. Antagonist L was shown to inhibit specific ^{125}I-GRP binding in a dose-dependent fashion, indicating that its effects were receptor mediated. In addition, early intracellular signals stimulated by bombesin, including Ca^{2+} mobilization and transmodulation of EGF-receptor binding (mediated by PKC activation) were inhibited by this antagonist.

A further specific bombesin antagonist was tested in Swiss 3T3 cells. N-acetyl-GRP(20–26) (antagonist N, Table 5.1) was found, like antagonist L, to act at the bombesin receptor to block bombesin/GRP-stimulated mitogenesis. It was about four-fold less potent than antagonist L.

Testing bombesin antagonists in SCLC

The compounds characterized as broad-spectrum and specific antagonists in Swiss 3T3 cells were tested as inhibitors of bombesin-mediated signals and growth in SCLC cell lines. Because SCLC is a heterogeneous group of tumours, each compound was tested in several cell lines. All five antagonists reversibly inhibited GRP-stimulated Ca^{2+} mobilization in cells loaded with the fluorescent indicator fura-2/AM, confirming that they could act as competitive antagonists of the bombesin receptor on SCLC. As expected, the specific antagonists L and N had no effect on Ca^{2+} mobilization stimulated by other ligands, but the broad-spectrum antagonists A, D and G inhibited Ca^{2+} mobilization stimulated by GRP, vasopressin, bradykinin, cholecystokinin and galanin in different cell lines (Trepel et al., 1988a; Woll & Rozengurt, 1989a, 1990).

SCLC cell lines grow as floating aggregates and are also able to form colonies in semisolid medium. Indeed, there is a positive correlation between cloning efficiency of the cells and the histological involvement and invasiveness of the tumour in specimens taken from SCLC (Carney et al., 1980). The antagonists were tested for growth inhibitory effects in both liquid and semisolid media. The specific bombesin antagonists L and N failed to inhibit SCLC growth in liquid medium, but they have been reported to inhibit colony formation in soft agar in two cell lines (Trepel et al., 1988a; Mahmoud et al., 1989). In contrast, the broad-spectrum antagonists A, D and G inhibited the growth of all nine SCLC cell lines tested, in liquid and semisolid media (Woll & Rozengurt, 1988a, 1990; Sethi & Rozengurt, 1991). Antagonists D and G were equipotent, with half-maximal effect at about 20 μM, whereas antagonist A was five-fold less potent.

The important difference in biological activity between specific and broad-spectrum antagonists is emphasized in the experiment depicted in Fig. 5.2, using the SCLC cell line H345 which is known to produce and respond to GRP. The broad-spectrum antagonists (D and G) caused a dramatic decrease of the cloning efficiency of these cells, whereas specific antagonist L had no detectable effect. However, addition of L blocked the ability of GRP to increase clonal growth, indicating that this specific

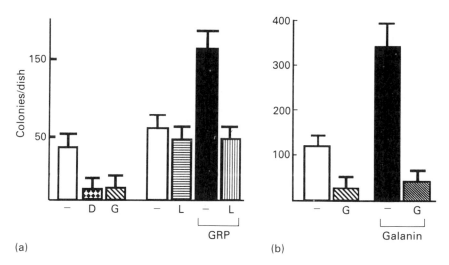

(a)   (b)

Fig. 5.2. The effect of specific and broad-spectrum antagonists on colony formation
in H345 (a) and H69 (b) small cell lung cancer cells. Cells 3–5 days postpassage
were washed and resuspended in serum-free medium. Cells were then disaggregated
into an essentially single cell suspension, judged by microscopy, by passing the cells
through a 19-gauge needle and then through a 15 μm nylon gauze. Viability was
judged by trypan blue exclusion on a standard haemocytometer. Cell number was
determined using a Coulter counter and approximately 10^4 viable cell/ml were sus-
pended in culture medium and 0.3% agarose. 1 ml of the mixture was plated in five
replicates in 35-mm plastic dishes containing a base layer of 0.5% agarose in culture
medium that had hardened. Both layers contained antagonist with or without
neuropeptide at the same concentration. Cultures were incubated at 37°C in a
humidified atmosphere of 5% CO_2/95% air. Colonies represent aggregates of cells
greater than 120 μm counted under a microscope after 21 days. The concentrations
of D, G, L (abbreviations as in Table 5.1), gastrin-releasing peptide and galanin
were 20 μM, 20 μM, 1 μM, 10 nM and 50 nM, respectively. Each bar represents the
mean ± SEM ($n = 10$).

antagonist was biologically active in the assay. Broad-spectrum antagonists also decrease clonal growth in the presence of neuropeptide stimulation. For example, Fig. 5.2b shows that antagonist G profoundly inhibited
the clonal growth of SCLC H69 cells in the absence of any exogenously
added peptide, as well as blocking the stimulation of colony growth
produced by addition of the neuropeptide galanin. The striking finding
that antagonists D and G inhibit the basal and stimulated clonal growth
of so many cell lines, regardless of positivity for bombesin receptors,
suggests that broad-spectrum antagonists could be more useful anticancer
drugs than ligand-specific growth factor antagonists. As a first step
towards testing this possibility, the effect of antagonist G on the growth
of a H69 SCLC xenograft has been examined. This antagonist profoundly
inhibited the growth of the tumour, compared with the control and the
inhibitory effect was clearly maintained beyond the duration of adminis-

tration (Sethi *et al.*, 1992). These results demonstrate that antagonist G can inhibit SCLC growth *in vivo* as well as *in vitro*.

Development strategies

The bombesin antagonists described above are now entering preclinical studies *in vivo*. Because of the increasing interest in growth factor antagonists, many researchers are working to improve existing compounds. Further analogues of antagonists L and N have been produced and shown to be bombesin-specific, with enhanced potency compared with their prototypes. They have been tested in fibroblasts and pancreatic cells, but studies in tumour cells are not yet available (Coy *et al.*, 1989; Heimbrook *et al.*, 1989; Saari *et al.*, 1989).

Additional structure–function studies have confirmed the importance of the carboxy terminal of the bombesin molecule in receptor recognition, by examining the effects of substitutions in position 12, and deletion of the C-terminal methionine. The analogues obtained are potent bombesin antagonists *in vitro* and *in vivo* but have not been tested in SCLC (Camble *et al.*, 1989; Saeed *et al.*, 1989; Wang *et al.*, 1990). The use of different antagonists has already permitted receptor subtypes to be distinguished; we expect that a clear classification of the various receptors will soon emerge (von Schrenk *et al.*, 1990).

Interestingly, reduction of peptide bonds in substance P analogues to yield pseudopeptide derivatives appears to enhance their specificity for substance P and make them relatively less potent antagonists of bombesin and other peptides (Qian *et al.*, 1989). Additional structural changes could be introduced to make the antagonists less irritant or cardioactive (Ljungqvist *et al.*, 1988).

An interesting class of compounds has been developed as gastrin/ cholecystokinin antagonists. They have a non-peptidal, benzodiazepine-like structure and are orally bioavailable (Chang & Lotti, 1986; Evans *et al.*, 1986; Huang *et al.*, 1989; Lotti & Chang, 1989). These compounds have been used to study pancreatic secretion *in vivo* in rats and dogs (Anderson & Dockray, 1988; Konturek *et al.*, 1989). Because cholecystokinin receptors have been demonstrated in SCLC, cholecystokinin (CCK) antagonists may prove useful for treatment (Yoder & Moody, 1987; Mailleux & Vanderhaeghen, 1990; but see Staley *et al.*, 1990). There is a considerable body of evidence implicating gastrin and CCK as growth factors for tumours of the stomach and colon (Woll, 1991). Gastrin/CCK antagonists may therefore be of most interest in gut tumours, and earlier antagonists have been shown to inhibit the growth of cultured colon tumour cells *in vitro* (Hoosein *et al.*, 1990). The development of further orally active antagonists to neuropeptide receptors (e.g. renin, Morishima *et al.*, 1989; substance P, Snider *et al.*, 1991) will allow clinical testing of the role of growth factors in cancer.

The only neuropeptide growth factor antagonist to have entered clinical trials to date is the gastrin antagonist proglumide (Harrison *et al.*, 1990). It is a weak antagonist with partial agonist activity, and no benefit was seen in patients with gastric cancer receiving 800 mg orally, four times daily.

It is not yet clear whether growth factor antagonists should be considered as cytotoxic or cytostatic drugs. Conventional strategies for testing new anticancer drugs in patients with advanced disease may be inappropriate. They might be better used in the adjuvant or maintenance setting. Similarly, maximal tolerated doses may not be optimal for growth regulation, and new approaches will be required to monitor treatment. For example, doses of bombesin/GRP antagonists that achieve suppression of gastric acid secretion may not be those required to suppress tumour growth.

Finally, it should be noted that the neuropeptide-stimulated mitogenesis can be blocked by down-regulation of receptors (Millar & Rozengurt, 1990b) or by interrupting the signal transduction process at various postreceptor levels (Fig. 5.1). Thus, prolonged treatment with vasopressin causes heterologous desensitization to the mitogenic action of bombesin in the absence of bombesin receptor down-regulation (Millar & Rozengurt, 1989). The target of this heterologous desensitization is the release of arachidonic acid rather than the activation of phospholipase C-mediated events (Millar & Rozengurt, 1990a). Other downstream components of the mitogenic signalling cascade can be attacked by specific inhibitors, such as guanosine diphosphate (GDP) analogues and protein kinase C blockers (Fig. 5.1) (Woll & Rozengurt, 1989b). These approaches have the advantage of affecting signals from many mitogens. It might be thought that attacking such ubiquitous targets would have toxic effects throughout the body, but this must not be assumed. The calcium channel blockers, including nifedipine and verapamil, have demonstrated that specific pharmaceutical effects can be obtained with such apparently blunt instruments.

Conclusion

Studies of the biology of cancer have identified many new potential targets for cancer chemotherapy. Increased understanding of tumour growth factors and their modes of action has already opened novel avenues of research. The effects of blocking signal pathways utilized by many growth factors and hormones are unpredictable and can only be determined by *in vivo* testing. However, the emerging model of multiple autocrine and paracrine growth factors in many types of cancer suggests that broad-spectrum antagonists will be the most promising group.

References

Alexander, R.W., Upp, J.R., Poston, G.J., Gupta, V., Townsend, C.M. & Thompson, J.C. (1988). Effects of bombesin on growth of human small cell lung carcinoma *in vivo*. *Cancer Research* **48**, 1439–1441.

Anderson, L. & Dockray, G.J. (1988). The cholecystokinin antagonist L-364,718 inhibits the action of cholecystokinin but not bombesin on rat pancreatic secretion *in vivo*. *European Journal of Pharmacology* **146**, 307–311.

Arai, H., Hori, S., Aramori, I., Ohkubo, H. & Nakanishi, S. (1990). Cloning and expression of a cDNA encoding an endothelin receptor. *Nature* **348**, 730–732.

Battey, J.F., Way, J.M., Corjay, M.H., Shapira, H., Kusano, K., Harkins, R., Wu, J.M., Slattery, T., Mann, E. & Feldman, R.I. (1990). Molecular cloning of the bombesin/GRP receptor from Swiss 3T3 cells. *Proceedings of the National Academy of Sciences USA* **88**, 395–399.

Birnbaumer, M., Seibold, A., Gilbert, S., Ishido, M., Barberis, C., Antaramian, A., Brabet, P. & Rosenthal, W. (1992). Molecular cloning of the receptor for human antidiuretic hormone. *Nature* **357**, 333–335.

Bishop, J.M. (1991). Molecular themes in oncogenesis. *Cell* **64**, 235–248.

Brooks, S.F., Erusalimsky, J.D., Totty, N.F. & Rozengurt, E. (1990). Purification and internal amino acid sequence of the 80 kDa protein kinase C substrate from Swiss 3T3 fibroblasts. *FEBS Letters* **268**, 291–295.

Brooks, S.F., Herget, T., Erusalimsky, J.D. & Rozengurt, E. (1991). Protein kinase C activation potently down-regulates the expression of its major substrate, 80 K in Swiss 3T3 cells. *EMBO Journal* **10**, 2497–2505.

Bunn, P.A., Dienhart, D.G., Chan, D., Puck, T.T., Tagawa, M., Jewett, P.B. & Braunschweiger, E. (1990). Neuropeptide stimulation of calcium flux in human lung cancer cells: delineation of alternative pathways. *Proceedings of the National Academy of Sciences USA* **87**, 2162–2166.

Camble, R., Cotton, R., Dutta, A.S., Garner, A., Hayward, C.F. Moore, V.E. & Scholes, P.B. (1989). *N*-isobutyryl-His-Trp-Ala-Val-D-Ala-His-Leu-NHMe (ICI 216140) a potent *in vivo* antagonist analogue of bombesin/gastrin releasing peptide (BN/GRP) derived from the C-terminal sequence lacking the final methionine residue. *Life Sciences* **45**, 1521–1527.

Carney, D.N. Cuttitta, F., Moody, T.W. & Minna, J.D. (1987). Selective stimulation of small cell lung cancer clonal growth by bombesin and gastrin-releasing peptide. *Cancer Research* **47**, 821–825.

Carney, D.N., Gazdar, A.F. & Minna, J.D. (1980). Positive correlation between histological tumor involvement and generation of tumor cell colonies in agarose in specimens taken directly from patients with small cell lung carcinoma of the lung. *Cancer Research* **40**, 1820–1823.

Chang, R.S.L. & Lotti, V.J. (1986). Biochemical and pharmacological characterization of an extremely potent and selective nonpeptide cholecystokinin antagonist. *Proceedings of the National Academy of Sciences USA* **83**, 4923–4926.

Coffer, A., Fabregat, I., Sinnett-Smith, J. & Rozengurt, E. (1990a). Solubilization of the bombesin receptor from Swiss 3T3 cells membranes: functional association to a guanine nucleotide regulatory protein. *FEBS Letters* **263**, 80–84.

Coffer, A., Sinnett-Smith, J. & Rozengurt, E. (1990b). Bombesin receptor from Swiss 3T3 cells: affinity chromatography and reconstitution into phospholipid vesicles. *FEBS Letters* **275**, 159–164.

Coy, D.H., Heinz-Erian, P., Jiang, N.-Y., Sasaki, Y., Taylor, J., Moreau, J.-P., Wolfrey, W.T., Gardner, J.D. & Jensen, R.T. (1988). Probing peptide backbone function in bombesin: a reduced peptide bond analogue with potent and specific receptor antagonist activity. *Journal of Biological Chemistry* **263**, 5056–5060.

Coy, D.H., Taylor, J.E., Jiang, N.-Y., Kim, S.H., Wang, L.H., Huang, S.C., Moreau, J.-P., Gardner, J.D. & Jensen, R.T. (1989). Short-chain pseudopeptide bombesin receptor antagonists with enhanced binding affinities for pancreatic acinar and Swiss 3T3 cells display strong antimitotic activity. *Journal of Biological Chemistry* **264**, 14691–14697.

Cross, M. & Dexter, T.M. (1991). Growth factors in development, transformation, and tumorigenesis. *Cell* **64**, 271–280.

Cuttitta, F., Carney, D.N., Mulshine, J., Moody, T.W., Fedorko, J., Fischler, A. & Minna, J.D. (1985). Bombesin-like peptides can function as autocrine growth factors in human small-cell lung cancer. *Nature* **316**, 823–826.

Davis, T.P., Burgess, H.S., Crowell, S., Moody, T.W., Culling-Berlund, A. & Liu, R.H. (1989). β-endorphin and neurotensin stimulate *in vitro* clonal growth of human SCLC cells. *European Journal of Pharmacology* **161**, 283–285.

Dunne, M.J., Bullett, M.J., Li, G.D., Wollheim, C.B. & Petersen, O.H. (1989). Galanin activates nucleotide-dependent K^+ channels in insulin-secreting cells via a pertussis toxin-sensitive G-protein. *EMBO Journal* **8**, 413–420.

Erisman, M.D., Linnoila, R.I., Hernandez, O., DiAugustine, R.P. & Lazarus, L.H. (1982). Human lung small-cell carcinoma contains bombesin. *Proceedings of the National Academy of Sciences USA* **79**, 2379–2383.

Erusalimsky, J.D., Brooks, S.F., Herget, T., Morris, C. & Rozengurt, E. (1991). Molecular cloning and characterization of the acidic 80-kDa protein kinase C substrate from rat brain. *Journal of Biological Chemistry* **266**, 7073–7080.

Erusalimsky, J.D., Friedberg, I. & Rozengurt, E. (1988). Bombesin, diacylglycerols and phorbol esters rapidly stimulate the phosphorylation of an $M_r = 80,000$ protein kinase C substrate in permeabilized 3T3 cells: effect of guanine nucleotides. *Journal of Biological Chemistry* **263**, 19188–19194.

Evans, B.E., Bock, M.G., Rittle, K.E., Dipardo, R.M., Whitter, W.L., Veber, D.F., Anderson, P.S. & Friedinger, R.M. (1986). Design of potent, orally effective, non-peptidal antagonists of the peptide hormone cholecystokinin. *Proceedings of the National Academy of Sciences USA* **83**, 4918–4922.

Fabregat, I. & Rozengurt, E. (1990). [DArg[1], DPhe[5], DTrp[7,9], Leu[11]] substance P, a neuropeptide antagonist, blocks binding, Ca^{2+}-mobilizing, and mitogenic effects of endothelin and vasoactive intestinal contractor in mouse 3T3 cells. *Journal of Cell Physiology* **145**, 88–94.

Feldman, R.I., Wu, J.M., Jenson, J.C. & Mann, E. (1990). Purification and characterization of the bombesin/gastrin releasing peptide receptor from Swiss 3T3 cells. *Journal of Biological Chemistry* **265**, 17364–17372.

Gil, J., Higgins, T. & Rozengurt, E. (1991). Mastoparan, a novel mitogen for Swiss 3T3 cells, stimulates pertussis toxin-sensitive arachidonic acid release without inositol phosphate accumulation. *Journal of Cell Biology* **113**, 943–950.

Goustin, A.S., Leof, E.B., Shipley, G.D. & Moses, H.L. (1986). Growth factors and cancer. *Cancer Research* **46**, 1015–1029.

Harrison, J.D., Jones, J.A. & Morris, D.L. (1990). The effect of the gastrin receptor antagonist proglumide on survival in gastric carcinoma. *Cancer* **66**, 1449–1452.

Heikkila, R., Trepel, J.B., Cuttitta, F., Neckers, L.M. & Sausville, E.A. (1987). Bombesin-related peptides induce calcium mobilization in a subset of human small cell lung cancer cell lines. *Journal of Biological Chemistry* **262**, 16456–16460.

Heimbrook, D.C., Saari, W.S., Balishin, N.L., Friedman, A., Moore, K.S., Rieman,

M.W., Kiefer, D.M., Rotberg, N.S., Wallen, J.W. & Oliff, A. (1989). Carboxyl-terminal modification of a gastrin releasing peptide derivative generates potent antagonists. *Journal of Biological Chemistry* **264**, 11258–11262.

Hoosein, N.M., Kiener, P.A., Curry, R.C. & Brattain, M.G. (1990). Evidence for autocrine growth stimulation of cultured colon tumor cells by a gastrin/cholecystokinin-like peptide. *Experimental Cell Research* **186**, 15–21.

Huang, S.C., Zhang, L., Chiang, H.C.V., Wank, S.A., Maton, P.N., Gardner, J.D. & Jensen, R.T. (1989). Benzodiazepine analogues L365,260 and L364,718 as gastrin and pancreatic CCK receptor antagonists. *American Journal of Physiology* **257**, G169–G174.

Issandou, M. & Rozengurt, E. (1990). Bradykinin transiently activates protein kinase C in Swiss 3T3 cells: distinction from activation by bombesin and vasopressin. *Journal of Biological Chemistry* **265**, 11890–11896.

Jensen, R.T., Jones, S.W., Folkers, K. & Gardner, J.D. (1984). A synthetic peptide that is a bombesin receptor antagonist. *Nature* **309**, 61–63.

Konturek, S.J., Tasler, J., Konturek, J.W., Cieszkowski, M., Szewczyk, K., Hładij, M. & Anderson, P.S. (1989). Effects of non-peptidal CCK receptor antagonist (L-364 718) on pancreatic responses to cholecystokinin, gastrin, bombesin, and meat feeding in dogs. *Gut* **30**, 110–117.

Kris, R.M., Hazan, R., Villines, J., Moody, T.W. & Schlessinger, J. (1987). Identification of the bombesin receptor on murine and human cells by cross-linking experiments. *Journal of Biological Chemistry* **262**, 11215–11220.

Lefkowitz, R.J. & Caron, M.G. (1988). Adrenergic receptors: models for the study of receptors coupled to guanine nucleotide regulatory proteins. *Journal of Biological Chemistry* **263**, 4993–4996.

Ljungqvist, A., Feng, D.-M., Hook, W., Shen, Z.-X., Bowers, C. & Folkers, K. (1988). Antide and related antagonists of luteinizing hormone release with long action and oral activity. *Proceedings of the National Academy of Sciences USA* **85**, 8326–8240.

Lotti, V.J. & Chang, R.S.L. (1989). A new potent and selective non-peptide gastrin antagonist and brain cholecystokinin receptor (CCK-B) ligand: L365,260. *European Journal of Pharmacology* **162**, 273–280.

McEachern, A.E., Shelton, E.R., Bhakta, S., Obernolte, R., Bach, C., Zuppan, P., Fujisaki, J., Aldrich, R.W. & Jarnagin, K. (1991). Expression cloning of a rat B_2 bradykinin receptor. *Proceedings of the National Academy of Sciences USA* **88**, 7724–7728.

Mahmoud, S., Palaszynski, E., Fiskum, G., Coy, D.H. & Moody, T.W. (1989). Small cell lung cancer bombesin receptors are antagonized by reduced peptide bond analogues. *Life Sciences* **44**, 367–373.

Mailleux, P. & Vanderhaeghen, J.-J. (1990). Cholestokinin receptors of A type in the human dorsal medulla oblongata and meningiomas, and of B type in small cell lung carcinomas. *Neuroscience Letters* **117**, 243–247.

Millar, J.B.A. & Rozengurt, E. (1988). Bombesin enhancement of cAMP accumulation in Swiss 3T3 cells: evidence of a dual mechanism of action. *Journal of Cell Physiology* **137**, 214–222.

Millar, J.B.A. & Rozengurt, E. (1989). Heterologous desensitization of bombesin-induced mitogenesis by prolonged exposure to vasopressin: a post-receptor signal transduction block. *Proceedings of the National Academy of Sciences USA* **86**, 3204–3208.

Millar, J.B.A. & Rozengurt, E. (1990a). Arachidonic acid release by bombesin: a novel post-receptor target for heterologous mitogenic desensitization. *Journal of Biological Chemistry* **265**, 19973–19979.

Millar, J.B.A. & Rozengurt, E. (1990b). Chronic desensitization to bombesin by progressive down-regulation of bombesin receptors in Swiss 3T3 cells. *Journal of Biological Chemistry* **20**, 12052–12058.

Moody, T.W., Murphy, A., Mahmoud, S. & Fiskum, G. (1987). Bombesin-like peptides elevate cytosolic calcium in small cell lung cancer cells. *Biochemical and Biophysical Research Communications* **147**, 189–195.

Moody, T.W., Pert, C.B., Gazdar, A.F., Carney, D.N. & Minna, J.D. (1981). High levels of intracellular bombesin characterize human small-cell lung carcinoma. *Science* **214**, 1246–1248.

Morishima, H., Koike, Y., Nakano, M., Atsuumi, S., Tanaka, S., Funabashi, H., Hashimoto, J., Sawasaki, Y., Mino, N. & Nakano, M. (1989). A novel nonpeptidic, orally active renin inhibitor. *Biochemical and Biophysical Research Communications* **159**(3), 999–1005.

Qian, J.-M., Coy, D.H., Jiang, N.-Y., Gardner, J.D. & Jensen, R.T. (1989). Reduced peptide bond pseudopeptide analogues of substance P: a new class of substance P receptor antagonists with enhanced specificity. *Journal of Biological Chemistry* **264**, 16667–16671.

Rozengurt, E. (1983). Growth factors, cell proliferation and cancer: an overview. *Molecular Biology and Medicine* **1**, 169–181.

Rozengurt, E. (1985). The mitogenic response of cultured 3T3 cells: integration of early signals and synergistic effects in a unified framework. In Cohen, P. & Houslay, M. (eds) *Molecular Mechanisms of Transmembrane Signalling*, Vol. 4, pp. 429–452. Elsevier Science Publishers, Amsterdam.

Rozengurt, E. (1986). Early signals in the mitogenic response. *Science* **234**, 161–166.

Rozengurt, E. (1991). Neuropeptides as cellular growth factors: role of multiple signalling pathways. *European Journal of Clinical Investigation* **21**, 123–134.

Rozengurt, E. & Sinnett-Smith, J. (1983). Bombesin stimulation of DNA synthesis and cell division in cultures of Swiss 3T3 cells. *Proceedings of the National Academy of Sciences USA* **80**, 2936–2940.

Rozengurt, E. & Sinnett-Smith, J. (1988). Early signals underlying the induction of the c-*fos* and c-*myc* genes in quiescent fibroblasts: studies with bombesin and other growth factors. *Progress in Nucleic Acid Research and Molecular Biology* **35**, 261–295.

Rozengurt, E. & Sinnett-Smith, J. (1990). Bombesin stimulation of fibroblast mitogenesis: specific receptors, signal transduction and early events. *Philosophical Transactions of the Royal Society of London, B* **327**, 209–221.

Rozengurt, E., Erusalimsky, J., Mehmet, H., Morris, C., Nånberg, E. & Sinnett-Smith, J. (1988). Signal transduction in mitogenesis: further evidence for multiple pathways. *Cold Spring Harbor Symposia on Quantitative Biology* **53**, 945–954.

Saari, W.S., Helmbrook, D.C., Friedman, A., Fisher, T.W. & Oliff, A (1989) A gastrin-releasing peptide antagonist containing a *psi* (CH$_2$O) amide bond surrogate. *Biochemical and Biophysical Research Communications* **165**, 114–117.

Saeed, Z.A., Huang, S.C., Coy, D.H., Jiang, N.-Y., Heinz-Erian, P., Mantey, S., Gardner, J.D. & Jensen, R.T. (1989). Effect of substitutions in position 12 of bombesin on antagonist activity. *Peptides* **10**, 597–603.

Sager, R. (1989). Tumor suppressor genes: the puzzle and the promise. *Science* **246**, 406–412.

Sethi, T. & Rozengurt, E. (1991a). Galanin stimulates Ca^{2+} mobilization, inositol phosphate accumulation and clonal growth in small cell lung cancer cells. *Cancer Research* **51**, 1674–1679.

Sethi, T. & Rozengurt, E. (1991b). Multiple neuropeptides stimulate clonal growth of small cell lung cancer: effects of bradykinin, vasopressin, cholecystokinin, galanin and neurotensin. *Cancer Research* **51**, 3621–3623.

Sethi, T., Langdon, S., Smyth, J. & Rozengurt, E. (1992). Growth of small cell lung cancer cells: stimulation by multiple neuropeptides and inhibition by broad spectrum antagonists *in vitro* and *in vivo*. *Cancer Research*, **52** (Suppl.), 2737S–2742S.

Sinnett-Smith, J., Lehmann, W. & Rozengurt, E. (1990). Bombesin receptor in membranes from Swiss 3T3 cells. Binding characteristics, affinity labelling and modulation by guanine nucleotides. *Biochemical Journal* **265**, 485–493.

Sinnett-Smith, J., Zachary, I. & Rozengurt, E. (1988). Characterization of a bombesin receptor on Swiss mouse 3T3 cells by affinity cross-linking. *Journal of Cellular Biochemistry* **38**, 237–249.

Snider, R.M., Constantine, J.W., Lowe, J.A. III, Longo, K.P., Lebel, W.S. Woody, H.A., Drozda, S.E., Desai, M.C., Vinick, F.J., Spender, R.W. & Hess, H.-J. (1991). A potent nonpeptide antagonist of the substance P (NK$_1$) receptor. *Science* **251**, 435–437.

Söderdahl, G., Betsholtz, C., Johansson, A., Nilsson, K. & Bergh, J. (1988). Differential expression of platelet-derived growth factor and transforming growth factor genes in small- and non-small-cell lung carcinoma cell lines. *International Journal of Cancer* **41**, 636–641.

Sporn, M.B. & Roberts, A.B. (1985). Autocrine growth factors and cancer. *Nature* **313**, 745–747.

Staley, J., Fiskum, G., Davis, T.P. & Moody, T.W. (1989a). Neurotensin elevates cytosolic calcium in small cell lung cancer cells. *Peptides* **10**, 1217–1221.

Staley, J., Fiskum, G. & Moody, T.W. (1989b). Cholecystokinin elevates cytosolic calcium in small cell lung cancer cells. *Biochemical and Biophysical Research Communications* **163**, 605–610.

Staley, J., Jensen, R.T. & Moody, T.W. (1990). CCK antagonists interact with CCK-B receptors on human small cell lung cancer cells. *Peptides* **11**, 1033–1036.

Suzuki, M., Yamaguchi, K., Abe, K., Adachi, N., Nagasaki, K., Asanuma, F., Adachi, I., Kimura, S., Terada, M., Taya, Y., Matsuzaki, J. & Miki, K. (1987). Detection of gastrin-releasing peptide mRNA in small cell lung carcinomas using synthetic oligodeoxyribonucleotide probes. *Japanese Journal of Clinical Oncology* **17**, 157–163.

Takuwa, N., Takuwa, Y., Ohue, Y., Mukai, H., Endoh, K., Yamashita, K., Kumada, M. & Munekata, E. (1990). Stimulation of calcium mobilization but not proliferation by bombesin and tachykinin neuropeptides in human small cell lung cancer cells. *Cancer Research* **50**, 240–244.

Tateishi, M., Ishida, T., Mitsudomi, T., Kaneko, S. & Sugimachi, K. (1990). Immunohistochemical evidence of autocrine growth factors in adenocarcinoma of the human lung. *Cancer Research* **50**, 7077–7080.

Trepel, J.B., Moyer, J.D., Cuttitta, F., Frucht, H., Coy, D.H., Natale, R.B., Mulshine, J.L., Jensen, R.T. & Sausville, E.A. (1988a). A novel bombesin receptor antagonist inhibits autocrine signals in a small cell lung carcinoma cell line. *Biochemical and Biophysical Research Communications* **156**, 1383–1389.

Trepel, J.B., Moyer, J.D., Heikkila, R. & Sausville, E.A. (1988b). Modulation of bombesin-induced phosphatidylinositol hydrolysis in a small-cell lung-cancer cell line. *Biochemical Journal* **255**, 403–410.

Veale, D., Kerr, N., Gibson, G.J. & Harris, A.L. (1989). Characterization of epidermal growth factor receptor in primary human non-small cell lung cancer. *Cancer Research* **49**, 1313–1317.

von Schrenk, T., Wang, L.-H., Coy, D.H., Villanueva, M.L., Mantey, S. & Jensen, R.T. (1990). Potent bombesin receptor antagonists distinguish receptor subtypes. *American Journal of Physiology* **259**, G468–G473.

Wang, L.-H., Coy, D.H., Taylor, J.E., Jiang, N.-Y., Kim, S.H., Moreau, J.-P., Huang, S.C., Mantey, S.A., Frucht, H. & Jensen, R.T. (1990). Desmethionine alkylamide bombesin analogues: a new class of bombesin receptor antagonists with potent antisecretory activity in pancreatic acini and antimitotic activity in Swiss 3T3 cells. *Biochemistry* **29**, 616–622.

Woll, P.J. (1991a). Neuropeptide growth factors and cancer. *British Journal of Cancer* **63**, 469–475.

Woll, P.J. (1991b). Growth factors and lung cancer. *Thorax* **46**, 924–929.

Woll, P.J. & Rozengurt, E. (1988a). [DArg^1, DPhe^5, DTrp^{7,9} Leu^{11}]substance P a potent bombesin antagonist in murine Swiss 3T3 cells, inhibits the growth of human small cell lung cancer cells *in vitro*. *Proceedings of the National Academy of Sciences USA* **85**, 1859–1863.

Woll, P.J. & Rozengurt, E. (1988b) [Leu^{13}-*psi*(CH$_2$NH) Leu^{14}]bombesin is a specific bombesin receptor antagonist in Swiss 3T3 cells. *Biochemical and Biophysical Research Communications* **155**, 359–365.

Woll, P.J. & Rozengurt, E. (1988c). Two classes of antagonist interact with receptors for the mitogenic neuropeptides bombesin, bradykinin and vasopressin. *Growth Factors* **1**, 75–83.

Woll, P.J. & Rozengurt, E. (1989a). Multiple neuropeptides mobilise calcium in small cell lung cancer: effects of vasopressin, bradykinin, cholecystokinin, galanin and neurotensin. *Biochemical and Biophysical Research Communications* **164**, 66–73.

Woll, P.J. & Rozengurt, E. (1989b). Therapeutic implications of growth factors in small cell lung cancer. *Lung Cancer* **5**, 287–295.

Woll, P.J. & Rozengurt, E. (1990). A neuropeptide antagonist that inhibits the growth of small cell lung cancer *in vitro*. *Cancer Research* **50**, 3968–3973.

Wood, S.M., Wood, J.R., Ghatei, M.A., Lee, Y.C., O'Shaughnessy, D. & Bloom, S.R. (1981). Bombesin, somatostatin and neurotensin-like immunoreactivity in bronchial carcinoma. *Journal of Clinical Endocrinology and Metabolism* **53**, 1310–1312.

Yoder, D.G. & Moody, T.W. (1987). High affinity binding of cholecystokinin to small cell lung cancer cells. *Peptides* **8**, 103–107.

Zachary, I. & Rozengurt, E. (1985). High-affinity receptors for peptides of the bombesin family in Swiss 3T3 cells. *Proceedings of the National Academy of Sciences USA* **82**, 7616–7620.

Zachary, I. & Rozengurt, E. (1986). A substance P antagonist also inhibits the specific binding and mitogenic effects of vasopressin and bombesin-related peptides in Swiss 3T3 cells. *Biochemical and Biophysical Research Communications* **137**, 135–141.

Zachary, I. & Rozengurt, E. (1987). Identification of a receptor for peptides of the bombesin family in Swiss 3T3 cells by affinity cross-linking. *Journal of Biological Chemistry* **262**, 3947–3950.

Zachary, I., Gil, J., Lehmann, W., Sinnett-Smith, J. & Rozengurt, E. (1991). Bombesin, vasopressin and endothelin rapidly stimulate tyrosine phosphorylation in intact Swiss 3T3 cells. *Proceedings of the National Academy of Sciences USA* **88**, 4577–4581.

Zachary, I., Sinnett-Smith, J.W. & Rozengurt, E. (1986). Early events elicited by bombesin and structurally related peptides in quiescent Swiss 3T3 cells. I. Activation of protein kinase C and inhibition of epidermal growth factor binding. *Journal of Cell Biology* **102**, 2211–2222.

Zachary, I., Woll, P.J. & Rozengurt, E. (1987). A role for neuropeptides in the control of cell proliferation. *Developmental Biology* **124**, 295–308.

Chapter 6
Ether lipids in experimental cancer chemotherapy

Larry W. Daniel

Introduction

The search for effective anticancer treatments has traditionally targeted DNA replication and the cell nucleus. This approach led to the development of many useful drugs and will continue to be a primary focus of new drug development. However, new strategies for drug development are being sought with the rationale that drugs directed toward non-DNA targets may be useful as single agents or in combination with existing drugs. The pathways of proliferative signal transduction are now known in considerable detail and offer numerous potential targets for pharmacological intervention. The cell membrane has also been suggested as a target for drug development (Powis, *et al.*, 1990; Tritton & Hickman, 1990). However, drugs directed towards membrane interactions will ultimately have effects on signal transduction pathways and it may be more productive to consider these areas as one. Overall, the proliferative signal transduction pathways provide a unifying hypothesis that the mechanism of action of diverse oncogenes in producing neoplastic transformation share common signal transduction pathways. Therefore, inhibition of these signalling pathways would be effective in cells transformed by diverse mechanisms.

One group of membrane-active drugs are synthetic derivatives of naturally occurring ether-linked lipids. The compound 1-*O*-octadecyl-2-

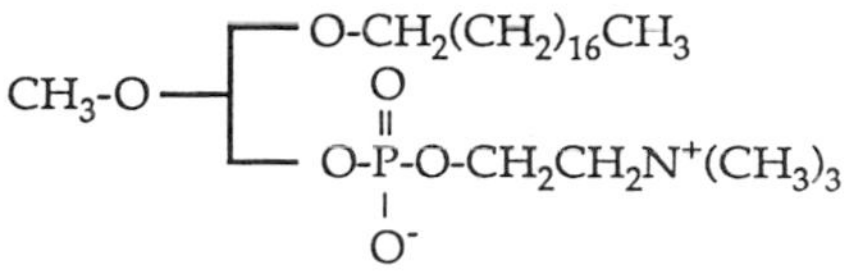

$$CH_3-O-\begin{cases} O-CH_2(CH_2)_{16}CH_3 \\ \overset{O}{\underset{O^-}{O-\overset{\|}{P}-O-CH_2CH_2N^+(CH_3)_3}} \end{cases}$$

ET-18-OCH$_3$ (edelfosine)

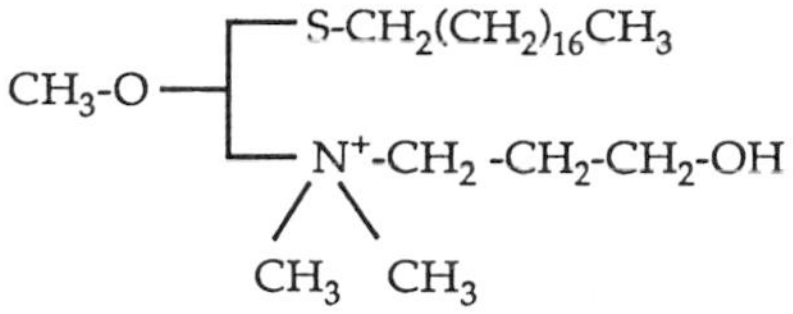

$$CH_3-O-\begin{cases} S-CH_2(CH_2)_{16}CH_3 \\ N^+-CH_2-CH_2-CH_2-OH \\ \diagup\;\diagdown \\ CH_3\quad CH_3 \end{cases}$$

CP-10

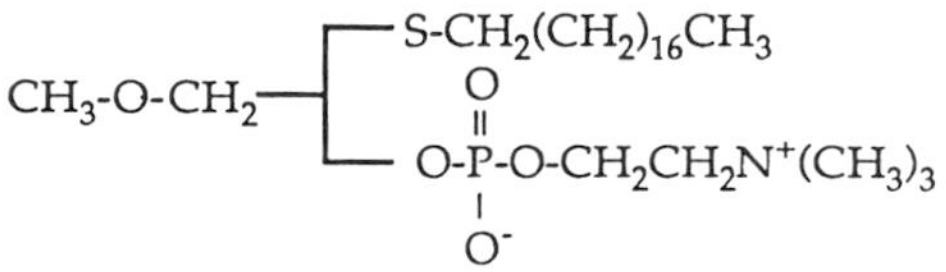

$$CH_3-O-CH_2-\begin{cases} S-CH_2(CH_2)_{16}CH_3 \\ \overset{O}{\underset{O^-}{O-\overset{\|}{P}-O-CH_2CH_2N^+(CH_3)_3}} \end{cases}$$

BM 41.440 (ilmofosine)

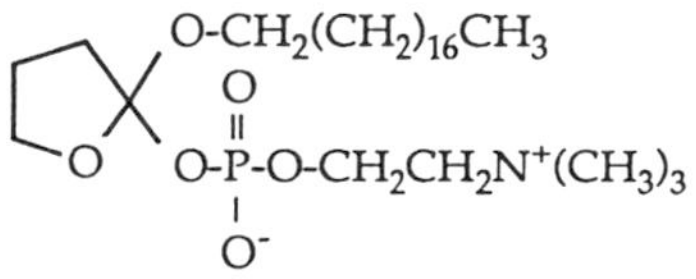

$$\begin{array}{l} O-CH_2(CH_2)_{16}CH_3 \\ \overset{O}{\underset{O^-}{O-\overset{\|}{P}-O-CH_2CH_2N^+(CH_3)_3}} \end{array}$$

SRI 62-834

$$H_3C(CH_2)_{14}-CH_2-O-\overset{\overset{\displaystyle O}{\|}}{\underset{\underset{\displaystyle O^-}{|}}{P}}-O-CH_2CH_2N^+(CH_3)_3$$

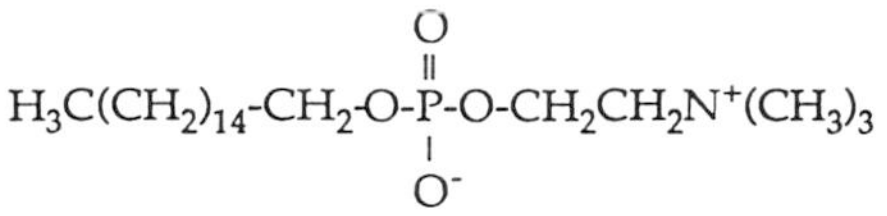

HePC (miltefosine)

Fig. 6.1. Structures of representative ether-linked lipids. ET-18-OCH$_3$ (1-O-octadecyl-2-O-methyl-rac-glycero-3-phosphocholine) is the most widely studied of the antineoplastic ether-linked lipids and has been the prototype for further drug development. Compounds with structural modifications at all three positions of the glycerol backbone have been synthesized and evaluated. The long chain alkyl group (O or S-linked) at position 1 is an important structural feature of all active compounds. A variety of modifications at position 2 indicates that the 2-O-methyl group is not required for activity (i.e. BM 41.440). Substantial modifications of the backbone (for example, SRI 62-834) or removal of the glycerol backbone have resulted in active compounds (e.g. hexadecylphosphocholine, HePC). In addition, alterations of the phosphocholine at position 3 are possible with the retention of antineoplastic activity (CP-10). ET-18-OCH$_3$, BM 41.440, SRI 62-834 and HePC are currently in clinical trials.

O-methyl-rac-glycero-3-phosphocholine (ET-18-OCH$_3$) (Fig. 6.1) is representative of the first generation of ether lipids tested preclinically and in phase I and phase II clinical trials (Berdel, 1990, 1991). ET-18-OCH$_3$ is selectively cytotoxic to neoplastic cells, both *in vivo* and *in vitro*, and has been the basis of many mechanistic studies. The critical target for ET-18-OCH$_3$ is not known; however, the compound interferes with proliferative signal transduction at multiple sites. ET-18-OCH$_3$ inhibits inositol lipid turnover in intact cells and phosphatidylinositol-specific phospholipase C (PI-PLC) *in vitro*. Protein kinase C (PKC), a key enzyme in proliferative signal transduction, may also be involved in the mechanism of action of ET-18-OCH$_3$ (Daniel, 1990). PKC is inhibited both in cell-free assays and in intact cell systems by ET-18-OCH$_3$ and other active ether lipid ana-logues (Helfman et al., 1983; Parker et al., 1987; Marx et al., 1988; Marasco et al., 1990). Thus, ET-18-OCH$_3$ is an important prototype for mechanistic studies of membrane-active agents which interfere with signal transduction pathways and is the basis for the development of a second generation of compounds now in clinical trials.

Ether-linked lipids in mammalian cells

Many types of normal cells contain ether-linked phospholipid species. The relative amounts of ether lipids are characteristic of the cell type and species, indicating that the cellular content of these components is highly regulated. Two subclasses of ether-linked phospholipids are common in mammalian cells (Fig. 6.2). 1-O-alkyl-linked (alkyl-) species are found in both the ethanolamine (PE) and the choline-phospholipid (PC) classes of many tissues. The content of alkyl-PC varies among tissues from very low in liver (0–2.4% of total PC) to high in polymorphonuclear leucocytes (16.4–50.2%) (Sugiura & Waku, 1987). In contrast, 1-O-alk-1'-enyl-linked (alkenyl-) species are found almost exclusively in the PE fraction. A notable exception is heart tissue in which alkenyl-PC may comprise 33–52% of the total PC (Sugiura & Waku, 1987).

Alkyl-lipids are synthesized by the same general sequence of reactions required for synthesis of 1,2-diacyl-linked species. The only enzyme unique to alkyl-lipid synthesis is alkyl-dihydroxyacetone phosphate (alkyl-DHAP) synthase which catalyses the exchange of a long chain alcohol and the fatty acid moiety of acyl-DHAP (Hajra 1970; Wykle et al., 1972b). The only additional enzymatic requirement for alkenyl-PE synthe-sis is a cytochrome b$_5$-dependent mixed function oxidase (alkyl de-saturase) (Wykle et al., 1972a). This enzyme is specific for the desaturation of alkyl-PE which may explain the low content of alkenyl-PC in most tissues.

In spite of the progress in defining their synthesis, the biological roles of ether lipids remain relatively obscure. The ether phospholipids of many cell types, such as neutrophils, are enriched in arachidonic acid, a precur-sor for bioactive molecules including prostaglandins and leucotrienes (Mueller et al., 1982). Therefore, the ether-linked group may provide the basis for selective metabolism of certain molecular species (i.e. ara-chidonate containing) of phospholipids, in response to cell stimulation. The ether-linked species are also a storage site for arachidonic acid in times of dietary essential fatty acid deficiency (Blank et al., 1973). These observations indicate that ether-linked phospholipids are important in cell function.

Identification of the most specific function known for ether lipids came with the structural characterization of the inflammatory mediator platelet-

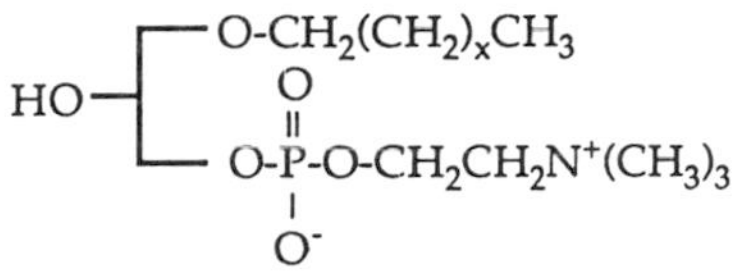

O-CH$_2$(CH$_2$)$_x$CH$_3$

HO—[
O
‖
O-P-O-CH$_2$CH$_2$N$^+$(CH$_3$)$_3$
|
O$^-$

1-O-alkyl-2-lyso-sn-glycero-3-phosphocholine
(an alkyllysophospholipid)

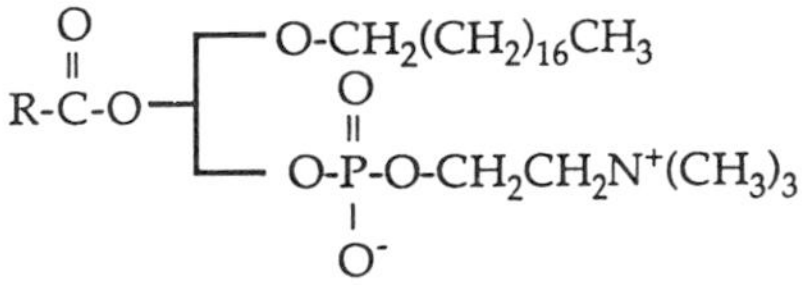

O
‖
R-C-O—[
O-CH$_2$(CH$_2$)$_{16}$CH$_3$
O
‖
O-P-O-CH$_2$CH$_2$N$^+$(CH$_3$)$_3$
|
O$^-$

1-O-alkyl-2-acyl-sn-glycero-3-phosphocholine

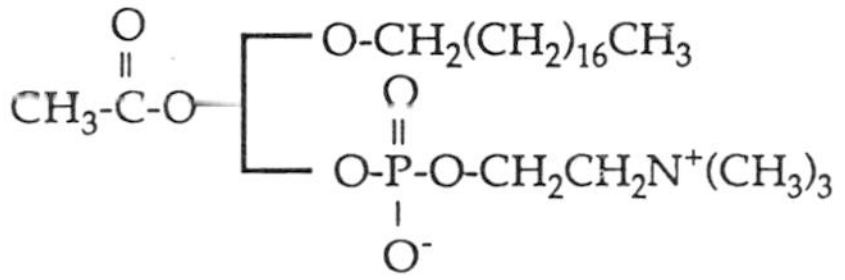

O
‖
CH$_3$-C-O—[
O-CH$_2$(CH$_2$)$_{16}$CH$_3$
O
‖
O-P-O-CH$_2$CH$_2$N$^+$(CH$_3$)$_3$
|
O$^-$

1-O-alkyl-2-acetyl-sn-glycero-3-phosphocholine
(platelet activating factor)

O
‖
R-C-O—[
O-CH=CH(CH$_2$)$_x$-CH$_3$
O
‖
O-P-O-CH$_2$CH$_2$NH$_3$$^+$
|
O$^-$

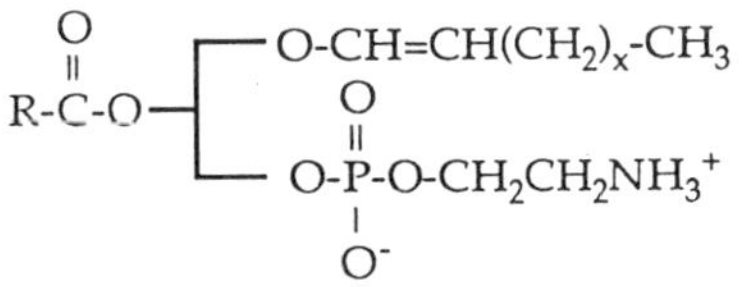

1-O-alk-1'-enyl-2-acyl-sn-glycero-3-phosphoethanolamine
(an ethanolamine plasmalogen)

Fig. 6.2. Structures of naturally occurring ether-linked lipids. Most mammalian cell types contain significant amounts of ether-linked phospholipid species. The ether bond at position 1 can be either alkyl or alkenyl. The alkyl bond is common in choline-phospholipids and the alkenyl-bond is found predominantly in ethanolamine-phospholipids. The other examples shown are: 1-O-alkyl-2-lyso-sn-glycero-3-phosphocholine, an intermediate in the synthesis of platelet-activating factor and prostaglandins; 1-O-alkyl-2-acetyl-sn-glycero-3-phosphocholine, platelet-activating factor.

activating factor (PAF, 1-O-alkyl-2-acetyl-sn-glycero-3-phosphocholine). PAF has potent and diverse biological functions in numerous systems and was the first biologically active phospholipid to be identified (for reviews see Hanahan, 1986; O'Flaherty & Wykle, 1989; Prescott et al., 1990). Like many biologically active compounds, PAF has a high degree of structural specificity and is quickly metabolized. The sn-1 alkyl chain, sn-2 short chain acyl moiety and the natural stereochemical configuration are all required for PAF activity. Degradation of PAF is rapid in most cell types. The sn-2 acetyl group is first removed by an acetyl hydrolase and the resultant alkyl-lyso-PC is acylated to form the inactive metabolite alkyl-PC. Alternatively, alkyl-lyso-PC can be degraded by alkyl-glycerol mono-oxygenase to yield a fatty aldehyde and glycero-3-phosphocholine. The strict structural specificity and rapid metabolism of PAF will be discussed in relation to ET-18-OCH$_3$ in a later section.

Overall, ether-linked phospholipids are important structural and functional components of most mammalian cells. The function and metabolism of these compounds will be an important focus for future research.

Ether-linked lipids as antineoplastic agents

The synthesis and testing of alkyl-linked lipids as antineoplastic agents began by a circuitous route (reviewed by Westphal, 1987). The initial observation that complement-fixing immune reactions are accompanied by phospholipase A$_2$ activation and accumulation of lyso-PC led to the proposal that lyso-PC was a biologically active mediator of immune reactions. A number of synthetic lyso-PC analogues were synthesized by the group of Westphal at the Max-Plank-Institut in Freiburg, Germany, during the late 1960s. These investigators concentrated on alkyl-lysophospholipids (ALP) because of their greater metabolic stability compared to acyl phospholipids. One of the analogues, ET-18-OCH$_3$ (Fig. 6.1), proved of interest and has become the prototype of the class of drugs collectively referred to as ALP analogues. (The usage of lyso in the term ALP has caused some confusion since true lyso compounds are generally inactive. Therefore, the term ALP will be used here for historical purposes only. The terms AMG-PC, OM-GPC, alkylmethoxy-GPC and others have been used to describe the compound originally referred to as ET-18-OCH$_3$. For clarity, the original abbreviation ET-18-OCH$_3$ will be used).

Soon after the initial synthesis of ET-18-OCH$_3$, it was shown to inhibit the growth of allogeneic Ehrlich ascites tumour cells in mice (Munder *et al.*, 1977). The compound also was protective against metastases of the Lewis lung carcinoma when administered after surgical removal of the primary tumour (Berdel *et al.*, 1980). Similar effects observed in several other transplantable and chemically induced *in vivo* systems have been attributed, in part, to macrophage activation (reviewed by Berdel, 1990). However, ET-18-OCH$_3$ and related analogues also selectively inhibit the growth of neoplastic cells in culture indicating direct cellular effects (Andreesen, *et al.*, 1978; Runge *et al.*, 1980; Berdel & Munder, 1987). The mechanism of the antineoplastic and cytotoxic effects of ET-18-OCH$_3$ has been studied in a number of systems but remains to be fully understood. Cytotoxicity by a direct detergent effect upon cell membranes has been

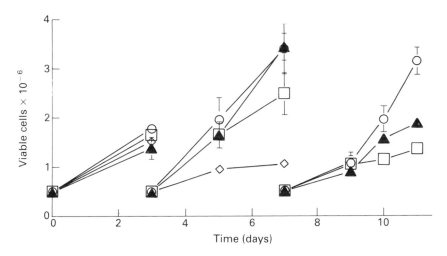

Fig. 6.3. HL-60 cell growth inhibition by ET-18-OCH$_3$. The HL-60 cells (5 × 10^5/ml) were incubated with ET-18-OCH$_3$ (0–1.5 μM) and viable cell numbers determined by hemocytometer counting in the presence of trypan blue. At 3–4 day intervals, the cells were harvested and resuspended (5 × 10^5 cell/ml) in the same concentration of ET-18-OCH$_3$ as in the previous incubation mixture. These experiments indicate that repeated incubations with low concentrations of drug increase the effectiveness of ET-18-OCH$_3$. The experiment also demonstrates that low concentrations of ET-18-OCH$_3$ (c.1 μM) are cytostatic. ○, control; ◇, 1.5 μM ET-18-OCH$_3$; □, 1.0 μM ET-18-OCH$_3$; ▲, 0.5 μM ET-18-OCH$_3$.

suggested and destruction of tumour cell membranes has been observed at relatively high concentrations of drug (Noseda *et al.*, 1989). However, at lower concentrations ET-18-OCH$_3$ is cytostatic rather than cytotoxic (Fig. 6.3). In the experimental protocol used, HL-60 cells were incubated with ET-18-OCH$_3$ (0–1.5 μM) and cell viability was measured by trypan blue dye exclusion. At 3–4 day intervals the cells were subcultured (5 × 10^5 cell/ml) in the original drug concentration. This experiment suggests that ET-18-OCH$_3$ is cytostatic at non-lytic concentrations and suggests a mechanism of action other than a direct detergent effect. The protocol of repeated exposure to low concentrations of drug led to increased cytostatic activity suggesting that the sensitive cells accumulate ET-18-OCH$_3$ until a cytostatic level is reached. This observation may have clinical significance in enhancing the activity of repeated low drug concentrations to minimize toxicity.

Cellular uptake and metabolism of ET-18-OCH$_3$

Differences in the uptake and metabolism of ET-18-OCH$_3$ among sensitive and resistant cells could explain the differential sensitivities. Soodsma *et al.* (1970, 1972) observed that the levels of alkyl-cleavage enzyme activity in Morris hepatoma cells were lower than in normal livers. This observation led to the hypothesis that tumour cells accumulate ET-18-OCH$_3$ because of lower alkyl-cleavage enzyme activity (Berdel et al., 1983b). However, studies of the substrate specificity of the alkyl-cleavage enzyme indicated that a free hydroxyl group at position 2 of the glycerol moiety was required (Snyder et al., 1973; Lee, et al., 1981). Therefore, ET-18-OCH$_3$ is not a substrate for the enzyme (Hoffman et al., 1986; Kötting et al., 1987). Further studies with HL-60 cells which are sensitive and K562 cells which are resistant to ET-18-OCH$_3$ (Tidwell et al., 1981) found no significant difference in the alkyl-cleavage enzyme activity among these cell types (Hoffman et al., 1986). Therefore, degradation of ET-18-OCH$_3$ by the alkyl-cleavage enzyme is not a factor in determining drug sensitivity.

The alkylphospholipid-specific lysophospholipase D (Wykle et al., 1977, 1980) is also a potential detoxification mechanism. However, Wilcox et al. (1987) demonstrated that ET-18-OCH$_3$ is not a substrate for lyso-phospholipase D. Neither HL-60 cells nor K562 cells metabolize a significant amount of the incorporated ET-18-OCH$_3$ even upon prolonged incubation (Hoffman, et al., 1986; Wilcox et al., 1987). After 24 h of incubation, the majority of incorporated ET-18-OCH$_3$ was intact in both the HL-60 and K562 cells, 93 and 91% respectively (Hoffman et al., 1986). In HL-60 cells, the major metabolite of ET-18-OCH$_3$ is the corresponding diglyceride, 1-O-octadecyl-2-O-methyl-glycerol (Wilcox et al., 1987). van Blitterswijk et al. (1987b) also observed this metabolite in ET-18-OCH$_3$-treated MO$_4$ cells. These authors suggest that the glyceride metabolite may contribute to the cellular effects of ET-18-OCH$_3$. However, this seems unlikely due to the small amounts of metabolite formed (Hoffman et al., 1986; Wilcox et al., 1987) and the relatively lower activity of the metabolite compared to the parent compound (L.W. Daniel et al., unpublished data).

Differences in cellular incorporation could also determine sensitivity to ET-18-OCH$_3$. The sensitive cell line HL-60 has been shown to incorporate more ET-18-OCH$_3$ than the relatively resistant cell line K562 (377 versus 188 pmol/10^7 cell) (Hoffman et al., 1986). However, MDCK cells which are relatively resistant to ET-18-OCH$_3$ (Parker et al., 1987) incorporate more ET-18-OCH$_3$ than either K562 or HL-60 cells (Wilcox et al., 1987). In both the experiments to measure drug uptake described above, trace amounts of [^{3}H]ET-18-OCH$_3$ were used. Further experiments comparing the uptake of [^{3}H]ET-18-OCH$_3$ by HL-60 and K562 cells using cytostatic drug concentrations reveal markedly enhanced incorporation by the sensitive cells (Daniel et al., 1990). Bazill and Dexter (1990) have shown that inhibitors of endocytosis protect cells from the cytotoxic actions of ET-18-OCH$_3$. These data suggest that endocytosis is a major route for uptake of ET-18-OCH$_3$ and related analogues. Therefore, drug uptake may contribute to determining differential sensitivity. Further studies to correlate the degree of cellular growth inhibition with the cellular content of ET-18-

OCH_3 will be useful in clarifying the importance of incorporation in determining selectivity.

In addition to drug uptake, differences in cell membrane composition may contribute to ET-18-OCH_3 sensitivity. HL-60 cells contain relatively more endogenous ether-linked phospholipids than K562 cells (Chabot et al., 1989). To determine if the cellular content of endogenous ether lipids was related to ET-18-OCH_3 sensitivity, Chabot et al. (1989) grew K562 cells in the presence of 1-O-hexadecyl-sn-glycerol. This protocol increased the endogenous content of both alkyl- and alkenyl-PC and PE to levels comparable with those observed in HL-60 cells. This alteration resulted in increased sensitivity of the supplemented cells to ET-18-OCH_3. However, the cells were still relatively resistant when compared to HL-60 cells. This observation implies that the endogenous content of ether-linked lipids may play a role in determining sensitivity to ET-18-OCH_3; however, other factors including drug incorporation are also important. The studies of Chabot et al. (1989) also indicate that there may be a critical balance between endogenous ether-linked and diacyl-linked phospholipids which can be disrupted by exogenous ether lipids. The alkyl-cleavage enzyme may have a role in determining sensitivity to ET-18-OCH_3, not by the mechanism originally proposed, but by regulating the endogenous content of ether lipids. The observation that many tumour cells have higher contents of ether lipids than normal cells (Snyder & Wood, 1968, 1969) may help to explain the selectivity of ET-18-OCH_3 for neoplastic cells. It is also of interest that the degree of tumour cell metastasis can be directly correlated with the ether lipid content of the cells (Friedberg et al., 1986; Calorini et al., 1987, 1989).

The cellular content of cholesterol has also been shown to affect the sensitivity of cells to growth inhibition by ether lipids (Malewicz & Baumann, 1988). Diomede et al. (1990) measured cholesterol levels in cells sensitive (HL-60) and resistant to growth inhibition by ET-18-OCH_3 and found an inverse correlation between cholesterol content and sensitivity. Supplementation of sensitive cells with exogenous cholesterol decreased [^{3}H]ET-18-OCH_3 uptake and sensitivity (Diomede et al., 1990). Conversely, depleting cells of cholesterol increases sensitivity to ET-18-OCH_3 (L. Diomede, personal communication). Therefore, manipulation of ether lipid and cholesterol may be valuable in increasing the effectiveness of ether lipid analogues.

Fujiwara et al. (1989) have studied the effects of heat on the sensitivity of tumour cells to ET-18-OCH_3 and found that the two are supra-additive. At 42°C, human ovarian carcinoma cells were sensitized to low concentrations of ET-18-OCH_3 (less than 5 μM). Since the doses of heat and drug are achievable clinically, the use of heat could be adapted to clinical protocols especially in bone marrow purging.

Inhibition of metastasis

Early studies indicated that ET-18-OCH$_3$ inhibited the spread of tumour cells from the site of inoculation and prolonged the survival of animals after surgical removal of the primary tumour (discussed above). In later studies, Storme *et al.* (1985) used an elegant model of tumour cell invasion *in vitro* to characterize this antimetastatic effect. ET-18-OCH$_3$ was found to inhibit MO$_4$ cell infiltration into chick embryonic lung fragments. Interestingly, the concentration of ET-18-OCH$_3$ (5 μM) which completely inhibited tumour cell invasion decreased tumour cell growth by only 25%. This observation indicated that the inhibition of metastasis was not due to simple growth inhibition, but to alterations in cellular properties. The anti-invasive effect of ET-18-OCH$_3$ was accompanied by alterations in membrane fluidity and may indicate that the cell membrane is the target for the anti-invasive activity (van Blitterswijk *et al.*, 1987a). Further studies indicate that modifications of cell surface carbohydrate content may be related to the antimetastatic effects of ET-18-OCH$_3$ (Storme *et al.*, 1987; Bolscher *et al.*, 1988). However, no specific carbohydrate alterations have been correlated with inhibition of metastatic activity. Similar observations were made recently by Engebraaten *et al.* (1991). In this study, ET-18-OCH$_3$ was demonstrated to inhibit the invasion of a glioma cell line into cultured brain spheroids. The anti-invasive effect could be demonstrated at non-toxic concentrations, further indicating that the antimetastatic effect is not due to cytotoxicity alone.

Bone marrow purging

The technique of bone marrow transplantation in acute leukaemia allows aggressive treatment and subsequent reconstitution of normal haematopoietic cells. Autologous transplantation of bone marrow cells obtained during remission offers great promise, if residual leukaemic cells can be eliminated (Beutler *et al.*, 1982). The observations that leukaemic cells were more sensitive to ET-18-OCH$_3$ than normal haematopoietic cells (Andreesen *et al.*, 1978; Berdel *et al.*, 1982) led to the testing of ET-18-OCH$_3$ in bone marrow purging experiments (Glasser *et al.*, 1984). Simulated remission marrow was prepared by mixing normal murine marrow cells with 2% WEHI-3B leukaemic cells. These cells were treated *in vitro* with ET-18-OCH$_3$ and injected into mice following whole body irradiation. This procedure resulted in significantly prolonged survival of the mice receiving the treated cells (Glasser *et al.*, 1984). Thus, ET-18-OCH$_3$ eliminated leukaemic cells from the mixture while sparing a sufficient number of normal stem cells to allow haematological reconstitution. This approach was later extended to a human *in vitro* model using normal bone marrow and a human leukaemia cell line (HL-60) (Vogler *et al.*, 1987). In this model system, a 4-h exposure to ET-18-OCH$_3$ was sufficient to inhibit HL-60 cell viability while sparing normal progenitor cells. Similar results were obtained using the human B-cell leukaemia cell line Daudi (Okamoto *et al.*, 1987).

The encouraging animal studies and *in vitro* studies of bone marrow purging have been followed by clinical trials with promising initial results (Berdel *et al.*, 1989a; Vogler *et al.*, 1990a,b). Purging with ET-18-OCH$_3$ did not reduce the total marrow progenitor cells or sensitize the cells to cryopreservation (Vogler *et al.*, 1990a). Therefore, ET-18-OCH$_3$ appears to be safe for use in autologous bone marrow transplantation and may be less toxic to normal stem cells than compounds currently in use. However, Verdonck *et al.* (1990) have screened 56 leukaemia patients and found that there is a heterogeneous response of the leukaemic cells to growth inhibition by ET-18-OCH$_3$. These data suggest that in some patients the dose required to inhibit leukaemic cells may be too toxic for normal marrow cells. Further studies to determine the optimum protocol for purging should determine the efficacy of ET-18-OCH$_3$ and second-generation analogues for clinical use.

Induction of differentiation

Neoplastic transformation of bone marrow stem cells leads to blocks in cell maturation at distinct stages of development. Thus, cells remain in the proliferative pool and accumulate rapidly. This failure to differentiate is central to the pathology of the disease and agents capable of inducing maturation *in vivo* could be of profound clinical importance (Koeffler, 1983). Leukaemia cell lines capable of differentiating *in vitro* provide a useful model system for the study of differentiating agents. HL-60, an acute myelogenous leukaemia cell line (Collins *et al.*, 1977), is frequently used because the cells are multipotent and capable of differentiation in either the monocytic or granulocytic lineage. This capability for multi-lineage differentiation has been utilized to identify compounds capable of inducing specific programmes of differentiation. Tumour necrosis factor (Squinto *et al.*, 1989; Kim *et al.*, 1991) and 12-*O*-tetradecanoyl phorbol 13-acetate (TPA) (Rovera *et al.*, 1979) induce differentiation to monocytes and macrophages. However, dimethylsulphoxide (Collins *et al.*, 1978) or retinoic acid (Breitman *et al.*, 1980) induce granulocytic differentiation. Many other compounds have also been shown to induce HL-60 cell differentiation. For example, Langdon and Hickman (1987) have shown that any of a variety of polar organic compounds including methanol and ethanol induce granulocytic differentiation. A generalization from these studies is that the optimum concentration for the induction of differentiation causes a 50% reduction in cell numbers compared to control cells (Koeffler, 1983; Langdon & Hickman, 1987). This reduction in cell numbers is primarily due to cytostatic effects at the concentrations optimum for induction of differentiation (Fig. 6.3). In spite of the large number of agents capable of inducing differentiation in cultured cells, differentiation *in vivo* has been difficult to pursue. TPA, one of the most active compounds, cannot be used because of its observed tumour-promoting activity. Other compounds including dimethylsulphoxide and ethanol require high concentrations for activity (*c*.1%, v/v). However, recent reports indicate that all *trans* retinoic acid induces maturation of leukaemic bone marrow promyelocytes *in vitro* (Huang *et al.*, 1987) and induces complete remissions of acute promyelocytic leukaemia (Huang *et al.*, 1988, 1989; Chomienne, *et al.*, 1986).

Therefore, differentiation therapy could become an important clinical tool for the treatment of leukaemia (Degos, 1990a, b) as new agents with enhanced activities are identified. Honma *et al.* (1981) have shown that ET-18-OCH$_3$ and related alkyl lipids induce differentiation of both HL-60 and M1 murine myeloid leukaemia cells *in vitro*. The concentration of ET-18-OCH$_3$ required for optimum differentiating activity resulted in an approximate 50% reduction in cell growth as observed with other differentiating agents. Choline-containing analogues were most effective in this system, but ethanolamine analogues were also somewhat active. Neither phosphatidic acid analogues nor phosphatidylserine analogues were active (Honma *et al.*, 1981). In this study, the ether lipid treated HL-60 cells became morphologically and functionally more mature. However, the lineage of differentiation is unclear in the studies by Honma *et al.* In some experiments, granulocytes and macrophages are reported in a single category of 'morphological change'. It is stated that HL-60 cells differentiate morphologically into mature granulocytes when treated with ET-18-OCH$_3$ (Honma *et al.*, 1981). It is our experience that ether lipid treatment of HL-60 cells induces morphological changes similar to cells of the granulocytic lineage (Rogers *et al.*, 1990). However, the ET-18-OCH$_3$ treated cells are not morphologically or functionally equivalent to the more mature granulocyte-like cells induced by dimethylsulphoxide (L.W. Daniel *et al.*, unpublished data). Therefore, different agents may result in varying degrees of granulocytic differentiation. This differential effect is not surprising since TPA induces more complete differentiation of HL-60 cells in the monocyte/macrophage lineage than other monocyte differentiating agents.

Subsequent studies with related ethylene-glycophospholipids (Honma *et al.*, 1983a), also observed morphological and functional differentiation of HL-60 and M1 cells *in vitro*. These experiments were continued in a syngeneic mouse model to demonstrate increased survival times due to drug treatment (Honma *et al.*, 1983b). Therefore, ether lipids may be useful agents for differentiation therapy of leukaemia. Current compounds should be useful in determining the biochemical targets relevant to the induction of differentiation and provide a basis for new drug synthesis.

Proliferative signal transduction pathways as targets for cancer chemotherapy

The pathways of signal transduction leading to cell proliferation have been the subject of intense investigation from many perspectives. During the past 10 years, the major pathways have been outlined and current research is rapidly adding details on the regulation, integration and complexities of the pathways involved. The overall pathways of proliferative signal transduction are outlined in Fig. 6.4. Several recent reviews provide excellent coverage of these topics (Berridge, 1987; Heldin, *et al.*, 1987; Hunter, 1987, 1991; Nishizuka, 1988; Macara, 1989; Vogt & Bos, 1989; Pelech *et al.*, 1990; Bishop, 1991; Cross & Dexter, 1991; Cantley *et al.*, 1991; Lewin, 1991) and the current discussion will focus upon points of potential therapeutic intervention.

Proliferative signal transduction begins at the cell membrane with binding of growth factors to the cognate receptor. Growth factor binding stimulates the activity of receptor-type tyrosine kinases that interact with guanosine triphosphate (GTP)-binding proteins and activate phospholipase C (PLC). Hydrolysis of phosphatidylinositol 4,5-bisphosphate (PtdIns(4,5)P$_2$) by PLC yields two bioactive messengers, inositol 1,4,5-trisphosphate (Ins(1,4,5)P$_3$) and diacylglycerol (DAG). (Ins(1,4,5)P$_3$) functions to increase intracellular Ca^{2+} and DAG stimulates PKC. The activation of PKC leads to a multitude of cellular responses which are dependent upon the cell type. In many cells PKC activation induces the expression of transcription factors including AP-1 and NF-κB. Collectively, these factors have been referred to as TPA-responsive elements since TPA can activate PKC independent of the normal pathways (Nishizuka, 1988). Although some of the genes regulated by these transcriptional factors are known, many details of the role of transcriptional regulation after growth factor stimulation remain to be determined. The signal transduction pathways presented in Fig. 6.4 provide a simplified outline of the factors involved. Inappropriate expression of several key components results in oncogenic transformation and oncogene products corresponding to four classes of normal cellular proteins have been identified (Fig. 6.4, shown in italics). Therefore, the overall importance of the proliferative signal transduction pathways in maintaining normal growth control is evident. Both PLC and PKC are key factors in producing messengers and transducing their signals, and are thus attractive targets for drug development. ET-18-OCH$_3$ has been shown to inhibit PLC, both in whole cell assay systems (Seewald *et al.*, 1990), and in a cell-free assay system (Perrella *et al.*, 1990; Powis *et al.*, 1991). PKC is also inhibited by ET-18-OCH$_3$ and related

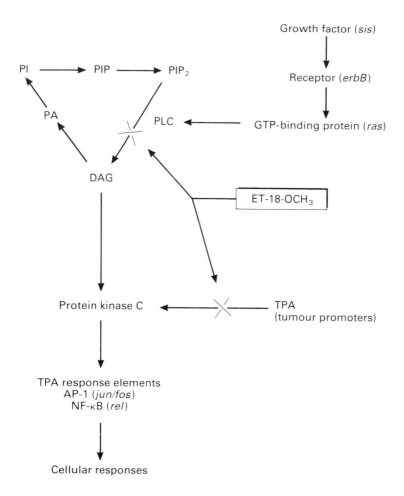

Fig. 6.4. Summary of proliferative signal transduction pathways. The pathways of proliferative signal transduction consist of a sequence of signals and second messengers. Four functionally defined classes of oncogenes with homology to growth factors, growth factor receptors, guanosine triphosphate (GTP)-binding proteins and DNA-binding proteins have been identified. Alterations in the function of any of these classes of oncogenes can result in neoplastic transformation. Representative oncogenes whose products are homologous to the components of the signal transduction pathways are shown in italics. Two important control points are phospholipase C (PLC) and protein kinase C (PKC). ET-18-OCH$_3$ inhibits both PLC and PKC and these activities may be related to the growth inhibitory properties of the compounds. DAG, 1,2-diacylglycerol: PA, phosphatidic acid; PI, phosphatidylinositol; PIP, phosphatidylinositol 4-phosphate; PIP$_2$, phosphatidylinositol 4,5-bisphosphate; TPA, 12-O-tetradecanoylphorbol-13-acetate.

analogues in cell-free assays (Helfman *et al.*, 1983; Parker *et al.*, 1987). In addition, ET-18-OCH$_3$ antagonizes a number of biochemical effects of PKC stimulation by TPA (Daniel *et al.*, 1987; Parker *et al.*, 1987; Daniel, 1990). Therefore, the ether lipids may have multiple antagonistic effects on the pathways of proliferative signal transduction.

Seewald *et al.* (1990) have used mitogen-stimulated Swiss 3T3 fibroblasts to determine the effects of ET-18-OCH$_3$ on cellular Ca^{2+} signalling. The concentration of ET-18-OCH$_3$ required to inhibit growth by 50% was 19 μM. In this model, ET-18-OCH$_3$ (10 μM) caused an 81% reduction in platelet-derived growth factor (PDGF) stimulated inositol phosphate formation. ET-18-OCH$_3$ (5 μM) also inhibited PDGF stimulated Ca^{2+} release (95%) without affecting resting Ca^{2+} concentrations (Seewald *et al.*, 1990). Both effects are within the concentration range of ET-18-OCH$_3$ that inhibits growth of the 3T3 cells indicating that alterations in inositol phospholipid metabolism may play a role in the growth inhibitory effects of ET-18-OCH$_3$. Additional studies by Powis *et al.* (1991) found that ET-18-OCH$_3$ directly inhibits the hydrolysis of [^{3}H]PIP$_2$ by PLC. In two cell lines, the PLC content was directly correlated with drug resistance, further implicating PLC in the mechanism of action of ET-18-OCH$_3$. Further studies in additional cell lines should clarify this association.

PKC inhibition by ET-18-OCH$_3$

The central role of PKC in cellular functions has made it a popular focus of drug development. Several classes of compounds have been shown to inhibit PKC, including staurosporine (Tamaoki *et al.*, 1986), 1-(5-isoquinoline-sulphonyl)-piperazine (C1) (Gerard *et al.*, 1986), sphingolipids (Hannun *et al.*, 1986), palmitoylcarnitine (Katoh *et al.*, 1981b), and Adriamycin (Katch *et al.*, 1981a). Helfman *et al.* (1983) were the first to demonstrate inhibition of PKC by ET-18-OCH$_3$. These authors found that ET-18-OCH$_3$ inhibits PKC, but not cyclic adenosine monophosphate (cAMP)-dependent protein kinase or cyclic guanosine monophosphate (cGMP)-dependent protein kinase. ET-18-OCH$_3$ remains one of the most specific PKC inhibitors known, due to its interaction with the regulatory domain of PKC (Helfman *et al.*, 1983; Kuo *et al.*, 1986). In contrast, other compounds including staurosporine (Tamaoki *et al.*, 1986) and C1 (Gerard *et al.*, 1986) are competitive inhibitors at the adenosine triphosphate (ATP) binding-site and, therefore, inhibit other protein kinases.

The tumour promoter TPA stimulates PKC directly (Castagna *et al.*, 1982) and is a useful tool for defining PKC-dependent cellular events. Therefore, TPA has also been used to study the effectiveness of PKC inhibitors in intact cells (Daniel *et al.*, 1987). In this model system, cells are incubated with TPA and ET-18-OCH$_3$ (Fig. 6.4) and the cellular effects are determined. Parker *et al.* (1987) have used this protocol with Madin Darby canine kidney (MDCK) cells to demonstrate a dose-dependent inhibition of TPA-induced phosphorylation of 40 and 48 kDa proteins by ET-18-OCH$_3$. In addition, ET-18-OCH$_3$ inhibited TPA-stimulated arachidonic acid release and prostaglandin synthesis. The concentration dependence for inhibition of both protein phosphorylation and prostaglandin synthesis was similar. In contrast, ET-18-OCH$_3$ did not inhibit arachidonic acid release or prostaglandin synthesis in response to the calcium ionophore A23187, a process not requiring PKC. These data indicate that ET-18-OCH$_3$ can inhibit the activation of PKC and inhibit the effects of TPA in intact cells. MDCK cells also increase the turnover of PC in response to TPA (Daniel *et al.*, 1987). This effect is a combination of both increased PC synthesis (Daniel *et al.*, 1987) and PC breakdown (Daniel *et al.*, 1986). Both the synthesis and breakdown of PC are inhibited by ET-18-OCH$_3$. However, synthesis of PC is more sensitive to inhibition by ET-18-OCH$_3$ than degradation (Daniel *et al.*, 1987). At present, there is no satisfactory explanation for this observation. TPA stimulates the activity of cytidine triphosphate (CTP)-cholinephosphate cytidylyltransferase (CT), the rate-limiting step in PC synthesis (Paddon & Vance, 1980; Vance, 1989). The stimulation is apparently dependent upon PKC since pretreatment of cells (down-regulation of PKC) abolishes the activity (Kolesnick, 1987). However, the relevant substrates for PKC phosphorylation have not been identified. ET-18-OCH$_3$ inhibits TPA-stimulated PC synthesis by inhibiting the activity of CT in intact cells (L.W. Daniel *et al.*, unpublished data), but does not inhibit purified CT (R. Cornell, personal communication). Therefore, the mechanism of TPA stimulation and ET-18-OCH$_3$ inhibition of CT remains to be determined. ET-18-OCH$_3$ may be a useful tool in identifying the mechanism of CT regulation by PKC. TPA also stimulates PC turnover by phospholipase D and subsequent phosphatidic acid phosphohydrolase to yield diglycerides (reviewed by Pelech & Vance, 1989; Exton, 1990). In MDCK cells, TPA stimulation results in the formation of both alkyl- and acyl-diglycerides (Daniel *et al.*, 1986) and degradation of approximately 10–15% of the cellular PC pool (L.W. Daniel, unpublished observations). The TPA-stimulated phospholipase D has not been purified or characterized in detail. Therefore, the mechanism of stimulation by TPA or inhibition by ET-18-OCH$_3$ remains to be determined.

In addition to PC degradation and synthesis, ET-18-OCH$_3$ inhibits oleic acid incorporation into PC. The inhibition of oleic acid incorporation by ET-18-OCH$_3$ in eight cell lines was correlated with the sensitivity of the cells to growth inhibition (Herrmann, 1985). Further studies by Herrmann and Neumann (1986) compared oleoyl:CoA-1-acyl-*sn*-glycero-3-phosphocholine acyl transferase activity (acyl transferase) in sensitive (Meth A fibrosarcoma) and resistant cells (bone marrow-derived murine macrophages). The sensitive cells had less acyl-transferase activity (1.05 nmol/min/mg) than the resistant cells (2.98 nmol/min/mg) and the enzyme from sensitive cells was more sensitive to inhibition by ET-18-OCH$_3$ (K_i = 13 μM versus 423 μM).

Another frequently studied effect of TPA is the macrophage-induced differentiation of HL-60 cells (Rovera et al., 1979). Several lines of evidence indicate the importance of PKC in HL-60 cell differentiation. TPA causes translocation of PKC from the cytoplasm to the plasma membrane and later to the nuclear membrane during HL-60 cell differentiation (Kiss et al., 1988). The translocation results in PKC activation and phosphorylation of specific sets of cellular proteins (Kiss et al., 1988). HL-60 cells resistant to TPA-induced differentiation exhibit a decreased expression of PKCβ (Nishikawa et al., 1990) indicating that distinct isoforms of PKC may control differentiation. Nakaki et al. (1984) have used the PKC inhibitor palmitoylcarnitine to determine the requirement for PKC in HL-60 cell differentiation. They found that palmitoylcarnitine inhibited TPA-induced differentiation, even when added 1–2 days after TPA stimulation. Neither palmitic acid nor carnitine inhibited the effect of TPA. Kiss et al. (1987) have also shown that ET-18-OCH$_3$ inhibits TPA-induced HL-60 cell differentiation and phosphorylation of specific proteins. Therefore, TPA-induced macrophage differentiation appears to require PKC activation. Other inducers of HL-60 cell differentiation may also require stimulation of PKC activity. Obeid et al. (1990) have shown that 1,25-(OH)$_2$-vitamin D$_3$, another inducer of monocytic differentiation, increases the level of PKCβ mRNA and increases enzymatic activity. This increased activity of PKC results in enhanced phosphorylation of HL-60 cell proteins without increased levels of diglycerides. Therefore, various differentiating agents may have different cellular targets. However, PKC activation appears to be critical for the induction of HL-60 cells in the monocytic lineage. The relevant targets for PKC phosphorylation during the induction of differentiation are unknown. Although phosphorylation of several specific proteins has been observed in TPA stimulated HL-60 cells, the functional significance is not known (Kiss et al., 1987; Morin et al., 1987; Warren et al., 1988; Obeid et al., 1990).

TPA-induced monocytic differentiation of both HL-60 and U-937 cells is accompanied by the induction of both fos and jun (Sherman et al., 1990; Verma et al., 1991). Together, the products of these oncogenes form a heterodimeric complex. The active dimer regulates transcription of several specific genes containing the AP-1 consensus sequence (TGACTCA) (Vogt & Bos, 1989). Both of these gene products are regulated by transcriptional activation. TPA also stimulates activation of the transcription factor NF-κB during HL-60 cell differentiation (Griffin et al., 1989). NF-κB is present in unstimulated cells as an inactive complex with an inhibitory protein IκB (Bauerle & Baltimore, 1988). Phosphorylation of IκB by PKC releases the active NF-κB complex (Ghosh & Baltimore, 1990). Therefore, these PKC-induced transcription factors are associated with HL-60 cell differentiation. To investigate if NF-κB activation was required, the authors have measured NF-κB activity during TPA-induced differentiation (Rogers *et al.*, 1991). HL-60 cells were transfected with a plasmid containing binding sites for NF-κB linked to a chloramphenicol acetyltransferase (CAT) gene. TPA induced NF-κB activity concomitant with HL-60 cell differentiation as detemined by cellular adhesion. ET-18-OCH$_3$ inhibited the induction of NF-κB and cellular adhesion by TPA. The concentration dependencies for both effects were strikingly similar, indicating that NF-κB expression is required for differentiation. The inhibition of NF-κB expression by ET-18-OCH$_3$ and other PKC inhibitors indicates that the nuclear oncogenes may be targets in the mechanism of action of ET-18-OCH$_3$.

Drug development

Interest in ET-18-OCH$_3$ as a selective antineoplastic agent led to the search for more effective and specific agents. Many chemical modifications of the basic ET-18-OCH$_3$ structure have been synthesized and tested. The structural requirements for inhibition of cell growth are not rigid compared with PAF, another bioactive phospholipid. In spite of their similar structures, PAF and ET-18-OCH$_3$ (Figs 6.1 & 6.2) have very dissimilar biological activities. ET-18-OCH$_3$ has relatively little PAF activity and both isomers of ET-18-OCH$_3$ inhibit HL-60 cell growth (Kudo *et al.*, 1987). [The isomers of ET-18-OCH$_3$ and PAF will be referred to as L-, 1-*O*-alkyl-2-*O*-methyl(acetyl)-*sn*-glycero-3-phosphocholine, natural isomer; or D-, 3-*O*-alkyl-2-*O*-methyl(acetyl)-*sn*-glycero-1-phosphocholine.] In contrast, only the L-PAF isomer has PAF activity, indicating strict stereochemical specificity. D-PAF, the unnatural isomer, inhibits HL-60 cell growth and is as potent as ET-18-OCH$_3$ (Hoffman *et al.*, 1984a,b). Acyl-PC analogues and L-PAF are relatively ineffective inhibitors of HL-60 cell growth. The growth inhibiting effects of D-PAF are probably due to the inability of cellular enzymes to metabolize the unnatural isomer. However, this has not been directly tested.

In summary, the strict structural requirements for PAF activity imply a receptor-mediated mechanism of action. However, the relative lack of specificity for cell growth inhibition implies that this effect is not coupled to a specific receptor. Further, these data indicate that the PAF receptor is not involved in the growth inhibitory effects of ET-18-OCH$_3$ (Berdel *et al.*, 1987a). This conclusion is supported by the observations that HL-60 cells do not have specific PAF receptors until differentiated to granulocytes (O'Flaherty *et al.*, 1989) and when differentiated to granulocytes, the HL-60 cells become more resistant to ET-18-OCH$_3$ (Vallari *et al.*, 1988). ET-18-OCH$_3$ does not compete with [^{3}H]PAF for binding to the PAF receptor (Vallari *et al.*, 1990). Therefore, the PAF receptor does not appear to be involved in determining the antineoplastic activity of the ether lipids and synthetic strategies directed towards new antineoplastic agents should be directed away from compounds with PAF activity.

Structural modifications at position 1—sulphur-containing analogues

Substitutions of sulphur for oxygen in the 1-alkyl chain of ET-18-OCH$_3$ have been reported by two groups (Morris-Natschke *et al.*, 1986; Bosies *et al.*, 1987). Piantadosi and coworkers reported the synthesis of five sulphur-containing analogues of ET-18-OCH$_3$. These included 1-*S*-octadecyl-, 1-*S*-hexadecyl, 2-*O*-methyl and 2-*O*-ethyl analogues. All of the compounds were as active as ET-18-OCH$_3$ in HL-60 growth inhibition assays and had reduced PAF activity compared to the oxygen-containing analogue (Morris-Natschke *et al.*, 1986). The sulphur containing homologue of ET-18-OCH$_3$ was also an active inhibitor of HL-60 cell derived PKC *in vitro* (Daniel *et al.*, 1990). Therefore, the sulphur substitution is useful in lowering PAF activity without affecting cell growth inhibition or PKC inhibition.

The Boehringer Mannheim group has also used a thioether substitution to develop a series of analogues of which BM 41.440 (proprietary name, Ilmofosine) (Fig. 6.2) was found to be most active (Berdel *et al.*, 1983a). BM 41.440 has been shown to inhibit the growth of leukaemic cells and solid tumours *in vitro* (Berdel *et al.*, 1983a; Fromm *et al.*, 1987). Herrmann and Neumann (1987) have used a clonogenic assay system to determine that 34 of 64 human malignant cell types tested were sensitive to BM 41.440. The *in vivo* efficacy of BM 41.440 in preventing the growth and spread of experimental tumours has been demonstrated in some (Berdel *et al.*, 1980) but not all systems tested (Leder *et al.*, 1987).

The mechanism of action of BM 41.440 may be similar to ET-18-OCH$_3$ because the drugs seem to have similar biochemical effects upon cells. BM 41.440 inhibits PKC and is competitive with the phosphatidylserine cofactor (Shoji *et al.*, 1988). Also, like ET-18-OCH$_3$, BM 41.440 inhibits TPA-induced HL-60 cell differentiation and inhibits phosphorylation of several proteins associated with the differentiated phenotype (Shoji *et al.*, 1988). The inhibition of PKC may be related to the observed synergy of BM 41.440 with *cis*-diammine-dichloroplatinum (*cis*-DDP) (Hofmann *et al.*, 1989) since synergy of *cis*-DDP with other PKC inhibitors has been reported (Hofmann *et al.*, 1988). BM 41.440, like the other thioether phospholipids discussed above, does not inhibit PAF binding to the PAF receptor and has been used to demonstrate that PAF binding and antineoplastic activity are not correlated (Berdel *et al.*, 1987c).

Alkylamide and phytanyl analogues

To determine further the structural requirements at position 1, Marx *et al.*

(1988) synthesized a series of alkylamide analogues of ET-18-OCH$_3$. This series included C16 and C18 alkylamide analogues and both were found to be equally active in growth inhibition assays (Noseda et al., 1987; Marx et al., 1988). The alkylamide analogues were also active inhibitors of PKC in in vitro assays but were less effective than ET-18-OCH$_3$. These analogues have not been tested in vivo. These data indicate that a variety of position 1 modifications are possible without a loss of activity. However, the long chain alkyl moiety or other metabolically stable hydrophobic group is required for activity.

Hoffman et al. (1984b) reported the synthesis and testing of a number of 1-phytanyl analogues of ET-18-OCH$_3$. These analogues were useful in further defining the structural requirements for position 1. However, the 20-carbon branch-chain phytanyl moiety resulted in decreased potency in the HL-60 cell model and higher toxicity to normal cells, and this modification has not been useful in further drug treatment.

Structural modifications at position 2 and modifications of the glycerol moiety

Few systematic studies of position 2 modifications have been attempted. However, relatively minor modifications at position 2 appear to have little effect on growth inhibition or PKC inhibition. For example, methoxy, ethoxy or methoxymethyl analogues are approximately equally active (Morris-Natschke et al. 1986). Kudo et al. (1987) have tested compounds with longer alkyl chains at position 2 (C8–C16) and found that all the analogues were much less active than ET-18-OCH$_3$ in an assay using mouse P388 leukaemia cells. An acetoacetyl analogue was also inactive in this system.

These data indicate that a specific functional group is not required at position 2. The analogue ET-18-H has a methylene group at position 2 and although slightly less active than ET-18-OCH$_3$, is still an active growth inhibitor (Berdel et al., 1983b). Honma et al. (1983a) have shown that ethyleneglycophospholipids inhibit HL-60 cell growth and induce HL-60 cell differentiation. Therefore, the 3-carbon glycerol backbone is not required for activity.

Hexadecylphosphocholine (HePC)

Eibl (1984) and Eibl et al. (1986) have synthesized a series of compounds to determine the minimum structural requirements for cell growth inhibition and found that the glycerol moiety can be deleted without loss of activity. These studies led to the identification of HePC (Fig. 6.1) as an active compound (Eibl et al., 1986; Muschiol et al., 1987; Scherf et al., 1987). Mechanistically, HePC seems to resemble ET-18-OCH$_3$ (Grunicke *et al.*, 1990). K562 cells are resistant to ET-18-OCH$_3$ and are comparably resistant to HePC (Danhauser-Reidl *et al.*, 1990b). HePC, like ET-18-OCH$_3$, inhibits PKC and HL-60 cell differentiation (Kuo *et al.*, 1990). The inhibition of PKC by HePC like ET-18-OCH$_3$ is competitive at the phosphatidylserine binding-site (Shoji *et al.*, 1991).

HePC is active against a variety of tumours *in vitro* and *in vivo* (Muschiol *et al.*, 1987; Scherf *et al.*, 1987). The compound is active in cell lines resistant to methotrexate or colchicine (Himmelmann *et al.*, 1990; Danhauser-Riedl *et al.*, 1990b). Although HePC is somewhat less active than ET-18-OCH$_3$ *in vitro* (Danhauser-Reidl *et al.*, 1990b), it may be a clinically useful drug. HePC is absorbed from the intestinal tract and is active when administered orally (Breiser *et al.*, 1987; Hilgard *et al.*, 1990b). Initial clinical trials indicate that HePC can be given orally and that serum levels comparable to the therapeutic levels in animals (100–200 μM) can be achieved (Berkovic *et al.*, 1990; Hilgard *et al.*, 1990a).

SRI 62-834

Houlihan *et al.* (1987) synthesized a tetrahydrofuran analogue of ET-18-OCH$_3$ referred to as SRI 62-834 (Fig. 6.1). This compound represents another interesting modification of the glycerol backbone that retains antitumour activity. The compound was initially shown to be as effective as ET-18-OCH$_3$ in a mouse Meth A sarcoma model (Houlihan *et al.*, 1987). Interestingly, the compound is effective in oral formulation.

SRI 62-834, at non-toxic concentrations, inhibits cell growth in response to PDGF. Although PDGF binding was inhibited by high concentrations of SRI 62-834, this does not appear to be relevant to the mechanism responsible for the antimitogenic effect (Houlihan *et al.*, 1987). SRI 62-834 does not have PAF activity at concentrations as high as 100 μM; however, it does inhibit [^{3}H]PAF binding to the human platelet receptor (IC$_{50}$ = 27.3 μM). Inhibitors of PAF binding inhibit the effects of SRI 62-834 and ET-18-OCH$_3$ on growth of WEHI-3B cells and it has been suggested that the PAF receptor may play a role in determining sensitivity to these agents (Bazill & Dexter, 1989). However, other observations, discussed previously, and subsequent studies by Bazill and Dexter (1990), argue against a role for the PAF receptor in the growth inhibition of ET-18-OCH$_3$.

Structural modifications at position 3

Several reports of structural modifications at position 3 of the glycerol backbone have been made. Most of the compounds retain the alkyl-glycerol phosphate of ET-18-OCH$_3$ and alter the head group. However, non-phosphorous analogues have been reported. Marasco *et al.* (1990)

synthesized a quaternary ammonium derivative of ET-18-OCH$_3$ which was as active as the parent compound in inhibiting PKC. Other analogues including 2-O-ethyl- and 1-thio- (CP-10, Fig. 6.1) were also active PKC inhibitors. However, a 1-naphthyl- substitution caused a loss of PKC and HL-60 cell growth inhibition (Marasco *et al.*, 1990; E.J. Modest, personal communication). The observed activities of these analogues indicate that structural modifications of the head group can be made without loss of either growth inhibition or PKC inhibition. This conclusion is also supported by the observations of Ishaq *et al.* (1989) that the choline head group could be replaced by inositol with the retention of PKC inhibitory activity. However, the inositol-containing analogues inhibit cell growth only at high concentrations. This may be due to a lack of uptake or due to metabolism of the compounds.

Guivisdalsky *et al.* (1990) have synthesized a group of interesting glycolipid analogues of ET-18-OCH$_3$. These compounds were designed to reduce the PAF activity of ET-18-OCH$_3$ and retain the growth inhibitory properties. These compounds retain the basic backbone structure of ET-18-OCH$_3$ and vary the phosphocholine moiety as glycero-α- and β-D-glucopyranosides, and glycero-1-thio-α and β-D-glucopyranosides. These analogues are growth inhibitory *in vitro* in the micromolar concentration range. As observed previously with other analogues, the stereoconfiguration of the glycerol did not appear critical for growth inhibition. However, the stereochemistry of the sugar group was an important determinant of activity.

Hong *et al.* (1986) and Berdel *et al.* (1988, 1989a) have collaborated in the synthesis and testing of a group of 1-β-D-arabinofuranosylcystosine (ara-C) conjugates of ether lipids. The rationale of these experiments was to combine two cytotoxic compounds in order to achieve additive or synergistic effects. These conjugates exhibited promising *in vitro* activities in six cell lines tested (Berdel *et al.*, 1987a). Some of the conjugates were active *in vivo* in a syngeneic Lewis lung carcinoma model, but no better than the parent compounds or equimolar mixtures of the lipids and ara-C. However, compounds were identified that were more active than the parent compounds as a single agent or in combination. Therefore, this approach appears promising and may lead to more active drugs. The mechanism of action or reason for synergy should be explored. For example, it is not known if the conjugates are the active form or if they are acting as prodrugs.

Kára *et al.* (1986) have identified a novel alkyl-phospholipid in a preparation referred to as crude anticancer phospholipids (cACPL). The active component 1-O-alkyl-2-acyl-*sn*-glycero-3-phospho-(N-acyl)-ethanolamine (PNAE) is selectively cytotoxic to tumour cells *in vitro* and *in vivo* in a mouse fibrosarcoma model (Kára *et al.*, 1986). The mechanism of action of this compound may be similar to ET-18-OCH$_3$. Mikhaevich *et al.* (1991) found that PNAE inhibits PKC competitively with respect to phosphatidylserine. Although PNAE was less active than ET-18-OCH$_3$ *in vitro*, the compounds are comparable in activity in intact cell assays. Therefore, the *N*-acyl modification may be useful in future structure–activity studies.

Clinical trials

The initial observations that synthetic ether lipids are selectively cytotoxic to neoplastic cells has led to the development of several new classes of active compounds. There are now four compounds in clinical trials (Fig. 6.1). Both ET-18-OCH$_3$ and BM 41.440 are in phase I and phase II trials in a variety of neoplastic diseases (Berdel *et al.*, 1987b; Herrmann *et al.*, 1987, 1989). HePC is currently being used in a topical formulation for the treatment of skin metastases in breast cancer patients (Unger *et al.*, 1988, 1989) and is in clinical trials as an oral formulation (Danhauser-Riedl *et al.*, 1990a). Clinical trials are also in progress using SRI 62-834 (Houlihan *et al.*, 1987).

To date, the results of clinical trials have not been impressive, possibly because only low plasma levels can be achieved using the drugs orally due to the limiting toxicity in the gastrointestinal tract at low doses (Berdel, 1987, 1990, 1991). New formulations or new compounds may be useful in increasing the clinical potential of the ether lipids. New strategies, including bone marrow purging, are also promising. Therefore, further clinical trials using new compounds and new strategies, such as intravenous dosing, should clarify the efficacy of these compounds.

Perspectives

ET-18-OCH$_3$ and derivatives should also be useful in defining relevant targets in the pathways of proliferative signal transduction. Further studies on the mechanism of selectivity and cell growth inhibition should be useful in developing new drugs that are both more effective and less toxic to normal cells. Knowledge of the mechanism of action of the ether lipids and other anticancer drugs should also lead to effective new combinations. For example, Adriamycin resistance may be due to increased PKC levels (Aquino *et al.*, 1988). Therefore, PKC inhibitors may be useful in combination with Adriamycin.

Further studies of the effects of ether lipids on gene expression should also lead to new targets and uses for the drugs. The observation that tumour necrosis factor activates both protective and destructive pathways may provide insight into other uses for ether lipid analogues (Larrick & Wright, 1990). Since the 'protective pathway' appears related to the activation of PKC and NF-κB (Osborn *et al.*, 1989), inhibitors of PKC (and

NF-κB expression) should increase the effectiveness of tumour necrosis factor. Therefore, ET-18-OCH$_3$ or other PKC inhibitors may prove useful in combination with tumour necrosis factor. NF-κB is also an important regulatory molecule in the activation of virus replication in cells latently infected with the human immunodeficiency virus (Nabel & Baltimore, 1987). Therefore, inhibition of NF-κB activation by ET-18-OCH$_3$ may have a role in the antiviral effects of ET-18-OCH$_3$ and related analogues. Kucera *et al.* (1990) recently reported that a variety of ether lipid analogues inhibit human immunodeficiency virus type 1 replication in a plaque assay system.

The ether lipids are therefore of interest as anticancer and antiviral drugs. They appear to have multiple targets in the pathways of cell growth and differentiation. This novel mechanism of action is of interest because the compounds have potential for use in combination with other mechanistically different agents. As the mechanism of action of the ether lipid analogues and other existing compounds are identified, new strategies for rational combinations of chemotherapeutic agents should follow.

Acknowledgements

The studies in my laboratory were supported by grants CA43297 and CA48995 from the National Cancer Institute and CH43520 from the American Cancer Society. I wish to thank my colleagues at Wake Forest University and our collaborators, especially Dr Ed Modest of Boston University and Dr Claude Piantadosi of the University of North Carolina; Chapel Hill, for their support and encouragement in these studies. These collaborators also include the authors listed in the following references: Chabot *et al.* (1989); Daniel *et al.* (1986, 1987, 1990); Ishaq *et al.* (1980); Kucera *et al.* (1990); Marasco *et al.* (1990); Marx *et al.* (1988); Morris-Natschke *et al.* (1986); Noseda *et al.* (1987, 1989); Parker *et al.* (1987); Rogers (1990, 1991); and Wilcox *et al.* (1987). I also wish to thank Drs Wolfgang Berdel, Ralph Vogler, Fred Snyder, Guy Storme and Luisa Diomede who contributed reprints, preprints and helpful suggestions; Dr Robert L. Wykle's comments on the manuscript, and Ginger Moore and Tommye Campbell's assistance are appreciated.

References

Andreesen, R., Modolell, M., Weltzien, H.U., Eibl, H., Common, H.H., Lohr, G.W. & Munder, P.G. (1978). Selective destruction of human leukemic cells by alkyl-lyso-phospholipids. *Cancer Research* **38**, 3894–3899.

Aquino, A., Hartman, K.D., Knode, M.C., Grant, S., Huang, K.P., Niu, C.H. & Glazer, R.I. (1988). Role of protein kinase C in phosphorylation of vinculin in adriamycin resistant HL-60 leukemia cells. *Cancer Research* **48**, 3324–3329.

Bauerle, P.A. & Baltimore, D. (1988). IκB: a specific inhibitor of the NF-κB transcription factor. *Science* **242**, 540–546.

Bazill, G.W. & Dexter, T.M. (1989). An antagonist to platelet activating factor counteracts the tumouricidal action of alkyl lysophospholipids. *Biochemical Pharmacology* **38**, 374–377.

Bazill, G.W. & Dexter, T.M. (1990). Role of endocytosis in the action of ether lipids on WEHI-3B, HL60, and FDCP-mix A4 cells. *Cancer Research* **50**, 7505–7512.

Berdel, W.E. (1987). Ether lipids and analogs in experimental cancer therapy. A brief review of the Munich experience. *Lipids* **22**, 970–973.

Berdel, W.E. (1990). Ether lipids and derivatives as investigational anticancer drugs. *Onkologie* **13**, 245–250.

Berdel, W.E. (1991). Membrane–interactive lipids as experimental anticancer drugs. *British Journal of Cancer* **64**, 208–211.

Berdel, W.E. & Munder, P.G. (1987). Antineoplastic actions of ether lipids related to platelet activating factor. In Snyder, F. (ed). *Platelet-Activating Factor and Related Lipid Mediators*, pp. 449–467. Plenum Press, New York.

Berdel, W.E., Bausert, W.R.E., Weltzien, H.U., Modolell, M.L., Widman, K.H. & Munder, P.G. (1980). The influence of alkyl-lysophospholipids and lysophospholipid-activated macrophages on the development of metastasis of 3-Lewis lung carcinoma. *European Journal of Cancer* **16**, 1119–1204.

Berdel, W.E. Danhauser, S., Hong, C., Schick, H.D., Reichert, A., Busch, R., Rastetter, J. & Vogler, W.R. (1988). Influence of 1-β-D-arabino-furanosylcytosine conjugates of lipids on the growth and metastasis of Lewis lung carcinoma. *Cancer Research* **48**, 826–829.

Berdel, W.E., Danhauser, S., Schick, H.D., Hong, C., West, C.R., Fromm, M., Fink, U., Reichert, A. & Rastetter, J. (1987a). Antineoplastic activity of conjugates of lipids and 1-β-D-arabinofuranosylcytosine. *Lipids* **22**, 943–946.

Berdel, W.E., Fink, U., Maubauch, P.A., Permametter, B. & Rastetter, J. (1982). Response of acute myelomonocytic leukemia to alkyl-lysophospholipids. *Blut* **44**, 177–186.

Berdel, W.E., Fink, U. & Rastetter, J. (1987b). Clinical phase I pilot study of the alkyl lysophospholipid derivative ET-18-OCH$_3$. *Lipids* **22**, 967–969.

Berdel, W.E., Fromm, M., Fink, U., Pahlke, W., Bicker, U., Reichert, A. & Rastetter, J. (1983a). Cytotoxicity of thioether-lysophospholipids in leukemia and tumours of human origin. *Cancer Research* **43**, 5538–5543.

Berdel, W.E., Greiner, E., Fink, U., Stavrou, D., Reichert, A., Rastetter, J., Hoffman, D.R. & Snyder, F. (1983b). Cytotoxicity of alkyl-lysophospholipid derivatives and low-alkyl-cleavage enzyme activities in rat brain tumor cells. *Cancer Research* **43**, 541–545.

Berdel, W.E., Korth R., Reichert, A., Houlihan, W.J., Bicker, U., Normura, H., Vogler, W.R., Benveniste, J. & Rastetter, J. (1987c). Lack of correlation between cytotoxicity of agonists and antagonists of platelet activating factor (paf-acether) in neoplastic cells and modulation of [^{3}H]-paf-acether binding to platelets from humans *in vitro*. *Anticancer Research* **7**, 1181–1188.

Berdel, W.E., Okamoto, S., Danhauser-Riedl, S., Hong, C.I., Winton, E.F., West, C.R., Rastetter, J. & Vogler, W.R. (1989a). Therapeutic activity of 1-β-D-arabinofuranosylcytosine conjugates of lipids in WEHI-3B leukemia in mice. *Experimental Hematology* **17**, 364–367.

Berdel, W.E., Okamoto, S., Reichert, A., Olson, A.C., Winton, E.F., Rastetter, J. & Vogler, W.R. (1989b). Studies on the role of ether lipids as purging agents in autologous bone marrow transplantation. In Kabara, J.J. (ed.) *The Pharmacological Effects of Lipids*, Vol. III, pp. 338–360. The American Oil Chemists Society (AOCS) Press, Illinios.

Berkovic, D., Fleer, E.A.M., Hilgard, P., Eibl, H. & Unger, C. (1990). Serum concentrations of hexadecylphosphocholine (He-PC) in the rat. *Proceedings of the American Association for Cancer Research* **31**, 413.

Berridge, M.J. (1987). Inositol trisphosphate and diacylglycerol: two interacting second messengers. *Annual Review of Biochemistry* **56**, 159–194.

Beutler, E. McMillan, R. & Spruce, W. (1982). The role of bone marrow transplantation in the treatment of acute leukemia in remission. *Blood* **59**, 1115–1117.

Bishop, J.M. (1991). Molecular themes in oncogenesis. *Cell* **64**, 235–248.

Blank, M.L., Wykle, R.L. & Snyder, F. (1973). The retention of arachidonic acid in ethanolamine plasmalogens of rat testes during essential fatty acid deficiency. *Biochimica et Biophysica Acta* **316**, 28–34.

Bolscher, J.G.M., Schallier, D.C.C., van Rooy, H., Storme, G.A. & Smets, L.A. (1988). Modification of cell surface carbohydrates and invasive behavior by an alkyl lysophospholipid. *Cancer Research* **48**, 977–982.

Bosies, E., Herrmann, D.B.J., Bicker, U., Gall, R. & Pahlke, W. (1987). Synthesis of thioether phosphocholine analogues. *Lipids* **22**, 947–951.

Breiser, A., Kim, D.-J., Fleer, E.A.M., Damenz, W., Drub, A., Berger, M., Nagel, G.A., Eibl, H. & Unger, C. (1987). Distribution and metabolism of hexadecylphosphocholine in mice. *Lipids* **22**, 925–926.

Breitman, T.R., Selonick, S.E. & Collins, S.J. (1980). Induction of differentiation of the human promyelocytic leukemia cell line (HL-60) by retinoic acid. *Proceedings of the National Academy of Sciences USA* **77**, 2936–2940.

Calorini, L., Fallani, A., Tombaccini, D., Barletta, E., Mugnal, G., Di Renzo, M.F., Comoglio, P.M. & Ruggieri, S. (1989). Lipid characteristics of RSV-transformed Balb/c 3T3 cell lines with different spontaneous metastatic potentials. *Lipids* **24**, 685–689.

Calorini, L., Fallani, A., Tombaccini, D., Mugnal, G. & Ruggieri, S. (1987). Lipid composition of cultured B16 melanoma cell variants with different lung-colonizing potential. *Lipids* **22**, 651–655.

Cantley, L.C., Auger, K.R., Carpenter, C., Duckworth, B., Graziani, A., Kapeller, R. & Soltoff, S. (1991). Oncogenes and signal transduction. *Cell* **64**, 281–302.

Castagna, M., Takai, Y., Kaibuchi, K., Sano, K., Kikkawa, U. & Nishizuka, Y. (1982). Direct activation of calcium-activated, phospholipid-dependent protein kinase by tumor-promoting phorbol esters. *Journal of Biological Chemistry* **257**, 7847–7851.

Chabot, M.C., Wykle, R.L., Modest, E.J. & Daniel, L.W. (1989). Correlation of ether lipid content of human leukemia cell lines and their susceptibility to 1-O-octadecyl-2-O-methyl-rac-glycero-3-phosphocholine. *Cancer Research* **49**, 4441–4445.

Chomienne, C., Baltitrand, N., Cost, H., Degos, L. & Abita, J.P. (1986). Structure–activity relationships of aromatic retinoids on the differentiation of the human histiocytic lymphoma cell line U-937. *Leukemia Research* **10**, 1301–1305.

Collins, S.J., Gallo, R.C. & Gallagher, R.E. (1977). Continuous growth and differentiation of human myeloid leukaemic cells in suspension culture. *Nature (London)* **270**, 347–349.

Collins, S.J., Ruscetti, F.W., Gallagher, R.E. & Gallo, R.C. (1978). Terminal differentiation of human promyelocytic leukemia cells induced by dimethyl-sulfoxide and other polar compounds. *Proceedings of the National Academy of Sciences USA* **75**, 2458–2462.

Cross, M. & Dexter, T.M. (1991). Growth factors in development, transformation, and tumorigenesis. *Cell* **64**, 271–280.

Danhauser-Riedl, S., Drozd, A., Bruntsch, U., Sinderman, H., Rastetter, J. & Berdel, W.E. (1990a). Phase I study of weekly oral Miltefosine (hexadecylphosphocholine) in patients with advanced malignant diseases. *Onkologie* **13**, 56.

Danhauser-Riedl, S., Himmelmann, A., Steinhauser, G., Busch, R., Vogler, W.R.,

Rastetter, J. & Berdel, W.E. (1990b). Cytotoxic effects of hexadecylphosphocholine in neoplastic cell lines including drug-resistant sublines *in vitro*. *Journal of Lipid Mediators* **2**, 271–280.

Daniel, L.W. (1990). Protein kinase C inhibition by alkyl-linked lipids. In Kabara, J.J. (ed.) *The Pharmacological Effects of Lipids* Vol. III, pp. 90–96. The American Oil Chemists Society, Illinois.

Daniel, L.W., Etkin, L.A., Morrison, B.T., Parker, J., Morris-Natschke, S., Surles, J.R. & Piantadosi, C. (1987). Ether lipids inhibit the effects of phorbol diester tumor promoters. *Lipids* **22**, 851–855.

Daniel, L.W., Small, G.W. & Strum, J.C. (1990). Characterization of cells sensitive and resistant to ET-18-OCH$_3$. *Proceedings of the American Association for Cancer Research* **31**, 412.

Daniel, L.W., Waite, M. & Wykle, R.L. (1986). A novel mechanism of diglyceride formation. *Journal of Biological Chemistry* **261**, 9128–9132.

Degos, L. (1990a). Differentiating agents in the treatment of leukemia. *Leukemia Research* **14**, 717–719.

Degos, L. (1990b). Differentiating agents in the treatment of leukemia and myelodysplastic syndromes. *Leukemia Research* **14**, 731–733.

Diomede, L., Bizzi, A., Magistrelli, A., Modest, E.J., Salmona, M. & Noseda, A. (1990). Role of cell cholesterol in modulating antineoplastic ether lipid uptake, membrane effects and cytotoxicity. *International Journal of Cancer* **46**, 341–346.

Eibl, H. (1984). Phospholipids as functional constituents of biomembranes. *Angewandte Chemie* **23**, 257–328.

Eibl, H., Unger, C., Fleer, E.A.M., Kim, D.J., Berger, M.R. & Nagel, G.A. (1986). Hexadecyl phosphocholine, a new antineoplastic agent: cytotoxic properties in leukemic cells. *Journal of Cancer Research and Clinical Oncology* **111**, 24.

Engebraaten, O., Bjerkvig, R. & Berens, M.E. (1991). Effect of alkyl-lysophospholipid on glioblastoma cell invasion into fetal rat brain tissue *in vitro*. *Cancer Research* **51**, 1713–1719.

Exton, J.H. (1990). Signaling through phosphatidylcholine breakdown. *Journal of Biological Chemistry* **265**, 1–4.

Friedberg, S.J., Smajdek, J. & Anderson, K. (1986). Surface membrane O-alkyl lipid concentration and metastasizing behavior in transplantable rat mammary carcinomas. *Cancer Research* **46**, 845–849.

Fromm, M., Berdel, W.E., Schick, H.D., Fink, U., Pahlke, W., Bicker, U., Reichert, A. & Rastetter, J. (1987). Antineoplastic activity of the thioether lysophospholipid derivative BM 41.440 *in vitro*. *Lipids* **22**, 916–918.

Fujiwara, K., Modest, E.J., Welander, C.E. & Wallen, C.A. (1989). Cytotoxic interactions of heat and an ether lipid analogue in human ovarian carcinoma cells. *Cancer Research* **49**, 6285–6289.

Gerard, C., McPhail, L.C., Marfat, A., Stimler-Gerard, N.P., Bass, D.A. & McCall, C.E. (1986). Role of protein kinases in stimulation of human polymorphonuclear leukocyte oxidative metabolism by various agonists: differential effects of a novel protein kinase inhibitor. *Journal of Clinical Investigation* **77**, 61–65.

Ghosh, S. & Baltimore, D. (1990). Activation *in vitro* of NF-κB by phosphorylation of its inhibitor IκB. *Nature* **344**, 678–682.

Glasser, L., Somberg, L.B. & Vogler, W.R. (1984). Purging murine leukemic marrow with alkyl-lysophospholipids. *Blood* **64**, 1288–1291.

Griffin, G.E., Leung, K., Folks, T.M., Kunkel, S. & Nabel, G.J. (1989). Activation of HIV gene expression during monocyte differentiation by induction of NF-κB. *Nature* **339**, 70–73.

Grunicke, H., Hofmann, J., Oberhuber, H., Uberall, F., Zaknun, J., Voegeli, R. &

Hilgard, P. (1990). Hexadecylphosphocholine inhibits protein kinase C and depresses the inositol phosphate response in NIH 3T3 fibroblasts. *Journal of Cancer Research and Clinical Oncology* **116**, 889.

Guivisdalsky, P.N., Bittman, R., Smith, Z., Blank, M.L., Snyder, F., Howard, S. & Salari, H. (1990). Synthesis and antineoplastic properties of ether-linked thioglycolipids. *Journal of Medicinal Chemistry* **33**, 2614–2621.

Hajra, A.K. (1970). Acyl dihydroxyacetone phosphate: precursor of alkyl ethers. *Biochemical and Biophysical Research Communication* **39**, 1037–1044.

Hanahan, D.J. (1986). Platelet activating factor: a biologically active phosphoglyceride. *Annual Review of Biochemistry* **55**, 483–509.

Hannun, Y.A., Loomis, C.R., Merrill, A.H. Jr & Bell, R.M. (1986). Sphingosine inhibition of protein kinase C activity and of phorbol dibutyrate binding *in vitro* and in human platelets. *Journal of Biological Chemistry* **261**, 12604–12609.

Heldin, C.H., Betsholtz, C., Claesson-Welch, L. & Westermark, B. (1987). Subversion of growth regulatory pathways in malignant transformation. *Biochimica et Biophysica Acta* **907**, 219–244.

Helfman, D.M., Barnes, K.C., Kinkade, J.M. Jr, Vogler, W.R., Shoji, M. & Kuo, J.F. (1983). Phospholipid-sensitive Ca^{2+}-dependent protein phosphorylation system in various types of leukemic cells from human patients and in human leukemic cell lines HL60 and K562, and its inhibition by alkyl-lysophospholipid. *Cancer Research* **43**, 2955–2961.

Herrmann, D.B.J. (1985). Changes in cellular lipid synthesis of normal and neoplastic cells during cytolysis induced by alkyl lysophospholipid analogues. *Journal of the National Cancer Institute* **75**, 423–430.

Herrmann, D.B.J. & Neumann, H.A. (1986) Cytotoxic ether phospholipids. *Journal of Biological Chemistry* **261**, 7742–7747.

Herrmann, D.B.J. & Neumann, H.A. (1987). Cytotoxic activity of the thioether phospholipid analogue BM 41.440 in primary human tumor cultures. *Lipids* **22**, 955–957.

Herrmann, D.B.J., Neumann, H.A., Berdel, W.E., Heim, M.E., Fromm, M., Boerner, D. & Bicker, U. (1987). Phase I trial of the thioether phospholipid analogue BM 41.440 in cancer patients. *Lipids* **22**, 962–966.

Herrmann, D.B.J., Neumann, H.A., Heim, M.E., Berdel, W.E., Fromm, M., Andreesen, R., Queiber, W., Doerner, D., Sterz, R., Besenfelder, E. & Bicker, U. (1989). Short- and long-term tolerability study of the thioether phospholipid derivative Ilmofosine in cancer patients. *Contributions to Oncology: New Drugs in Oncology* **37**, 236–247.

Hilgard, P., Eibl, H. & Unger, C. (1990a). Serum concentrations of hexadecyl-phosphocholine (He-PC) in the rat. *Proceedings of the American Association for Cancer Research* **31**, 413.

Hilgard, P., Stekar, J., Sindermann, H., Peukert, M. & Unger, C. (1990b). Antineoplastic activity of alkylphosphocholines *in vivo*. *Journal of Cancer Research and Clinical Oncology* **116**, 889.

Himmelmann, A.W., Danhauser-Riedl, S., Steinhauser, G., Busch, R., Modest, E.J., Noseda, A., Rastetter, J., Vogler, W.R. & Berdel, W.E. (1990). Cross-resistance pattern of cell lines selected for resistance towards different cytotoxic drugs to membrane-toxic phospholipids *in vitro*. *Cancer Chemotherapy and Pharmacology* **26**, 437–443.

Hoffman, D.R., Hajdu, J. & Snyder F. (1984a). Cytotoxicity of platelet activating factor and related alkyl-phospholipid analogs in human leukemia cells, polymorphonuclear neutrophils, and skin fibroblasts. *Blood* **63**, 545–552.

Hoffman, D.R., Hoffman, L.H. & Snyder, F. (1986). Cytotoxicity and metabolism of alkyl phospholipid analogues in neoplastic cells. *Cancer Research* **46**, 5803–5809.

Hoffman, D.R., Stanley, J.D., Berchtold, R. & Snyder, F. (1984b). Cytotoxicity of ether-linked phytanyl phospholipid analogs and related derivatives in human HL-60 leukemia cells and polymorphonuclear neutrophils. *Research Communications in Chemical Pathology and Pharmacology* **44**, 293–306.

Hofmann, J., Doppler, W., Jakob, A., Maly, K., Posch, L., Uberall, F. & Grunicke, H. (1988). Enhancement of the antiproliferative effect of *cis*-diamminedichloroplatinum (II) and nitrogen mustard by inhibitors of protein kinase C. *International Journal of Cancer* **42**, 382–388.

Hofmann, J., Uberall, F., Posch, L., Maly, K., Herrmann, D.B.J. & Grunicke, H. (1989) Synergistic enhancement of the antiproliferative activity of *cis*-diamminedichloroplatinum (II) by the ether lipid analogue BM41440, an inhibitor of protein kinase C. *Lipids* **24**, 312–317.

Hong, C.I., An, S.H., Buchheit, D.J., Nechaev, A., Kirisits, A.J., West, C.R. & Berdel, W.E. (1986). Nucleoside conjugates. 7. Synthesis and antitumor activity of 1-β-D-arabinofuranosylcytosine conjugates of ether lipids. *Journal of Medicinal Chemistry* **29**, 2038–2044.

Honma, Y., Kasukabe, T., Hozumi, M., Tsushima, S. & Nomura, H. (1981). Induction of differentiation of cultured human and mouse myeloid leukemia cells by alkyl-lyso-phospholipids. *Cancer Research* **41**, 3211–3216.

Honma, Y., Kasukabe, T., Okabe-Kado, J., Hozumi, M., Tsushima, S. & Nomura, H. (1983a). Antileukemic effect of alkyl phospholipids. I. Inhibition of proliferation and induction of differentiation of cultured myeloid leukemia cells by alkyl ethyleneglyco-phospholipids. *Cancer Chemotherapy and Pharmacology* **11**, 73–76.

Honma, Y., Kasukabe, T., Okabe-Kado, J., Hozumi, M., Tsushima, S. & Nomura, H. (1983b). Prolongation of survival times of leukemic mice by alkyl ethylene-glyco-phospholipids. *Cancer Chemotherapy and Pharmacology* **11**, 77–79.

Houlihan, W.J., Lee, M.L., Munder, P.G., Nemecek, G.M., Handley, D.A., Winslow, C.M., Happy, J. & Jaeggi, C. (1987). Antitumor activity of SRI 62-834, a cyclic ether analog of ET-18-OCH₃. *Lipids* **22**, 884–890.

Huang, M., Ye, Y., Chen, S., Chai, J., Lu, J., Zhao, L., Gu, L. & Wang, Z. (1988). Use of all-*trans* retinoic acid in the treatment of acute promyelocytic leukemia. *Blood* **72**, 567–572.

Huang, M., Ye, Y., Chen, S., Chai, J., Lu, J., Zhao, L., Gu, L. & Wang, Z. (1989). Use of all-*trans* retinoic acid in the treatment of acute promyelocytic leukemia. *Hematologic und Bluttransfusion* **32**, 88–96.

Huang, M., Ye, Y., Chen, S., Zhao, J., Gu, L., Cai, J., Zhao, L., Xie, J., Shen, Z. & Wang, Z (1987). All-*trans* retinoic acid with or without low dose cytosine arabinoside in acute promyelocytic leukemia. *Chinese Medical Journal* **100**(12), 949–953.

Hunter, T. (1987). A thousand and one protein kinases. *Cell* **50**, 823–829.

Hunter, T. (1991). Cooperation between oncogenes. *Cell* **64**, 249–270.

Ishaq, K.S., Capobianco, M., Piantadosi, C., Noseda, A., Daniel, L.W. & Modest, E.J. (1989). Synthesis and biological evaluation of ether-linked derivatives of phosphatidylinositol. *Pharmaceutical Research* **6**, 216–224.

Kára, J., Borovicka, M., Liebl, V., Smolíková & Ubik, K. (1986). A novel nontoxic alkyl-phospholipid with selective antitumor activity, plasmanyl-(*N*-acyl)-ethanolamine (PNAE), isolated from degenerating chick embryonal tissues and from an anticancer biopreparation cACPL. *Neoplasma* **33**, 187–205.

Katoh, N., Wise, B.C., Wrenn, R.W. & Kuo, J.F. (1981a). Inhibition by adriamycin of calmodulin-sensitive and phospholipid-sensitive calcium-dependent phosphorylation of endogenous proteins from heart. *Biochemical Journal* **198**, 199–205.

Katoh, N., Wrenn, R.W., Wise, B.C., Shoji, M. & Kuo, J.F. (1981b). Substrate proteins for calmodulin-sensitive and phospholipid-sensitive calcium-dependent protein kinase in heart, and inhibition of their phosphorylation by palmitoylcarnitine. *Proceedings of the National Academy of Sciences USA* **78**, 4813–4817.

Kim, M.Y., Linardic, C., Obeid, L. & Hannun, Y. (1991). Identification of sphingomyelin turnover as an effector mechanism for the action of tumor necrosis factor α and γ-interferon. *Journal of Biological Chemistry* **266**, 484–489.

Kiss, Z., Deli, E. & Kuo, J.F. (1988). Temporal changes in intracellular distribution of protein kinase C during differentiation of humas leukemia HL60 cells induced by phorbol ester. *FEBS Letters* **231**, 41–46.

Kiss, Z., Deli, E., Vogler, W.R. & Kuo, J.F. (1987). Antileukemic agent alkyl-lysophospholipid regulates phosphorylation of distinct proteins in HL-60 and K562 cells and differentiation of HL-60 cells promoted by phorbol ester. *Biochemical and Biophysical Research Communications* **142**, 661–666.

Koeffler, H.P. (1983). Induction of differentiation of human acute myelogenous leukemia cells: therapeutic implications. *Blood* **62**, 709–721.

Kolesnick, R.N. (1987). Thyrotropin-releasing hormones and phorbol esters induce phosphatidylcholine synthesis in GH_3 pituitary cells. Evidence for stimulation via protein kinase C. *Journal of Biological Chemistry* **262**, 14525–14530.

Kötting, J., Unger, C. & Eibl, H. (1987). Substrate specificity of *O*-alkyl-glycerol monooxygenase. *Lipids* **22**, 831–835.

Kucera, L.S., Iyer, N., Leake, E., Raben, A., Modest, E.J., Daniel, L.W. & Piantadosi, C. (1990). Novel membrane-interactive ether lipid analogs that inhibit infectious HIV-1 production and induce defective virus formation. *AIDS Research and Human Retroviruses* **6**, 491–501.

Kudo, I., Nojima, S., Chang, H.W., Yanoshita, R., Hayashi, H., Kondo, E., Nomura, H. & Inoue, K. (1987). Antitumor activity of synthetic alkyl-phospholipids with or without paf activity. *Lipids* **22**, 862–867.

Kuo, J.F., Shoji, M., Girard, P.R., Mazzei G.J., Turner, R.S. & Su, H.-D. (1986). Phospholipid/calcium-dependent protein kinase (protein kinase C) system: a major site of bioregulation. *Advances in Enzyme Regulation* **25**, 387–400.

Kuo, J.F., Zheng, B., Shoij, M., Vogler, W.R. & Eibl, H. (1990). Inhibition of protein kinase C, Na, K-ATPase and HL-60 cell differentiation by alkyl-phosphocholine and alkylammonium bromide derivatives. *Journal of Cancer Research and Clinical Oncology* **116**, 889.

Langdon, S.P. & Hickman, J.A. (1987). Correlation between the molecular weight and potency of polar compounds which induce the differentiation of HL-60 human promyelocytic leukemia cells. *Cancer Research* **47**, 140–144.

Larrick, J.W. & Wright, S.C. (1990). Cytotoxic mechanism of tumor necrosis factor-α. *FASEB Journal* **4**, 3215–3223.

Leder, G.H., Fiebig, H.H., Wallbrecher, E., Winterhalter, B.R. & Lohr, G.W. (1987). *In vitro* and *in vivo* cytotoxicity of alkyl lysophospholipid ET-18-OCH_3 and thioether lipid BM 41.440. *Lipids* **22**, 958–961.

Lee, T.-C., Blank, M.L., Fitzgerald, V. & Snyder, F. (1981). Substrate specificity in the biocleavage of the *O*-alkyl bond: 1-alkyl-2-acetyl-*sn*-glycero-3-phosphocholine (a hypotensive and platelet-activating lipid) and its metabolites. *Archives of Biochemistry and Biophysics* **208**, 353–357.

Lewin, B. (1991). Oncogenic conversion by regulatory changes in transcription factors. *Cell* **64**, 303–312.

Macara, I.G. (1989). Oncogenes and cellular signal transduction. *Physiological Reviews* **69**, 797–820.

Malewicz, B. & Baumann, W.J. (1988). The cytoxicity and antiproliferative effects of lysophosphatidylcholine and alkyl lysophospholipids are modulated by cholesterol. *Journal of the American Oil Chemists Society* **65**, 532.

Marasco, C.J., Piantadosi, C., Meyer, K.L., Morris-Natschke, S., Ishaq, K.S., Small, G.W. & Daniel, L.W. (1990). Synthesis and biological activity of novel quaternary ammonium derivatives of alkylglycerols as potent inhibitors of protein kinase C. *Journal of Medicinal Chemistry* **33**, 985–992.

Marx, M.H., Piantadosi, C., Noseda, A., Daniel, L.W. & Modest, E.J. (1988). Synthesis and evaluation of neoplastic cell growth inhibition of 1-*N*-alkyl-amide analogues of glycero-3-phosphocholine. *Journal of Medicinal Chemistry* **31**, 858–863.

Mikhaevich, I.S., Gerasimova, G.K. & Kára, J. (1991). Inhibition of protein kinase C by semisynthetic phospholipid plasmanyl-(*N*-acyl)-ethanolamine, a nontoxic antitumor preparation. *Biochemistry International* **23**, 215–220.

Morin, M.J., Kreutter, D., Rasmussen, H. & Sartorelli, A.C. (1987). Disparate effects of activators of protein kinase C on HL-60 promyelocytic leukemia cell differentiation. *Journal of Biological Chemistry* **262**, 11758–11763.

Morris-Natschke, S., Surles, J.R., Daniel, L.W., Berens, M.E., Modest, E.J. & Piantadosi, C. (1986). Synthesis of sulfur analogues of alky lyso-phospholipid and neoplastic cell growth inhibitory properties. *Journal of Medicinal Chemistry* **29**, 2114–2117.

Mueller, H.W., O'Flaherty, J.T. & Wykle, R.L. (1982). Ether lipid content and fatty acid distribution in rabbit polymorphonuclear neutrophil phospholipids. *Lipids* **17**, 72–77.

Munder, P.G., Weltzien, H.U. & Modolell, M. (1977). Lysolecithin and the action of complement. *Immunology* **7**, 411–424.

Muschiol, C., Berger, M.R., Schuler, B., Scherf, H.R., Garzon, F.T., Zeller, W.J., Unger, C., Eibl, H.J. & Schmahl, D. (1987). Alkyl phosphocholines: toxicity and anticancer properties. *Lipids* **22**, 930–934.

Nabel, G. & Baltimore, D. (1987). An inducible transcription factor activates expression of human immunodeficiency virus in T cells. *Nature (London)* **326**, 711–713.

Nakaki, T., Mita, S., Yamamoto, S., Nakadate, T. & Kato, R. (1984). Inhibition by palmitoylcarnitine of adhesion and morphological changes in HL-60 cells induced by 12-*O*-tetradecanoylphorbol-13-acetate. *Cancer Research* **44**, 1908–1912.

Nishikawa, M., Komada, F., Uemura, Y., Hidaka, H. & Shirakawa, S. (1990). Decreased expression of type II protein kinase C in HL-60 variant cells resistant to induction of cell differentiation by phorbol diester. *Cancer Research* **50**, 621–626.

Nishizuka, Y. (1988). The molecular heterogeneity of protein kinase C and its implications for cellular regulation. *Nature* **334**, 661–665.

Noseda, A., Berens, M.E., Piantadosi, C. & Modest, E.J. (1987). Neoplastic cell inhibition with new ether lipid analogs. *Lipids* **22**, 878–883.

Noseda, A., White, J.G., Godwin, P.L., Jerome, W.G. & Modest, E.J. (1989). Membrane damage in leukemic cells induced by ether and ester lipids: an electron microscopic study. *Experimental and Molecular Pathology* **50**, 69–83.

Obeid, L.M., Okazaki, T., Karolak, L.A. & Hannun Y.A. (1990). Transcriptional regulation of protein kinase C by 1,25-dihydroxyvitamin D_3 in HL-60 cells. *Journal of Biological Chemistry* **265**, 2370–2374.

O'Flaherty, J.T., Chabot, M.C., Redman, J. Jr, Jacobson, D. & Wykle, R.L. (1989). Receptor-independent metabolism of platelet-activating factor by myelogenous cells. *FEBS Letters* **250**, 341–344.

O'Flaherty, J.T. & Wykle, R.L. (1989). Platelet activating factor and human disease. In Barnes, P.J., Henson, P.M. & Page, C.P. (eds.) *Frontiers in Pharmacology and Therapeutics*, pp. 117–137, Blackwell Scientific Publications, Oxford.

Okamoto, S., Olson, A.C. & Vogler, W.R. (1987). Elimination of leukemic cells by the combined use of ether lipids *in vitro*. *Cancer Research* **47**, 2599–2603.

Osborn, L., Kunkel, S. & Nabel, G.J. (1989). Tumor necrosis factor and interleukin 1

stimulate the human immunodeficiency virus enhancer elements and regulate interleukin 2 receptor alpha-chain gene expression in primary human T lymphocytes.
Proceedings of the National Academy of Sciences USA **86**, 2336–2341.

Paddon, H.B. & Vance, D.E. (1980). Tetradecanoyl-phorbol acetate stimulates phosphatidylcholine biosynthesis in HeLa cells by an increase in the rate of the reaction
catalyzed by CTP:phosphocholine cytidylyltransferase. *Biochimica et Biophysica
Acta* **620**, 636–640.

Parker, J., Daniel, L.W. & Waite, M. (1987). Evidence of protein kinase C involvement
in phorbol diester-stimulated arachidonic acid release and prostaglandin synthesis.
Journal of Biological Chemistry **262**, 5385–5393.

Pelech, S.L. & Vance, D.E. (1989). Signal transduction via phosphatidylcholine cycles.
Trends in Biochemical Sciences **14**, 28–30.

Pelech, S.L., Sanghera, J.S. & Daya-Makin, M. (1990). Protein kinase cascades in
meiotic and mitotic cell cycle control. *Biochemistry and Cell Biology* **68**, 1297–1330.

Perrella, F.W., Piantadosi, C., Marasco, C.J. & Modest, E.J. (1990). Inhibition of
phospholipase C and cell growth by ether lipid analogues of phosphatidylinositol.
Proceedings of the American Association for Cancer Research **31**, 409.

Powis, G., Hickman, J., Workman, P., Tritton, T.R., Abita, J.P., Berdel, W.E.,
Gescher, A., Moses, H.L. & Nicolson, G.L. (1990). The cell membrane and cell
signals as targets in cancer chemotherapy. *Cancer Research* **50**, 2203–2211.

Powis, G., Seewald, M.J., Aksoy, I., Riebow, J. & Melder, D. (1991). Inhibition of
phosphatidylinositol specific phospholipase C (PIPLC) by ether lipid analogues.
Proceedings of the American Association for Cancer Research **32**, 399.

Prescott, S.M., Zimmerman, G.A. & McIntyre, T.M. (1990). Platelet-activating factor.
Journal of Biological Chemistry **265**, 17381–17384.

Rogers, M.A., Samples, L., Chabot, M.C., Marasco, C.J., Piantadosi, C. & Daniel,
L.W. (1990). Leukemic cell differentiation by ether-linked lipids: studies on quater-
nary ammonium alkylglycerols. *Proceedings of the American Association for Cancer
Research* **31**, 410.

Rogers, M.A., Small, G.W., Samples, L. & Daniel, L.W. (1991). Phorbol diester
stimulated HL-60 cell differentiation is associated with the activation of specific
DNA binding proteins. *Proceedings of the American Association for Cancer Research*
32, 295.

Rovera, A., Santoli, D. & Damsky, C. (1979). Human promyelocytic leukemia cells in
culture differentiate into macrophage-like cells when treated with a phorbol diester.
Proceedings of the National Academy of Sciences USA **76**, 2779–2783.

Runge, M.H., Andreesen, R., Pfleiderer, A. & Munder, P.G. (1980). Destruction of
human solid tumors by alkyl lysophospholipids. *Journal of the National Cancer
Institute* **64**, 1301–1306.

Scherf, H.R., Schuler, B., Berger, M.R. & Schmahl, D. (1987). Therapeutic activity of
ET-18-OCH$_3$ and hexadecylphosphocholine against mammary tumors in BD-VI
rats. *Lipids* **22**, 927–929.

Seewald, M.J., Olsen, R.A., Sehgal, I., Melder, D.C., Modest, E.J. & Powis, G. (1990).
Inhibition of growth factor-dependent inositol phosphate Ca^{2+} signaling by antitumor ether lipid analogues. *Cancer Research* **50**, 4458–4463.

Sherman, M.L., Stone, R.M., Datta, R., Bernstein, S.H. & Kufe, D.W. (1990). Transcriptional and post-transcriptional regulation of c-*jun* expression during monocytic
differentiation of human myeloid leukemic cells. *Journal of Biological Chemistry* **265**,
3320–3323.

Shoji, M., Raynor, R.L., Berdel, W.E., Vogler, W.R. & Kuo, J.F. (1988). Effects of
thioether phospholipid BM 41.440 on protein kinase C and phorbol ester-induced

differentiation of human leukemia HL60 and KG-1 cells. *Cancer Research* **48**, 6669–6673.

Shoji, M., Raynor, R.L., Fleer, E.A.M., Eibl, H., Vogler, W.R. & Kuo, J.F. (1991) Effects of hexadecylphosphocholine on protein kinase C and TPA-induced differentiation of HL60 cells. *Lipids* **26**, 145–149.

Snyder, F. & Wood, R. (1968). The occurrence and metabolism of alkyl and alk-1-enyl ethers of glycerol in transplantable rat and mouse tumors. *Cancer Research* **28**, 972–978.

Snyder, F. & Wood, R. (1969). Alkyl and alk-1-enyl ethers of glycerol in lipids from normal and neoplastic human tissues. *Cancer Research* **29**, 251–257.

Snyder, F., Malone, B. & Piantadosi, C. (1973). Tetrahydropterdine-dependent cleavage enzyme for *O*-alkyl lipids: substrate specificity. *Biochimica et Biophysica Acta* **316**, 259–265.

Soodsma, J.F., Piantadosi, C. & Snyder, F. (1970). The biocleavage of alkyl glyceryl ethers in Morris hepatomas and other transplantable neoplasms. *Cancer Research* **30**, 309–311.

Soodsma, J.F., Piantadosi, C. & Snyder, F. (1972). Partial characterization of the alkylglycerol cleavage enzyme system of rat liver. *Journal of Biological Chemistry* **247**, 3923–3929.

Squinto, S.P., Doucet, J.P., Block, A.L., Morrow, S.L. & Davenport, W.D. Jr (1989). Induction of macrophage-like differentiation of HL-60 leukemia cells by tumor necrosis factor-α: potential role of *fos* expression. *Molecular Endocrinology* **3**, 409–419.

Storme, G.A., Berdel, W.E., van Blitterswijk, W.J., Bruyneel, E.A., De Bruyne, G.K. & Mareel, M.M. (1985). Antiinvasive effect of racemic 1-*O*-octadecyl-2-*O*-methylglycero-3-phosphocholine on MO₄ mouse fibrosarcoma cells *in vitro*. *Cancer Research* **45**, 351–357.

Storme, G.A., Bruyneel, E.A., Schallier, D.C., Bolscher, J.G., Berdel, W.E. & Mareel, M.M. (1987). Effect of lipid derivatives on invasion *in vitro* and on surface glycoproteins of three rodent cell types. *Lipids* **22**, 847–850.

Sugiura, T. & Waku, K. (1987). Ether lipids in mammalian tissues. In Snyder, F. (ed.) *Platelet Activating Factor and Related Lipid Mediators*, p. 55. Plenum Press, New York.

Tamaoki, T., Nomoto, H., Takahashi, I., Kato, Y., Morimoto, M. & Tomita, F. (1986). Staurosporine, a potent inhibitor of phospholipid/Ca^{2+} dependent protein kinase. *Biochemical and Biophysical Research Communications* **135**, 397–402.

Tidwell, T., Guzman, G. & Vogler, W.R. (1981). The effects of alkyl-lysophospholipids on leukemic cell lines, HL60 and K562. *Blood* **57**, 794–797.

Tritton, T.R. & Hickman, J.A. (1990). How to kill cancer cells: membranes and cell signaling as targets in cancer chemotherapy. *Cancer Cells* **2**, 95–105.

Unger, C., Damenz, W., Fleer, E.A.M., Kimm, D.J., Breiser, A., Hilgard, P., Engel, J., Nagel, G. & Eibl, H. (1989). Hexadecylphosphocholine, a new ether lipid analogue: studies on the antineoplastic activity *in vitro* and *in vivo*. *Acta Oncologica* **28**, 213–217.

Unger, C., Eibl, H., Breiser, A., von Heyden, H.W., Engel, J., Hilgard, P., Peukent, M. & Nagel, G.A. (1988). Hexadecylphosphocholine (D 18506) in the topical treatment of skin metastases: a phase I trial. *Onkologie* **11**, 295–296.

Vallari, D.S., Austinhirst, R. & Snyder, F. (1990). Development of specific functionally active receptors for platelet-activating factor in HL-60 cells following granulocytic differentiation. *Journal of Biological Chemistry* **265**, 4261–4265.

Vallari, D.S., Smith, Z.L. & Snyder, F. (1988). HL-60 cells become resistant towards antitumor ether-linked phospholipids following differentiation into a granulocytic form. *Biochemical and Biophysical Research Communications* **156**, 1–8.

van Blitterswijk, W.J., Hilkmann, H. & Storme, G.A. (1987a). Accumulation of an alkyl lysophospholipid in tumor cell membranes affects membrane fluidity and tumor cell invasion. *Lipids* **22**, 820–823.

van Blitterswijk, W.J., van der Bend, R.L., Kramer, I.J.M., Verhoeven, A.J., Hilkmann, H. & de Widt, J. (1987b). A metabolite of an antineoplastic ether phospholipid may inhibit transmembrane signalling via protein kinase C. *Lipids* **22**, 842–846.

Vance, D.E. (1989). Regulatory and functional aspects of phosphatidylcholine metabolism. In D.E. Vance (ed.) *Phosphatidylcholine Metabolism*, pp. 225–239. CRC Press, Florida.

Verdonck, L.F., Witteveen, E.O., van Heugten, H.G., Rozemuller, E. & Rijksen, G. (1990). Selective killing of malignant cells from leukemic patients by alkyl-lysophospholipid. *Cancer Research* **50**, 4020–4025.

Verma, I.M., Mitchell, R.L., Kruijer, W., Van Beveren, C., Zokas, L., Hunter, T. & Cooper, J.A. (1991). Proto-oncogene *fos*: induction and regulation during growth and differentiation. *Cancer Cells* **3**, 275–287.

Vogler, W.R., Berdel, W.E. & Olson, A.C. (1990a). Ether lipids as purging agents for autologous bone marrow transplantation. *Cancer Research and Clinical Oncology* **116**, 994.

Vogler, W.R., Olson, A.C., Berdel, W.E., Okamoto, S. & Glasser, L. (1990b). Purging leukemia remission marrows with alkyl-lysophospholipids, preclinical and clinical results. In Gross, S., Gee, A.P. & Worthington-White, D. (eds.) *Progress in Clinical and Biological Research* Vol. 333, *Bone Marrow Purging and Processing*, pp. 1–20. Wiley-Liss, New York.

Vogler, W.R., Olson, A.C., Okamoto, S., Somberg, L.B. & Glasser, L. (1987). Experimental studies on the role of alkyl lysophospholipids in autologous bone marrow transplantation. *Lipids* **22**, 919–924.

Vogt, P.K. & Bos, T.J. (1989). The oncogene *jun* and nuclear signalling. *Trends in Biochemical Science* **14**, 172–175.

Warren, B.S., Kamano, Y., Pettit, G.R. & Blumberg, P.M. (1988). Mimicry of bryostatin 1 induced phosphorylation patterns in HL-60 cells by high phorbol ester concentrations. *Cancer Research* **48**, 5984–5988.

Westphal, O. (1987). Ether lipids in oncology-welcoming address. *Lipids* **22**, 787–788.

Wilcox, R.W., Wykle, R.L., Schmitt, J.D. & Daniel, L.W. (1987). The degradation of platelet activating factor and related lipids: susceptibility to phospholipases C and D. *Lipids* **22**, 800–807.

Wykle, R.L., Blank, M.L., Malone, B. & Snyder, F. (1972a). Evidence for a mixed function oxidase in the biosynthesis of ethanolamine plasmalogens from 1-alkyl-2-acyl-*sn*-glycero-3-phosphorylethanolamine. *Journal of Biological Chemistry* **247**, 5442–5447.

Wykle, R.L., Kraemer, W.F. & Schremmer, J.M. (1977). Studies of lysophospholipase D rat liver and other tissues. *Archives of Biochemistry and Biophysics* **184**, 149–155.

Wykle, R.L., Kraemer, W.F. & Schremmer, J.M. (1980). Specificity of lysophospholipase D. *Biochimica et Biophysica Acta* **619**, 58–67.

Wykle, R.L., Piantadosi, C. & Snyder, F. (1972b). The role of acyldihydroxy-acetone phosphate, NADH, and NADPH in biosynthesis of *O*-alkyl glycerolipids by microsomal enzymes of Ehrlich ascites tumor. *Journal of Biological Chemistry* **247**, 2944–2948.

Chapter 7
The role of protein kinase C and protein phosphorylation in multidrug resistance

Robert I. Glazer, Gang Yu, Flavia Borellini and
Shakeel Ahmad

Introduction

Since the discovery of Ca^{2+} - and phospholipid-dependent protein kinase or protein kinase C (PKC) almost a decade ago by Nishizuka *et al.* (Kikkawa *et al.*, 1982), and its identification as a major receptor for phorbol esters (Ashendel *et al.*, 1983; Kikkawa *et al.*, 1983), numerous studies have ascribed a multitude of signal transduction mechanisms to PKC that involve a variety of physiological and pharmacological agonists. The intense interest in PKC stems from its unique ability to be activated by diacylglycerol (and its phorbol ester mimetics), an effector whose formation is coupled to phospholipid turnover by the action of growth and differentiation factors. PKC is comprised of eight isoforms termed α, β_1, β_2, γ, δ, ε, ζ and η (Fig. 7.1), and thus, many of its functions are likely to be both isoform- and tissue-specific (Kikkawa *et al.*, 1989; Parker *et al.*, 1989). Because of these features, PKC undoubtedly occupies a central role in carrying out highly specialized signal transduction functions in response to physiological stimuli (Nishizuka, 1989). From a pharmacological standpoint, PKC has served as a focal point for the design of drugs with possible therapeutic efficacy in the treatment of cancer (Gescher & Dale, 1989), although at the present time, it is not clear whether PKC has a positive or negative proliferative effect in malignant cells (Choi *et al.*, 1990).

This chapter will describe some of the newer developments in cancer biology and pharmacology that are associated with PKC, particularly in the field of resistance to anticancer drugs. Evidence will be presented that directly implicates PKC as a modulator of multidrug resistance through a complex pattern of regulation that involves not only the drug efflux pump,

179

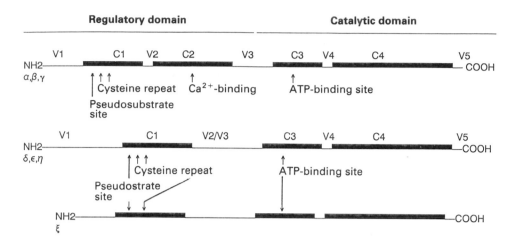

Fig. 7.1. Structural organization of the genes encoding the isoforms of protein kinase C (PKC). The gene of PKC is divided into a regulatory and a catalytic domain encompassing five variable (V1–V5) and four constant (C1–C4) regions. The Ca^{2+}- and phospholipid-dependent isoforms (α, β_1, β_2 and γ) differ from the Ca^{2+}-independent and phospholipid-dependent forms (δ, ε, ξ and η) by the presence of a Ca^{2+}-binding (C2) domain.

P-glycoprotein as a target substrate, but also proteins intimately involved with the transcriptional process such as topoisomerases and *trans*-activators of promoter elements. The regulation of these phosphoproteins by PKC may provide both short- and long-term regulation of drug resistance through transcriptional and post-translational mechanisms that may be associated with the acquisition and maintenance of the multidrug resistant (MDR) phenotype.

MDR and P-glycoprotein

MDR is associated with the elevated expression of the plasma membrane protein, P-glycoprotein, the product of the *mdr*1 gene (Beck, 1987; Croop *et al.*, 1988; Moscow & Cowan, 1988; Dickson & Gottesman, 1990). There is considerable genetic evidence in a wide variety of animal and human MDR cell lines that the *mdr*1 gene is amplified or overexpressed (Fojo *et al.*, 1985; Riordan *et al.*, 1985; Roninson *et al.*, 1986; Scotto *et al.*, 1986; Fairchild *et al.*, 1987). Transfection studies with both genomic and cDNA copies of the *mdr* gene have shown that it confers the MDR phenotype to the recipient cells (Debenham *et al.*, 1982; Gros *et al.*, 1986b; Shen *et al.*, 1986; Croop *et al.*, 1987; Sugimoto & Tsuruo, 1987; Ueda *et al.*, 1987b), although the degree of resistance is less than in drug-selected resistant cells. The expression of drug resistance through P-glycoprotein is believed to reside in its ability to function as an adenosine triphosphate (ATP)-dependent drug efflux pump. This conclusion is based on its protein sequence homology to a bacterial active transport protein (Chen *et al.*, 1986; Gerlach *et al.*, 1986; Gros *et al.*, 1986a), as well as by the ability of a monoclonal antibody to P-glycoprotein (MRK16) to partially restore drug sensitivity through enhancement of net drug uptake (Hamada & Tsuruo, 1986). Studies demonstrating that P-glycoprotein possesses adenosine triphosphatase (ATPase) activity (Hamada & Tsuruo, 1988), unidirectional drug transport (Kamimoto *et al.*, 1989) and ATP-dependent drug binding (Naito *et al.*, 1988) all provide evidence that this protein is an energy-dependent drug efflux pump. Although P-glycoprotein appears to be a major factor in MDR, there are relatively few studies addressing its regulation by post-translational modification.

PKC and MDR

The precise relationship of PKC activity to the MDR phenotype may be related to differences in the expression (activity and isoform) and regulation (intracellular distribution and activation) of PKC in various MDR cell lines. Cells selected for MDR contain increased levels of PKC (Palayoor *et al.*, 1987; Aquino *et al.*, 1988, 1990a; Fine *et al.*, 1988; Melloni *et al.*, 1989; O'Brian *et al.*, 1989; Posada *et al.*, 1989a,b), and in several instances, the elevated expression of PKC has been attributed to a specific isoform such as PKCα (Posada *et al.*, 1989a; O'Brian *et al.*, 1991) and PKCβ (Melloni *et al.*, 1989). Indeed, the appearance of PKCγ in Adriamycin (ADR)-resistant HL-60 cells, an isoform that is normally absent in wild-type cells (Aquino *et al.*, 1990b), suggests that it has a specific function in MDR (Fig. 7.2). The elevation of PKC activity appears to be a component of the MDR phenotype that is normally associated with differentiated cells. Friend erythroleukaemia cells displaying a low level of resistance to vincristine did not contain P-glycoprotein but did exhibit elevated PKCβ activity and reduced drug accumulation that was ameliorated by verapamil (Richon *et al.*, 1991). The elevation in PKCβ activity in the latter vincristine-resistant cell line correlated with their enhanced responsiveness to the differentiating agent, hexamethylene bisacetamide (Michaeli *et al.*, 1990). PKC activity is elevated in HL-60 cells undergoing differentiation in response to retinoic acid, dimethylsulphoxide or 1,25-dihydroxyvitamin D_3 (Zylber-Katz & Glazer, 1985), and these changes involve increases in the levels of PKCα and PKCβ, as well as the induction of PKCγ (Makowske *et al.*, 1988), a property also associated with ADR-resistant HL-60 cells (Aquino *et al.*, 1990b).

PKC inhibitors and activators

The majority of studies analysing the role of PKC in MDR cell lines have utilized pharmacological reagents which are known *in vitro* to either

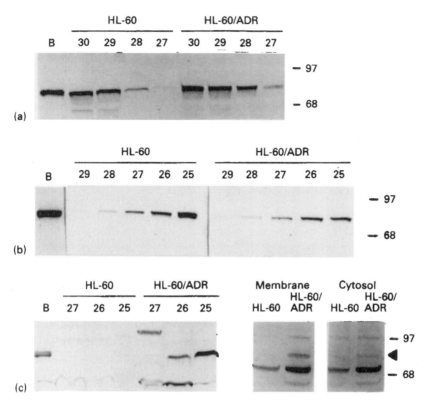

Fig. 7.2. Protein kinase C (PKC) isoforms in sensitive and Adriamycin-resistant HL-60 cells. Fractions from hydroxyapatite chromatography were immunoblotted with isoform-specific antibodies to PKC: (a) monoclonal antibody to PKCα; (b) monoclonal antibody to PKCβ; (c) polyclonal antibody to PKCγ. B, rat brain PKC (Aquino *et al.*, 1990b). Also shown is an immunoblot of membrane and cytosol extracts from HL-60 and HL-60/ADR cells using a polyclonal antibody to PKCγ. The arrowhead denotes the PKCγ holoenzyme.

stimulate or inhibit PKC. The protein kinase inhibitors, staurosporine and H-7 decreased resistance to ADR in S180 cells (Posada *et al.*, 1989a) and fibrosarcoma cells (O'Brian *et al.*, 1989) respectively. However, another study reported that staurosporine had no effect on ADR toxicity in wild type or MCF-7/ADR cells (Schwartz *et al.*, 1991). It is possible that the lack of sensitivity of some MDR cell lines to PKC inhibitors may reflect a high rate of proteolysis of PKC to its catalytic fragment, M-kinase, since the latter enzyme is insensitive to staurosporine and other inhibitors of PKC (Sauvage *et al.*, 1991). Nevertheless, the major obstacle to the use of PKC inhibitors is that they lack specificity for PKC (Meyer *et al.*, 1989) and produce cytotoxicity that may be unrelated to inhibition of protein kinase activity (Smith *et al.*, 1988). The effect of staurosporine is further complicated to its ability to complete for drug binding-sites on P-glyco-protein *in vitro* (Sato *et al.*, 1990).

Other studies have utilized phorbol esters as activators of PKC (Castagna *et al.*, 1982) to elucidate the role of this enzyme in resistance. Exposure of wild type or MDR B-cell leukaemia cell line MOLT-3 for 90 min to TPA increased membrane-associated PKC activity and increased trimetrexate (a lipophilic antifolate) resistance (Schwartz *et al.*, 1991). TPA mediated a rapid increase in resistance to colchicine in human B-cell leukaemia cells (O'Connor, 1985), and similar results were obtained after treating wild-type and ADR-resistant MCF-7 cells for 2 h with phorbol dibutyrate (Fine *et al.*, 1988). However, in one instance, treatment of wild-type S180 cells for 30 min with TPA resulted in reduced resistance to ADR coincident with enhanced PKC activity.

Long-term exposure to phorbol esters has also been used to modulate MDR through depletion or 'down-regulation' of PKC activity. Long-term exposure to TPA increased ADR resistance in wild-type and ADR-resistant S180 cells (Posada *et al.*, 1989b) and increased etoposide resistance in KB cells (Ferguson & Cheng, 1987); however, a similar regimen of TPA sensitized HeLa and A253 carcinoma cells to cisplatin (Basu *et al.*, 1990). Therefore, the majority of these studies implicate the involvement of PKC as a positive regulator of MDR. However, it is paradoxical that 'down-regulation' of PKC by prolonged exposure to phorbol esters produces the same effect as short-term exposure, and suggests that more than one mechanism is involved in the enhancement of resistance by these agents.

Proteolytic activation of PKC

The increase in resistance in MDR cells by exposure to phorbol esters may not only involve direct activation of PKC, but in specific instances may entail the activation of PKC by proteolysis to a Ca^{2+}- and phospholipid-independent form termed M-kinase (Inoue *et al.*, 1977; Takai *et al.*, 1977; Kishimoto *et al.*, 1983). In some cell lines, there is some evidence that the actual effector of phorbol ester action may be M-kinase *per se* (Melloni *et al.*, 1986; Murray *et al.*, 1987). HL-60/ADR cells contain high constitutive levels of M-kinase (Aquino *et al.*, 1988), as well as Ca^{2+}-dependent protease activity (Aquino *et al.*, 1990a). Vincristine-resistant Friend erythroleukaemia cells contain high levels of PKCβ compared to parental cells and exhibit higher and more sustained levels of M-kinase than wild-type cells after short-term exposure to TPA (Melloni *et al.*, 1989).

The differential sensitivity of various isoforms of PKC to Ca^{2+}-dependent neutral protease (calpain) also suggest that regulation of PKC via proteolysis may be physiologically relevant (Huang *et al.*, 1989; Kishimoto *et al.*, 1989). The phorbol ester-responsiveness of sensitive and resistant cells may be a function of the predominant isoform of PKC that is expressed in the cell and its sensitivity to proteolysis. PKCβ and PKCγ were 50- and 6-fold more sensitive, respectively, than PKCα to proteolysis by calpain I *in vitro* (Kishimoto *et al.*, 1989). Other studies have found that calpain produced similar rates of proteolysis of PKCα and -β to a catalytically stable form of M-kinase, whereas neutral serine protease destroyed PKC activity without generating M-kinase (Pontremoli *et al.*, 1990a). Treatment of human neutrophils with TPA or chemotactic peptide maximally generated M-kinase within 10 min (Pontremoli *et al.*, 1990b), a process that was abolished by the calpain inhibitor, leupeptin (Melloni *et al.*, 1986). In several cell lines treated with phorbol esters, PKCα was less susceptible to degradation than PKCβ (Ase *et al.*, 1988; Huang *et al.*, 1989; Pontremoli *et al.*, 1990b). Positive effectors of PKC activity such as diacylglycerol and phospholipid increased proteolysis of PKC by trypsin (Huang *et al.*, 1989; Newton & Koshland, 1989) and calpain (Imajoh *et al.*, 1986); Kishimoto *et al.*, 1989) and increased the susceptibility of PKCα to trypsin (Huang *et al.*, 1989). These results explain why membrane-associated PKCα is more sensitive to trypsin digestion than the soluble form of the enzyme (Newton & Koshland, 1989). Therefore, it is possible that the numerous effects attributed to phorbol esters may be mediated by the rapid proteolysis of PKC to M-kinase by calpain.

PKC and P-glycoprotein

Carlsen *et al.* (1977) was the first to note that P-glycoprotein existed as a phosphoprotein in colchicine-resistant but not in revertant cells. This finding has been corroborated in a variety of MDR cell lines (Center, 1983, 1985; Hamada *et al.*, 1987; Mellado & Horwitz, 1987; Myers *et al.*, 1989; Posada *et al.*, 1989a; Schurr *et al.*, 1989). A clue as to the origin of the protein kinase(s) responsible for this effect was provided by studies showing that phorbol ester activators of PKC could stimulate the phosphorylation of P-glycoprotein *in vivo* (Hamada *et al.*, 1987; Chambers *et al.*, 1990a). The involvement of PKC in this process was further supported by studies demonstrating that P-glycoprotein is a substrate for PKC *in vitro* (Chambers *et al.*, 1990b) and that stimulation of P-glycoprotein phosphorylation by phorbol esters *in vivo* leads to reduced drug accumulation in vincristine-resistant KB cells (Chambers *et al.*, 1990a).

Since many of the aforementioned studies strongly suggested a direct involvement of PKC in the MDR phenotype, our laboratory decided to directly address this question. MCF-7 cells were transfected with the human *mdr*-1 cDNA to produce a clonal cell line (BC-19 cells) that contained a level of P-glycoprotein as high as that present in the 200-fold ADR-resistant MDR cell line MCF-7/ADR (Fairchild *et al.*, 1990); however BC-19 cells were only 1/30 as sensitive to ADR as MCF-7/ADR (Fig. 7.3). When BC-19 cells were transfected with the cDNA encoding rabbit brain PKCα (Ohno *et al.*, 1987) two stable drug resistant isolates were obtained that were an order of magnitude more resistant than BC-19

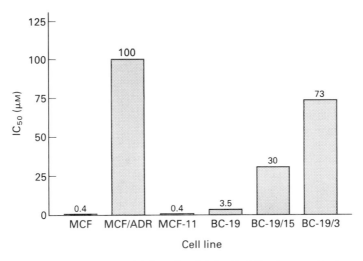

Fig. 7.3. Adriamycin sensitivity of MCF-7 cells following transfection with the *mdr* 1 and protein kinase Cα (PKCα) genes. Cells were exposed for 2 h to Adriamycin, washed and refed with drug-free medium. Cell number was determined after 4 days by staining with Gentian violet and measuring the absorbance in a microplate reader. The IC$_{50}$ was determined from semilogarithmic plots. MCF, wild type MCF-7 cells; MCF/ADR, Adriamycin-selected MCF-7 cells; MCF-11, a clone of MCF-7 cells transfected with PKCα; BC-19, MCF-7 cells transfected with *mdr* 1; BC-19/15 and BC-19/3, two clones of BC-19 cells transfected with PKCα.

cells (Fig. 7.3). The resistant clones contained 20–30-fold greater PKC activity than wild-type MCF-7 or BC-19 cells (Fig. 7.4). Endogenous phosphorylation of P-glycoprotein in the *mdr* 1/PKC-transfected cells was several-fold greater than in BC-19 cells and was stimulated further by phorbol dibutyrate (results not shown). Thus, overexpression of PKCα produced a positive regulatory effect on resistance characterized by increased phorbol ester-dependent resistance, increased P-glycoprotein phosphorylation and reduced drug accumulation (Fig. 7.5). Based on the phosphorylation consensus sequence for PKC, there are several potential phosphorylation sites in the intervening region between the two ATP binding-sites in the P-glycoprotein (Fig. 7.6). Therefore, it can be envisioned that phosphorylation can lead to conformational changes in the cytoplasmic domain of P-glycoprotein with accompanying changes in ATP and drug binding.

Other protein kinases and MDR

Still unanswered is the role of other protein kinases in the resistant phenotype. Center *et al.* (Staats *et al.*, 1990) have presented evidence that P-glycoprotein is phosphorylated *in vitro* by a Mn^{2+}- and phospholipid-dependent protein kinase associated with the plasma membrane of vincris-

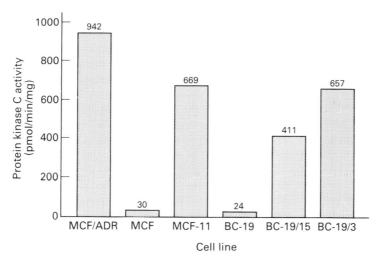

Fig. 7.4. Protein kinase C activity in *mdr*1- and PKCα-transfected cells. See Fig. 7.3 for a description of the cell lines.

tine-resistant HL-60 cells. It is unclear whether this enzyme is related to a Ca^{2+}-independent isoform of PKC (Fig. 7.1). On the other hand, some protein kinases may exert a negative regulatory effect on drug resistance. We recently observed that the cyclic adenosine monophosphate (cAMP) analogue, 8-Cl-cAMP, *sensitizes* two MDR HL-60 cell lines to ADR (Fig. 7.7). Although the mechanism for the effect of 8-chloro-cAMP is unknown, recent data suggest that this analogue specifically induces type II cAMP-dependent protein kinase (PKA) in MDR cells (unpublished results). Since P-glycoprotein is a substrate for PKA (Mellado & Horwitz, 1987), it is possible that PKA competes with PKC for similar phosphorylation domains in P-glycoprotein.

PKC and atypical drug resistance

Some forms of MDR are unrelated to expression of P-glycoprotein and have been termed atypical MDR (Beck, 1987). This type of resistance is believed to result from alterations in the activity or structure of topoisomerases (Beck, 1987, 1989). These nuclear enzymes are required for breaking and rejoining single (topoisomerase I) or double-stranded (topoisomerase II) DNA to facilitate such processes as transcription and DNA replication. Topoisomerase I is a specific target for the anticancer drug camptothecin (see Chapter 9), while topoisomerase II is believed to be a major target for ADR and etoposide (Ross, 1986). In camptothecin-resistant tumour cells, the level as well as the sensitivity of topoisomerase I to camptothecin is reduced (Andoh *et al.*, 1987; Sugimoto *et al.*, 1990). While the mechanism for this effect is unknown, two studies have suggested that this enzyme is regulated through phosphorylations. Durban *et al.* (1983)

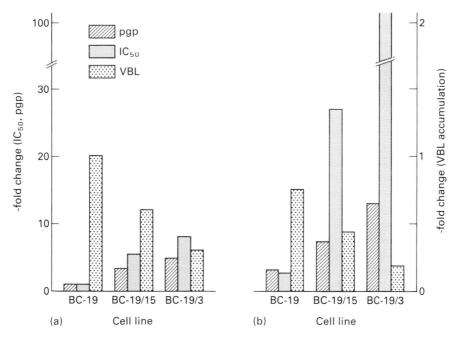

Fig. 7.5. Changes in [^{32}P]P-glycoprotein (pgp), Adriamycin cytotoxicity and vinblastine accumulation in the absence (a) and presence (b) of PDBU. The -fold changes in BC-19/15 and BC-19/3 cells in the absence or presence of PDBu are relative to untreated BC-19 cells = 1. pgp represents the radioactivity in two phorbol ester-sensitive tryptic phosphopeptides of P-glycoprotein. Adriamycin toxicity is based on its IC$_{50}$, and vinblastine (VBL) accumulation reflects drug retention over a 2 h period.

was the first to demonstrate that topoisomerase I is activated by phosphorylation *in vitro*. A recent study by Pommier *et al.* (1990) has shown that both the 100 kDa and 68 kDa forms of topoisomerase I from 9-hydroxyellipticine-resistant Chinese hamster cells are totally inactivated upon dephosphorylation but are fully reactivated by PKC. The reactivated forms of topoisomerase I behaved like the native enzyme with respect to the processivity of DNA relaxation and sequence selectivity of DNA cleavage in the presence of its specific inhibitor, camptothecin. That PKC may indeed be a regulator of topoisomerase I activity was also suggested by the stimulation of its activity in the HL-60 cells treated with TPA (Gorsky *et al.*, 1989). It remains to be determined whether reduced phosphorylation by PKC or 'down-regulation' of PKC is responsible for the decreased activity of topoisomerase I in camptothecin-resistant cells.

Topoisomerase II is also a substrate for PKC *in vitro* (Sayhoun *et al.*, 1986) and is phosphorylated *in vivo* (Heck *et al.*, 1989). However, treatment of HL-60 cells with TPA rapidly inhibits rather than stimulates etoposide-mediated DNA cleavage (Zwelling *et al.*, 1990). Etoposide resis-

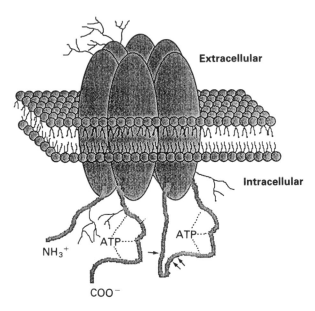

Fig. 7.6. Putative phosphorylation sites for protein kinase C (PKC) in P-glycoprotein. Arrows indicate phosphorylation consensus sequences for PKC in the intervening region between the two ATP-binding domains.

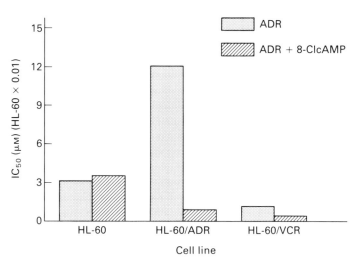

Fig. 7.7. Reversal of Adriamycin toxicity by 8-chloro-cyclic AMP in Adriamycin- and vincristine-resistant HL-60 cells. Cells were treated simultaneously with the IC_{10} for 8-chloro-cyclic AMP and varying concentrations of Adriamycin. After 48 h, cell viability was determined by trypan blue exclusion and cell number, and the IC_{50} for Adriamycin was determined from semilogarithmic plots. The IC_{50} value for HL-60 cells should be multiplied by 0.01.

tance is also associated with reduced PKC activity in P388 cells (Ido *et al.*, 1987). These data seem to suggest that 'down-regulation' of PKC may be associated with reduced topoisomerase II activity, but it is still premature to conclude that topoisomerase II is regulated directly by PKC (see Chapter 8).

PKC, *trans*-activation and MDR

A major characteristic of the MDR phenotype is the transcriptional activation of the *mdr*1 gene in cells selected for MDR (Fojo *et al.*, 1985; Riordan *et al.*, 1985; Roninson *et al.*, 1986; Scotto *et al.*, 1986; Fairchild *et al.*, 1987) and its decreased expression in revertant cell lines (Sugimoto *et al.*, 1987). The drug-dependent expression of the *mdr*1 gene (Kohno *et al.*, 1989; Chin *et al.*, 1990) may involve changes in the activity of DNA-binding proteins to their cognate regulatory elements within the promoter region of the *mdr*1 or other genes. The regulation of eukaryotic transcription occurs through specific *cis*-acting regulatory elements termed promoters or enhancers, which are composed of distinctive DNA sequence motifs (Johnson & McKnight, 1989; Mitchell & Tjian, 1989). Regulatory proteins interact with these elements in a highly specific and sometimes, cooperative manner, and determine which genes will be transcriptionally active. Many of the regulatory proteins are inducible factors (Maniatis *et al.*, 1987) that respond to such diverse factors as heavy metal ions (Karin *et al.*, 1984; Searle *et al.*, 1985), heat shock (Pelham, 1982), glucocorticoids (Chandler *et al.*, 1983), phorbol esters (Angel *et al.*, 1987), and anticancer drugs (Kohno *et al.*, 1989; Chin *et al.*, 1990). Therefore, the control of positive or negative *cis*-acting regulatory elements may be a function of inducible *trans*-activators in response to a selective environmental pressure such as exposure to anticancer drugs.

Both the human and murine *mdr*1 gene contain a major downstream promoter region within 300 bp of the transcription start site (Ueda *et al.*, 1987b; Hsu *et al.*, 1990; Raymond & Gros, 1990). The promoter region in the human *mdr*1 sequence contains binding elements for transcription factors Sp1, NF1/CTF and AP-1 (Fig. 7.8) while the mouse sequence contains additional binding sites for AP-2. The immediate promoter region in the 5′-untranslated region of the genomic PKCγ sequence also contains binding elements for transcription factors AP-1, AP-2 and Sp1 (Chen *et al.*, 1990) (Fig. 7.8). Of particular interest is the stimulation of AP-1 and AP-2 by phorbol esters and the stimulation of AP-2 by cAMP (Imagawa *et al.*, 1987). This suggests that the effects of these agents on resistance may involve a transcriptional as well as a post-translational component to their actions. Resistance to the protein kinase inhibitor, staurosporine, in yeast resulted in the elevation of an AP-1-like transcription factor that induced a 10-fold increase in protein kinase activity

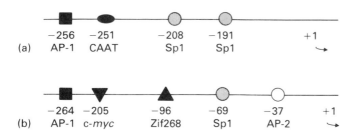

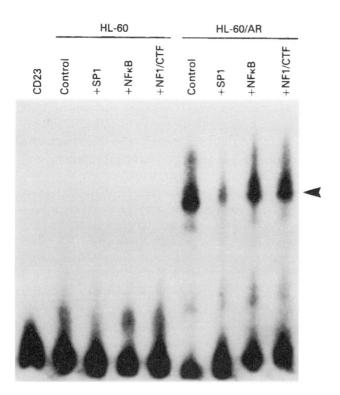

Fig. 7.8. Promoter elements in the 5′-untranslated region of (a) the MDR1 (human) and (b) protein kinase Cγ (rat liver) genes. The consensus binding sequences for transcription factors AP-1, c-myc, Zif268, Sp1, AP-2 and the CAAT-binding protein (NF1/CTF) are indicated. +1 indicates the transcription start site.

Fig. 7.9. Mobility shift assay of nuclear extracts from sensitive and Adriamycin-resistant HL-60 cells. Each lane represents 1.5 μg of protein in the absence (control) and presence of a 200-fold excess of competitor representing the binding consensus sequence for transcription factors Sp1, NFκB and NF1/CTF. The DNA probe (CD23) represents a 117 bp construct of the 5′-LTR of HIV-1 (Borellini *et al.*, 1990). CD23 represents the probe alone without nuclear extract. The arrowhead indicates the Sp1–DNA complex.

(Toda *et al.*, 1991). In HL-60/ADR cells (Bhalla *et al.*, 1985) that contain levels of PKCγ (Aquino *et al.*, 1990b), the level and DNA-binding activity of transcription factor Sp1 is greatly enhanced in comparison to sensitive cells (Fig. 7.9) (Borellini *et al.*, 1990). Recent studies have shown that M-kinase (Kishimoto *et al.*, 1983), but not the PKC holoenzyme, can activate TPA-responsive elements in the collagenase (Hata *et al.*, 1989) and c-*fos* (Muramatsu *et al.*, 1989) promoters. These data suggest that translocation of M-kinase to the nucleus in response to a metabolic stimulus may selectively activate *trans*-acting factors that differentially regulate transcription in MDR cells.

In a similar context, PKA may modulate the MDR phenotype through its catalytic subunit. Microinjection experiments have shown that AMP-responsive elements (CRE) in the c-*fos* promoter can be activated by the catalytic subunit of PKA but not by the cAMP-binding regulatory subunits, R_I and R_{II} (Riabowol *et al.*, 1988). This effect is presumably mediated by phosphorylation of the CRE-binding protein, CREB (Yamamoto *et al.*, 1988). The latter mechanism may explain the antagonistic effect of 8-chloro-cAMP on ADR toxicity in MDR HL-60 cells (Fig. 7.7). Type II PKA is induced by 8-chloro-cAMP (Cho-Chung, 1990) and its preferential induction in MDR cells could result in its translocation to the nucleus, where upon dissociation would phosphorylate and activate CREB. Activation of promoter elements containing a CRE could either induce the expression of genes that have a negative regulatory effect on MDR or activate a CRE that negatively regulates the expression of a gene that confers MDR.

Therefore, modulation of the MDR phenotype by PKC or PKA may be associated with the activity of *trans*-activators that exert a positive or negative regulatory effect on the transcription of P-glycoprotein and other genes, such as PKC and PKA, that may be necessary for its regulation (Fig. 7.10). It is conceivable that changes in the activity of *trans*-activators are responsible for the initiation of the resistant phenotype. A subpopulation of cells expressing higher *trans*-activator activity would have a selective advantage during induction of drug resistance. This could explain the heterogeneity in the expression of *mdr*1 or PKC among different MDR cell lines. Alternatively, enhanced expression of *trans*-activators may be a consequence of acquiring resistance and may represent a trait of the MDR phenotype. The identity of the target genes and promoter elements involved in MDR should give some insight into this hypothesis.

Conclusion

PKC appears to have a positive regulatory effect on MDR, and this effect may be operative at different levels. Drug resistance may be initiated via the activation by phosphorylation of *trans*-activators via PKC or M-

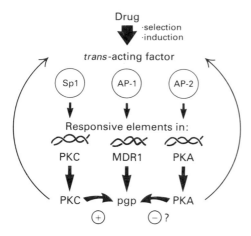

Fig. 7.10. Mechanisms by which *trans*-activators can affect drug resistance. The *trans*-activators are either induced directly by drug treatment (induction) or are constitutively abundant in a subpopulation that is resistant to drug treatment (selection). The *trans*-activators interact with their respective response elements synergistically to activate transcription of the protein kinase C (PKC), MDR1, protein kinase A (PKA) or other genes associated with resistance. A secondary level of regulation is the modulation of P-glycoprotein (pgp) and *trans*-activator activity by phosphorylation.

kinase to induce the transcription of MDR-specific genes such as *mdr* 1. PKC may also have a direct stimulatory effect on the activity of the *mdr* 1 gene product, P-glycoprotein, while PKA may produce an antagonistic effect. Understanding the role that phosphorylation plays in MDR at both the transcriptional and post-translational levels should help define the aetiology as well as the regulation of drug resistance in normal and malignant cells.

Acknowledgement

The work described emanating from this laboratory was supported, in part, by a grant from the Bristol-Myers Co.

References

Andoh, T., Ishii, K., Suzuki, Y., Okegami, Y., Kusunoki, Y., Takemoto, Y. & Okada, Y. (1987). Characterization of a mammalian mutant with a camptothecin-resistant DNA topoisomerase I. *Proceedings of the National Academy of Sciences USA* **84**, 5565–5569.

Angel, P., Imagawa, M., Chiu, R., Stein, B., Imbra, R.J., Rahmsdorf, H.J., Jonat, C., Herrlich, P. & Karin, M. (1987). Phorbol ester-inducible genes contain a common *cis*-element recognized by a TPA-modulated *trans*-acting factor. *Cell* **49**, 729–739.

Aquino, A., Hartman, K.D., Knode, M.C., Huang, K.-P., Niu, C.-H. & Glazer, R.I. (1988). Role of protein kinase C in phosphorylation of vinculin in Adriamycin-resistant HL-60 leukemia cells. *Cancer Research* **48**, 3324–3329.

Aquino, A., Johnson-Thompson, M. & Glazer, R.I. (1990a). Enhanced Ca^{2+}-dependent proteolysis associated with Adriamycin-resistant HL-60 cells. *Cancer Communications* **2**, 243–247.

Aquino, A., Warren, B., Omichinski, J., Hartman, K.D. & Glazer, R.I. (1990b). Protein kinase C-γ is present in Adriamycin-resistant HL-60 leukemia cells. *Biochemical and Biophysical Research Communications* **166**, 723–728.

Ase, K., Berry, N., Kikkawa, U., Kishimoto, A. & Nishizuka, Y. (1988). Differential down-regulation of protein kinase C subspecies in KM3 cells. *FEBS Letters* **236**, 396–400.

Ashendel, C.L., Staller, J.M. & Boutwell, R.K. (1983). Protein kinase activity associated with a phorbol ester receptor purified from mouse brain. *Cancer Research* **43**, 4333–4337.

Basu, A., Teicher, B.A. & Lazo, J.S. (1990). Involvement of protein kinase C in phorbol ester-induced sensitization of HeLa cells to *cis*-diamminechloroplatinum (II). *Journal of Biological Chemistry* **265**, 8451–8457.

Beck, W.T. (1987). The cell biology of multiple drug resistance. *Biochemical Pharmacology* **36**, 2879–2887.

Beck, W.T. (1989). Unknotting the complexities of multidrug resistance: the involvement of DNA topoisomerases in drug action and resistance. *Journal of the National Cancer Institute* **81**, 1683–1685.

Bhalla, K., Hindenburg, A., Traub, R.N. & Grant, S. (1985). Isolation and characterization of anthracycline-resistant human leukemic cell line. *Cancer Research* **45**, 3657–3662.

Borellini, F., Aquino, A., Josephs, S.F. & Glazer, R.I. (1990). Increased expression and DNA-binding activity of transcription factor Sp1 in Doxorubicin-resistant HL-60 leukemia cells. *Molecular and Cellular Biology* **10**, 5541–5547.

Carlsen, S.A., Till, J.E. & Ling, V. (1977). Modulation of drug permeability in Chinese hamster ovary cells. Possible role for phosphorylation of surface glycoproteins. *Biochimica et Biophysica Acta* **467**, 238–250.

Castagna, M., Takai, Y., Kaibuchi, K., Sano, K., Kikkawa, U. & Nishizuka, Y. (1982). Direct activation of calcium-activated, phospholipid-dependent protein kinase by tumour-promoting phorbol esters. *Journal of Biological Chemistry* **257**, 7847–7851.

Center, M.S. (1983). Evidence that Adriamycin resistance in Chinese hamster lung cells is regulated by phosphorylation of a plasma membrane glycoprotein. *Biochemical and Biophysical Research Communications* **115**, 159–166.

Center, M.S. (1985). Mechanisms regulating cell resistance to Adriamycin. Evidence that drug accumulation in resistant cells is modulated by phosphorylation of a plasma membrane glycoprotein. *Biochemical Pharmacology* **34**, 1471–1476.

Chambers, T.C., Chalikonda, I. & Eilon, G. (1990a). Correlation of protein kinase C translocation, P-glycoprotein phosphorylation and reduced drug accumulation in multidrug resistant human KB cells. *Biochemical and Biophysical Research Communications* **169**, 253–259.

Chambers, T.C., McAvoy, E.M., Jacobs, J.W. & Eilon, G. (1990b). Protein kinase C phosphorylates P-glycoprotein in multidrug resistant human KB carcinoma cells. *Journal of Biological Chemistry* **265**, 7679–7686.

Chandler, V.L., Maler, B.A. & Yamamoto, K.R. (1983). DNA sequences bound specifically by glucocorticoid receptor *in vitro* render a heterologous promoter responsive *in vivo*. *Cell* **33**, 489–499.

Chen, C.-J., Chin, J.E., Ueda, K., Clark, D.P., Pastan, I., Gottesman, M.M. & Roninson, I.B. (1986). Internal duplication and homology with bacterial transport proteins in the *mdr*1 (P-glycoprotein) gene from multidrug-resistant human cells. *Cell* **47**, 381–389.

Chen, K.-H., Widen, S.G., Wilson, S.H. & Huang, K.-P. (1990). Characterization of the 5′-flanking region of the rat protein kinase Cγ gene. *Journal of Biological Chemistry* **265**, 19961–19965.

Chin, K.-V., Chauhan, S.S., Pastan, I. & Gottesman, M.M. (1990). Regulation of *mdr* RNA levels in response to cytotoxic drugs in rodent cells. *Cell Growth and Differentiation* **1**, 361–365.

Cho-Chung, Y.S. (1990). Role of cyclic AMP receptor proteins in growth, differentiation, and suppression of malignancy: new approaches to therapy. *Cancer Research* **50**, 7093–7100.

Choi, P.M., Tchou-Wong, K.-M. & Weinstein, I.B. (1990). Overexpression of protein kinase C in HT29 colon cancer cells causes growth inhibition and tumor suppression. *Molecular and Cellular Biology* **10**, 4650–4657.

Croop, J.M., Gros, P. & Housman, D.E. (1988). Genetics of multidrug resistance. *Journal of Clinical Investigation* **81**, 1303–1309.

Croop, J.M., Guild, B.C., Gros, P. & Housman, D.E. (1987). Genetics of multidrug resistance: relationship of a cloned gene to the complete multidrug phenotype. *Cancer Research* **47**, 5982–5988.

Debenham, P.G., Kartner, N., Siminovitch, L., Riordan, J.R. & Ling, V. (1982). DNA-mediated transfer of multiple drug resistance and plasma membrane glycoprotein expression. *Molecular and Cellular Biology* **2**, 881–889.

Dickson, R.B. & Gottesman, M.M. (1990). Understanding of the molecular basis of drug resistance in cancer reveals new targets for chemotherapy. *Trends in Pharmacological Sciences* **11**, 305–307.

Durban, E., Mills, J.S., Roll, D. & Busch, H. (1983). Phosphorylation of purified Novikoff hepatoma topoisomerase I. *Biochemical and Biophysical Research Communications* **111**, 897–905.

Fairchild, C.R., Ivy, S.P., Kao-Shan, C.-S., Whang-Peng, J., Rosen, N., Israel, M.A., Melera, P.W., Cowan, K.H. & Goldsmith, M.E. (1987). Isolation of amplified and overexpressed DNA sequences from Adriamycin-resistant human breast cancer cell. *Cancer Research* **47**, 5141–5148.

Fairchild, C.R., Moscow, J.S., O'Brien, E.E. & Cowan, K.H. (1990). Multidrug resistance in cells transfected with human genes encoding a variant P-glycoprotein and glutathione-S-transferase-π. *Molecular Pharmacology* **37**, 801–809.

Ferguson, P.J. & Cheng, Y.-C. (1987). Transient protection of cultured human cells against antitumor agents by 12-O-tetradecanoylphorbol-13-acetate. *Cancer Research* **47**, 433–441.

Fine, R.L., Patel, J. & Chabner, B.A. (1988). Phorbol esters induce multidrug resistance in human breast cancer cells. *Proceedings of the National Academy of Sciences USA* **85**, 582–586.

Fojo, A.T., Whang-Peng, J., Gottesman, M.M. & Pastan, I. (1985). Amplification of DNA sequences in human multidrug-resistant KB carcinoma cells. *Proceedings of the National Academy of Sciences USA* **82**, 7661–7665.

Gerlach, J.H., Endicott, J.A., Juranka, P.F., Henderson, G., Sarangi, F., Deuchars, K.L. & Ling, V. (1986). Homology between P-glycoprotein and a bacterial haemolysin transport protein suggests a model for multidrug resistance. *Nature* **324**, 485–489.

Gescher, A. & Dale, I.L. (1989). Protein kinase C—a novel target for rational anticancer drug design? *Anticancer Drug Design* **4**, 93–105.

Gorsky, L.D., Cross, S.M. & Morin, M.J. (1989). Rapid increase in activity of DNA topoisomerase I, but not topoisomerase II, in HL-60 promyelocytic leukemia cells treated with a phorbol diester. *Cancer Communications* **1**, 83–92.

Gros, P., Croop, J. & Housman, D.E. (1986a). Mammalian multidrug resistance gene:

complete cDNA sequence indicates strong homology to bacterial transport proteins. *Cell* **47**, 371–380.

Gros, P., Neriah, Y.B., Croop, J.M. & Housman, D.E. (1986b). Isolation and expression of a complementary DNA that confers multidrug resistance. *Nature* **323**, 728–731.

Hamada, H. & Tsuruo, T. (1986). Functional role for the 170- to 180-kDa glycoprotein specific drug-resistant tumor cells as revealed by monoclonal antibodies. *Proceedings of the National Academy of Sciences USA* **83**, 7785–7789.

Hamada, H. & Tsuruo, T. (1988). Purification of the 170- to 180-kilodalton membrane glycoprotein associated with multidrug resistance. *Journal of Biological Chemistry* **263**, 1454–1458.

Hamada, H., Hagiwara, K-I., Nakajima, T. & Tsuruo, T. (1987). Phosphorylation of the M_r 170,000 to 180,000 glycoprotein specific to multidrug resistant cells: effects of verapamil, trifluoperazine, and phorbol esters. *Cancer Research* **47**, 2860–2865.

Hata, A., Akita, Y., Konno, Y., Suzuki, K. & Ohno, S. (1989). Direct evidence that the kinase activity of protein kinase C is involved in transcriptional activation through a TPA-responsive element. *FEBS Letters* **252**, 144–146.

Heck, M.M.S., Hittelman, W.N. & Earnshaw, W.C. (1989). *In vivo* phosphorylation of the 170-kDa form of eukaryotic DNA topoisomerase II. *Journal of Biological Chemistry* **264**, 15161–15164.

Hsu, S.I.-H, Cohen, D., Kirschner, L.S., Lothstein, I., Harstein, M. & Horwitz, S.B. (1990). Structural analysis of the mouse *mdr*1a (P-glycoprotein) promoter reveals the basis of differential transcript heterogeneity in multidrug-resistant J774.2 cells. *Molecular and Cellular Biology* **10**, 3596–3606.

Huang, F.L., Yoshida, Y., Cunha-Melo, J.R., Beaven, M.A. & Huang, K.-P. (1989). Differential down-regulation of protein kinase C isozymes. *Journal of Biological Chemistry* **264**, 4238–4243.

Ido, M., Sato, K., Sakurai, M., Inagaki, M., Saitoh, M., Watanabe, M. & Hidaka, H. (1987). Decreased phorbol ester receptor and protein kinase C in P388 murine leukemic cells resistant to etoposide. *Cancer Research* **47**, 3460–3463.

Imagawa, M., Chium R. & Karin, M. (1987). Transcription factor AP-2 mediates induction by two different signal-transduction pathways: protein kinase C and cAMP. *Cell* **51**, 251–260.

Imajoh, S., Kawasaki, H. & Suzuki, K. (1986). The amino-terminal hydrophobic region of the small subunit of calcium-activated neutral protease (CANP) is essential for its activation by phosphatidylinositol. *Journal of Biochemistry (Tokyo)* **99**, 1281–1284.

Inoue, M., Kishimoto, A., Takai, Y. & Nishizuka, Y. (1977). Studies on a cyclic nucleotide-independent protein kinase and its proenzyme in mammalian tissues II. Proenzyme and its activation by calcium-dependent protease from rat brain. *Journal of Biological Chemistry* **252**, 7610–7616.

Johnson, P.F. & McKnight, S.L. (1989). Eukaryotic transcriptional regulatory proteins. *Annual Review of Biochemistry* **58**, 799–839.

Kamimoto, Y., Gatmaitan, Z., Hsu, J. & Arias, I.M. (1989). The function of Gp170, the multidrug resistance gene product, in rat liver canalicular membrane vesicles. *Journal of Biological Chemistry* **264**, 11693–11698.

Karin, M., Haslinger, A., Holtgreve, H., Richards, R.I., Krauter, P., Westphal, H.M. & Beato, M. (1984). Characterization of DNA sequences through which cadmium and glucocorticoid hormones induce human metallothionein-II$_A$ gene. *Nature* **308**, 513–519.

Kikkawa, U., Kishimoto, A. & Nishizuka, Y. (1989). The protein kinase C family: heterogeneity and its implications. *Annual Review of Biochemistry* **58**, 31–44.

Kikkawa, U., Takai, Y., Minakuchi, R., Inohara, S. & Nishizuka, Y. (1982). Calcium-activated, phospholipid-dependent protein kinase from rat brain. Subcellular distribution, purification, and properties. *Journal of Biological Chemistry* **257**, 13341–13348.

Kikkawa, U., Takai, Y., Tanaka, Y., Miyake, R. & Nishizuka, Y. (1983). Protein kinase C as a possible receptor protein of tumor-promoting phorbol esters. *Journal of Biological Chemistry* **258**, 1142–1145.

Kishimoto, A., Kajikawa, N., Shiota, M. & Nishizuka, Y. (1983). Proteolytic activation of calcium-activated, phospholipid-dependent protein kinase by calcium-dependent neutral protease. *Journal of Biological Chemistry* **258**, 1156–1164.

Kishimoto, A., Mikawa, K., Hashimoto, K., Yasuda, I., Tanaka, S.-I., Tominaga, M., Kuroda, T. & Nishizuka, Y. (1989). Limited proteolysis of protein kinase C subspecies by calcium-dependent neutral protease (calpain). *Journal of Biological Chemistry* **264**, 4088–4092.

Kohno, K., Sato, S.-I., Takano, H., Matsuo, K.-I. & Kuwano, M. (1989). The direct activation of human multidrug resistance gene (MDR1) by anticancer agents. *Biochemical and Biophysical Research Communications* **165**, 1415–1421.

Makowske, M., Ballester, R., Cayre, Y. & Rosen, O.M. (1988). Immunochemical evidence that three protein kinase C isozymes increase in abundance during HL-60 differentiation induced by dimenthyl sulfoxide and retinoic acid. *Journal of Biological Chemistry* **263**, 3402–3410.

Maniatis, T., Goodbourn, S. & Fischer, J.A. (1987). Regulation of inducible and tisue-specific gene expression. *Science* **236**, 1237–1244.

Mellado, W. & Horwitz, S.B. (1987). Phosphorylation of the multidrug resistance associated glycoprotein. *Biochemistry* **26**, 6900–6904.

Melloni, E., Pontremoli, S., Michetti, M., Sacco, O., Sparatore, B. & Horecker, B.L. (1986). The involvement of calpain in the activation of protein kinase C in neutrophils stimulated by phorbol myristic acid. *Journal of Biological Chemistry* **261**, 4101–4105.

Melloni, E., Pontremoli, S., Viotti, P.L., Patrone, M., Marks, P.A. & Rifkind, R.A. (1989). Differential expression of protein kinase C isozymes and erythroleukemia cell differentiation. *Journal of Biological Chemistry* **264**, 18414–18418.

Meyer, T., Regenass, U., Fabbro, D., Alteri, E., Rosel, J., Muller, M., Caravatti, G. & Matter, A. (1989). A derivative of staurosporine (CGP 41 251) shows selectivity for protein kinase C inhibition and *in vivo* anti-tumour activity. *International Journal of Cancer* **43**, 851–856.

Michaeli, J., Lebedev, Y.B., Richon, V.M., Chen, Z.-X., Marks, P.A. & Rifkind, R.A. (1990). Conversion of differentiation inducer resistance to differentiation inducer sensitivity in erythroleukemia cells. *Molecular and Cellular Biology* **10**, 3535–3540.

Mitchell, P.J. & Tjian, R. (1989). Transcriptional regulation in mammalian cells by sequence-specific DNA binding proteins. *Science* **245**, 371–378.

Moscow, J.A. & Cowan, K.H. (1988). Multidrug resistance. *Journal of the National Cancer Institute* **80**, 14–20.

Muramatsu, M.-A., Kaibuchi, K. & Arai, K.-I. (1989). A protein kinase C cDNA without the regulatory domain is active after transfection *in vivo* in the absence of phorbol ester. *Molecular and Cellular Biology* **9**, 831–836.

Murray, A.W., Fournier, A. & Hardy, S.J. (1987). Proteolytic activation of protein kinase C: a physiological reaction? *Trends in Biological Sciences* **12**, 53–54.

Myers, M.B., Rittmann-Grauer, L., O'Brien, J.P. & Safa, A.R. (1989). Characterization of monoclonal antibodies recognizing a M_r 180,000 P-glycoprotein: differential expression of the M_r 180,000 and M_r 170,000 P-glycoproteins in multidrug-resistant human tumor cells. *Cancer Research* **49**, 3209–3214.

Naito, M., Hamada, H. & Tsuruo, T. (1988). ATP/Mg^{2+}-dependent binding of vincristine to the plasma membrane of multidrug-resistant K562 cells. *Journal of Biological Chemistry* **263**, 1187–11891.

Newton, A.C. & Koshland, D.E. Jr (1989). High cooperativity, specificity, and multiplicity in the protein kinase C-lipid interaction. *Journal of Biological Chemistry* **264**, 14909–14915.

Nishizuka, Y. (1989). Studies and prospectives of the protein kinase C family for cellular recognition. *Cancer* **10**, 1892–1903.

O'Brian, C.A., Fan, D., Ward, N.E., Dong, Z., Iwamoto, L., Gupta, K.P., Earnest, L.E. & Fidler, I.J. (1991). Transient enhancement of multidrug resistance by the bile acid deoxycholate in murine fibrosarcoma cells *in vitro*. *Biochemical Pharmacology* **41**, 797–806.

O'Brian, C.A., Fan, D., Ward, N.E., Seid, C. & Fidler, I.J. (1989). Level of protein kinase C activity correlates directly with resistance to Adriamycin in murine fibrosarcoma cells. *FEBS Letters* **246**, 78–82.

O'Connor, T.W.E. (1985). Phorbol ester-induced loss of colchicine ultrasensitivity in chronic lymphocytic leukaemia lymphocytes. *Leukemia Research* **9**, 885–895.

Ohno, S., Kawasaki, H., Imajoh, S. & Suzuki, K. (1987). Tissue-specific expression of three distinct types of rabbit protein kinase C. *Nature* **325**, 161–166.

Palayoor, S.T., Stein, J.M. & Hait, W.N. (1987). Inhibition of protein kinase C by antineoplastic agents: implications for drug resistance. *Biochemical and Biophysical Research Communications* **148**, 718–725.

Parker, P.J., Kour, G., Marais, R.M., Mitchell, F., Pears, C., Schaap, D., Stabel, S. & Webster, C. (1989). Protein kinase C—a family affair. *Molecular Cellular Endocrinology* **65**, 1–11.

Pelham, H.R.B. (1982). Regulatory upstream promoter element in the *Drosophila* Hsp70 heat shock gene. *Cell* **30**, 517–528.

Pommier, Y., Kerrigan, D., Hartman, K.D. & Glazer, R.I. (1990). Phosphorylation of mammalian DNA topoisomerase I and activation by protein kinase C. *Journal of Biological Chemistry* **265**, 9418–9422.

Pontremoli, S., Melloni, E., Sparatore, B., Michetti, M., Salamino, F. & Horecker, B.L. (1990a) Isozymes of protein kinase C in human neutrophils and their modification by two endogenous proteinases. *Journal of Biological Chemistry* **265**, 706–712.

Pontremoli, S., Michetti, M., Melloni, E., Sparatore, B., Salamino, F. & Horecker, B.L. (1990b). Identification of the proteolytically activated form of protein kinase C in stimulated human neutrophils. *Proceedings of the National Academy of Sciences USA* **87**, 3705–3707.

Posada, J.A., McKeegan, E.M., Worthington, K.F., Morin, M.J., Jaken, S. & Tritton, T.R. (1989a). Human multidrug resistant KB cells overexpress protein kinase C: involvement in drug resistance. *Cancer Communications* **1**, 285–292.

Posada, J.A., Vichi, P. & Tritton, T.R. (1989b). Protein kinse C in Adriamycin action and resistance in mouse sarcoma 180 cells. *Cancer Research* **49**, 6634–6639.

Raymond, M. & Gros, P. (1990). Cell-specific activity of *cis*-acting regulatory elements in the promoter of the mouse multidrug resistance gene *mdr*1. *Molecular and Cellular Biology* **10**, 6036–6040.

Riabowol, K.T., Fink, J.S., Gilman, M.Z., Walsh, D.A., Goodman, R.H. & Feramisco, J.R. (1988). The catalytic subunit of cAMP-dependent protein kinase induces expression of genes containing cAMP-responsive enhancer elements. *Nature* **336**, 83–86.

Richon, V.M., Weich, N., Leng, Kiyokawa, H., Ngo, L., Rifkind, R.A. & Marks, P.A. (1991). Characteristics of erythroleukemia cells selected for vincristine resistance that have accelerated inducer-mediated differentiation. *Proceedings of the National Academy of Sciences USA* **88**, 1666–1670.

Riordan, J.R., Duechars, K., Kartner, N., Alan, N., Trent, J. & Ling, V. (1985).

Amplification of P-glycoprotein genes in multidrug-resistant mammalian cell lines. *Nature* **316**, 817–819.

Roninson, I.B., Chin, J.E., Choi, K., Gros, P., Housman, D.E., Fojo, A., Shen, D.-W., Gottesman, M.M. & Pastan, I. (1986). Isolation of human *mdr* DNA sequences amplified in multidrug-resistant KB carcinoma cells. *Proceedings of the National Academy of Sciences USA* **83**, 4538–4542.

Ross, W.E. (1986). DNA topoisomerases as targets for cancer therapy. *Biochemical Pharmacology* **34**, 4191–4195.

Sayhoun, N., Wolf, M., Besterman, J., Hsieh, T.-S., Sander, M., LeVine, H. III, Chang, K.-J. & Cuatrecasas, P. (1986). Protein kinase C phosphorylates topoisomerase II: topoisomerase activation and its possible role in phorbol ester-induced differentiation of HL-60 cells. *Proceedings of the National Academy of Sciences USA* **83**, 1603–1607.

Sato, W., Yusa, K., Naito, M. & Tsuruo, T. (1990). Staurosporine, a potent inhibitor of C-kinase, enhances drug accumulation in multidrug-resistant cells. *Biochemical and Biophysical Research Communications* **173**, 1252–1257.

Sauvage, C., Cash, C.B. & Maitre, M. (1991). Isolation of human brain protein kinase C: evidence for kinase C catalytic fragment modulates G protein-GTPase activity. *Biochemical and Biophysical Research Communications* **174**, 593–599.

Schurr, E., Raymond, M., Bell, J.C. & Gros, P. (1989). Characterization of the multidrug resistance protein expressed in cell clones stably transfected with the mouse *mdr*1 cDNA. *Cancer Research* **49**, 2729–2734.

Schwartz, G.K., Arkin, H., Holland, J.F. & Ohnuma, T. (1991). Protein kinase C activity and multidrug resistance in MOLT-3 human lymphoblastic leukemia cells resistant to trimetrexate. *Cancer Research* **51**, 55–61.

Scotto, K.W., Biedler, J.L. & Melera, P.W. (1986). Amplification and expression of genes associated with multidrug resistance in mammalian cells. *Science* **232**, 751–755.

Searle, P.F., Stuart, G.W. & Palmiter, R.D. (1985). Building a metal-responsive promoter with synthetic regulatory elements. *Molecular and Cellular Biology* **5**, 1480–1489.

Shen, D.-W., Fojo, A., Roninson, I.B., Chin, J.E., Soffir, R., Pastan, I. & Gottesman, M.M. (1986). Multidrug resistance of DNA-mediated transformants is linked to transfer of the human *mdr*1 gene. *Molecular and Cellular Biology* **6**, 4039–4045.

Smith, C.D., Glickman, J.F. & Chang, K.-J. (1988). The antiproliferative effects of staurosporine are not exclusively mediated by inhibition of protein kinase C. *Biochemical and Biophysical Research Communications* **156**, 1250–1256.

Staats, J., Marquardt, D. & Center, M. (1990). Characterization of a member-associated protein kinase of multidrug-resistant HL60 cells which phosphorylates P-glycoprotein. *Journal of Biological Chemistry* **265**, 4084–4090.

Sugimoto, Y. & Tsuruo, T. (1987). DNA-mediated transfer and cloning of a human multidrug-resistant gene of Adriamycin-resistant myelogenous leukemia K562. *Cancer Research* **47**, 2620–2625.

Sugimoto, Y., Roninson, I.B. & Tsuruo, T. (1987). Decreased expression of the amplified *mdr*1 gene in revertants of multidrug-resistant human myelogenous leukemia K562 occurs without loss of amplified DNA. *Molecular and Cellular Biology* **7**, 4549–4552.

Sugimoto, Y., Tsukahara, S., Oh-hara, T., Isoe, T. & Tsuruo, T. (1990). Decreased expression of topoisomerase I in camptothecin-resistant tumour cell lines as determined by a monoclonal antibody. *Cancer Research* **50**, 6925–6930.

Takai, Y., Kishimoto, A., Inoue, M. & Nishizuka, Y. (1977). Studies on a cyclic nucleotide-independent protein kinase and its proenzyme in mammalian tissues I. Purification and characterization of an active enzyme from bovine cerebellum. *Journal of Biological Chemistry* **252**, 7603–7609.

Toda, T., Shimanuki, M. & Yanagida, M. (1991). Fission yeast genes that confer resistance to staurosporine encode an AP-1-like transcription factor and a protein kinase related to the mammalian ERK-/MAP2 and budding yeast *FUS3* and *KSS1* kinases. *Genes and Development* **5**, 60–73.

Ueda, K., Cardarelli, C., Gottesman, M.M. & Pastan, I. (1987a). Expression of full-length cDNA for the human '*MDR1*' gene confers resistance to colchicine, doxorubicin, and vinblastine. *Proceedings of the National Academy of Sciences USA* **84**, 3004–3008.

Ueda, K., Pastan, I. & Gottesman, M.M. (1987b). Isolation and sequence of the promoter region of the human multidrug-resistance (P-glycoprotein) gene. *Journal of Biological Chemistry* **262**, 17432–17436.

Yamamoto, K.K., Gonzalez, G.A., Biggs, W.H. III & Montminy, M.R. (1988). Phosphorylation-induced binding and transcriptional efficiency of nuclear factor CREB. *Nature* **334**, 494–498.

Zwelling, L.A., Hinds, M., Chan, D., Altschuler, E., Mayes, J. & Zipf, T.F. (1990). Phorbol ester effects on topoisomerase II activity and gene expression in HL-60 human leukemia cells with different proclivities toward monocytoid differentiation. *Cancer Research* **50**, 7116–7122.

Zylber-Katz, E. & Glazer, R.I. (1985). Phospholipid- and Ca^{2+}-dependent protein kinase activity and protein phosphorylation patterns in the differentiation of human promyelocytic leukemia cell line HL-60. *Cancer Research* **45**, 5159–5164.

Chapter 8
Resistance to topoisomerase II-directed anticancer agents

Amy L. Ellis and Leonard A. Zwelling

Introduction

DNA topoisomerase II (topo II) regulates the three-dimensional structure of DNA by binding to a DNA molecule, cleaving both strands of that DNA, and passing a second DNA duplex through the first before religating the cleavage site. Topo II is also the target of several structurally diverse classes of antineoplastic drugs. Some of these compounds bind to DNA (the anthracyline antibiotics, Adriamycin and daunorubicin; the anthracenedione, mitoxantrone; the aminoacridine, amsacrine) while others do not (epipodophyllotoxin derivatives, VM-26 and VP-16). The following articles are comprehensive reviews on topo II as a drug target: Zwelling, 1985; Glisson & Ross, 1987; Liu, 1989.

Drugs such as amsacrine or the epipodophyllotoxins appear to inhibit topo II after it cleaves DNA, but before the religation step (Osheroff, 1989). DNA cleavage cannot be visualized in the laboratory without enzyme denaturation and/or digestion. Topo II remains covalently bound to the 5′ end of DNA at the cleavage site, thus, the phrase 'stabilization of cleavable complex' is used to describe the drug-induced inhibition of topo II. Formation of cleavable complexes has been quantitatively associated with drug-induced cytotoxicity. At present, it is uncertain how the formation of cleavable complexes leads to cell death. However, the DNA of tumour cells which are resistant to drugs that target topo II has been shown to be resistant to cleavage stimulated by the drugs to which the cells are resistant, although this is not always the case. A recent review (Gewirtz, 1991) explores occasions, particularly in resistant cell lines, where DNA cleavage does not correlate with cytotoxicity. Such circumstances are not the focus of the current chapter.

This chapter will discuss how cellular resistance to topo II-reactive drugs may be a function of reduced enzyme levels or altered enzyme activity, including qualitative differences in the susceptibility of topo II to inhibitors.

Drug resistance due to reduced or altered enzyme activity

Goldenberg et al. (1986) described P388 murine leukaemia cells selected for Adriamycin resistance (ADR). At similar intracellular concentrations of drug, Adriamycin induced fewer DNA strand breaks (both single and double stranded) in resistant cells (P388/ADR) than in the drug-sensitive parent P388 line. The number of double-strand breaks correlated with the cytotoxicity of Adriamycin. Drug resistance in the P388/ADR cells appeared multifactorial (Deffie et al., 1988). The cells contained the P-glycoprotein efflux pump which can limit accumulation of Adriamycin and other drugs. The cells had elevated levels of glutathione transferase which can help detoxify free radical metabolites of compounds like the anthracycline antibiotics. However, the reduced strand cleavage in resistant cells, despite drug levels comparable to those producing cleavage in sensitive cells, indicated a potential role for topo II in the drug resistance phenotype. Also, the P388/ADR cells were crossresistant to the topo II inhibitor amsacrine (Seneviratne & Goldenberg, 1989). Although Adriamycin appears to have several potential mechanisms of cytotoxicity besides the inhibition of topo II (Myers et al., 1985), amsacrine is thought to exert its toxic effects on tumour cells primarily, if not exclusively, through topo II inhibition and its liphophilicity suggests that amsacrine is not a substrate for the P-glycoprotein transporter.

Nuclear extracts from sensitive and P388/ADR cells were analysed and compared for topo II catalytic and DNA cleavage activities (Deffie et al., 1989a). Topo II catalytic (strand passage) activity and drug-stimulated DNA cleaving potency were reduced in extracts derived from P388/ADR cells when compared with these activities in extracts from P388. Immunoblotting indicated that the level of topo II was reduced in extracts from drug-resistant P388 cells when compared with levels in the parent line. Subsequent experiments demonstrated a potential genetic basis for these observations. Southern blotting demonstrated that P388/ADR cells possessed two different alleles for the topo II gene—one the same as that found in DNA from drug-sensitive cells, but present at lower copy number, and another shortened version of the gene (Deffie et al., 1989b). P388/ADR cells contained less mRNA encoding topo II (a 6.6 kb message) than sensitive cells, as shown by northern blotting. The P388/ ADR cells also contained a truncated form of the topo II message which was not present in the sensitive cells. This is postulated to have been transcribed from the mutant allele of the topo II gene (Deffie et al., 1989b).

Similar observations have been made in other cell lines. The human small cell lung carcinoma, GLC4 was continuously exposed to gradually increasing concentrations of Adriamycin. The resulting cell population (GLC4/ADR) was 44-fold resistant to Adriamycin and crossresistant to VP-16 (38-fold). DNA cleavage and DNA–protein crosslink formation were greater in sensitive cells than in GLC4/ADR when both lines were exposed to the same intracellular concentration of Adriamycin (Zijlstra *et al.*, 1987). Cellular and nuclear extracts from GLC4/ADR had 2–3-fold lower topo II catalytic activity than extracts derived from GLC4, but contained nearly identical amounts of topo I activity (de Jong *et al.*, 1990). Five-fold higher concentrations of the topo II inhibitors VP-16 and amsacrine were required to stimulate the DNA cleavage produced by topo II in extracts from GLC4/ADR cells as compared to that produced by extracts derived from the drug sensitive GLC4 (de Jong *et al.*, 1990).

VP-16-resistant clones of KB (human nasopharyngeal carcinoma) cells were found to contain levels of topo II activity which were inversely proportional to the level of drug resistance, while topo I activity in each drug-resistant clone was slightly elevated (Ferguson *et al.*, 1988). Tan *et al.* (1989) observed this trend in P388 cells selected for amsacrine resistance. The decrease in topo II activity concomitant with increasing drug resistance seemed to be the result of a rearrangement found in one allele of the topo II gene in the amsacrine-resistant cells. This rearrangement may have inactivated the allele, for topo II mRNA levels were reduced in the resistant cells compared to the parental line (Tan *et al.*, 1989). As observed in the VP-16-resistant KB cells mentioned above, topo I levels were elevated in the P388 cells resistant to amsacrine. If this increase confers greater cell sensitivity to drugs which antagonize topo I, utilization of chemotherapeutic agents which interfere with topo I activity might be helpful in overcoming drug resistance in cancers treated initially with topo II antagonists.

If topo II activity is low in cells, there is a lower probability of the formation of the cleavable complexes associated with cytotoxicity. These cells would be resistant to inhibitors of topo II. Conversely, if tumour cells contain greater than average topo II activity, they may be hypersensitive to these drugs. Chinese hamster ovary (CHO-K1) cells were mutagenized with ethylmethane sulphonate and replica plated on plain agar and on agar containing a low level of Adriamycin. The clone ADR1 grew on plain agar, but did not grow when Adriamycin was present. The cells from this clone were not hypersensitive to vinca alkaloid microtubule inhibitors (substrates for the P-glycoprotein membrane efflux pump), but were hypersensitive to other topo II antagonistic drugs including VP-16, ellipticine, daunorubicin, amsacrine and mitoxantrone (Robson *et al.*, 1987). Accumulation of daunorubicin was similar in both CHO-K1 and ADR1 cells.

Drug-induced, topo II-mediated, protein-associated DNA cleavage was higher in the ADR1 cells than in CHO-K1 (Robson *et al.*, 1987). Amsacrine also stimulated more DNA strand cleavage in ADR1 cells than in CHO-K1 at equal concentrations of drug (Davies *et al.*, 1988). Topo II-containing nuclear extracts derived from ADR1 caused more DNA-protein crosslinking in the presence of amsacrine than did extracts from CHO-K1. Greater concentrations of amsacrine were necessary to inhibit decatenation of kDNA by equal amounts of nuclear protein (a measure of strand passage, i.e. topo II activity) from ADR1 than CHO-K1. Cleavage of substrate DNA stimulated by amsacrine was greater when ADR1 nuclear extract was used as the source of topo II, although sites of cleavage on DNA were the same as when CHO-K1 extract was utilized. These data were consistent with a greater amount of topo II in ADR1 cells as was demonstrated by immunoblotting.

Alterations in cellular topo II activity were not solely due to changed topo II levels. Chinese hamster lung cells (DC3F/9-OHE) selected for resistance to 9-hydroxyellipticine were crossresistant to the anthracyclines, vinca alkaloids, amsacrine and VP-16 (Salles *et al.*, 1982; Pommier *et al.*, 1986b). Although reduced accumulation of drug by DC3F/9-OHE cells may help explain tumour cell resistance to the vinca alkaloids and anthracylines, accumulation of amsacrine was similar in both sensitive and drug-resistant cells (Pommier *et al.*, 1986b). Furthermore, DNA single and double-strand cleavage and DNA–protein crosslinking were reduced in DC3F/9-OHE cells at equimolar concentrations of amsacrine and VP-16. DNA cleavage and protein crosslinking by amsacrine and VP-16 were also equal in isolated nuclei where cellular drug accumulation was not a factor (Pommier *et al.*, 1986b).

In nuclear extracts made from DC3F cells, amsacrine stimulated DNA-protein crosslinking activity. This activity was not stimulated by amsacrine in extract derived from the nuclei of DC3F/9-OHE cells, although baseline crosslinking in the absence of drug was greater using this extract (Pommier *et al.*, 1986a). Topo II activity was similar in extracts from both cell lines, but immunoblotting indicated that the number of DC3F/9-OHE topo II molecules in extracts was half that in DC3F extracts. However, this would not seem to account for the greater than 100-fold resistance to amsacrine of the drug-resistant cells. In contrast to the results using the nuclear extracts, results using purified topo II from DC3F and DC3F/9-OHE cells showed comparable amsacrine-induced DNA–protein crosslinking activity. The enzyme purification process revealed that DC3F/9-OHE extracts contained a previously undescribed DNA crosslinking activity that was not sensitive to stimulation by amsacrine, copurified with topo I activity, and could be related to topo I. The investigators hypothesized that this protein, which is not present in nuclear extracts of DC3F cells, may act as a modulating factor in DC3F/9-

OHE cells and nuclear extract, interfering with the topo II–drug interaction in the cell nucleus or nuclear extract (Pommier *et al.*, 1986a).

More than one isozyme of topo II can exist. A clone of P388 cells (A20) which had been selected for resistance to amsacrine was found to be crossresistant to a variety of drugs including other inhibitors of topo II such as VM-26, ellipticine and Adriamycin (Per *et al.*, 1987). VM-26 and amsacrine were found to induce more protein-associated DNA cleavage and DNA–protein crosslinking in wild-type P388 cells (wt20) than in A20. Accumulation of amsacrine was similar in both cell lines. Nuclear extracts from wt20 cells contained roughly twice the topo II catalytic activity as extracts derived from A20 nuclei. Immunoblotting of both nuclear extracts and whole cell lysates from wt20 and A20 demonstrated that topo II antibody detected two proteins—173 kDa and 164 kDa. The ratio of 164 kDa protein to 173 kDa protein was greater in wt20 than A20 (Per *et al.*, 1987). Topo II purified from both cell lines was in two antigenically distinct forms—170 kDa and 180 kDa that presumably correspond to the 164 kDa and 173 kDa immunoreactive cellular forms. Proteolytic cleavage patterns confirmed that the two enzymes were different (Drake *et al.*, 1987). Both enzymes had the same adenosine triphosphate (ATP) requirement, but strand passage activity of the p180 enzyme was less heat stable and had optimal activity at a higher salt concentration (Drake *et al.*, 1989). Catalytic activity differed between the two enzymes in that the p170 enzyme relaxed supercoiled DNA in a distributive fashion (relaxed one supercoil per DNA molecule before dissociating from DNA) and the p180 enzyme-relaxed supercoiled DNA in a processive manner (relaxed all supercoils in a DNA molecule before dissociating). Consequently, the p180 topo II may have a lower dissociation rate from DNA (Drake *et al.*, 1989).

Drug sensitivity of the topo II isozymes was also different. The p170 enzyme was more sensitive to the inhibition of catalytic activity and stimulation of DNA strand cleavage caused by VM-26. Although some VM-26-stimulated DNA cleavage sites were shared by both enzymes, there were other sites which were favoured by one isozyme of topo II over the other (Drake *et al.*, 1989).

Amounts of the p170 and p180 forms of topo II vary over the course of the cell cycle. Immunoblotting of lysates from U937 cells showed that the p170 enzyme was highest during logarithmic growth and fell as cell growth plateaued. Levels of p180 were highest during plateau and lowest during log phase (Drake *et al.*, 1989). Further studies using NIH3T3 cells demonstrated that the p170 isozyme of topo II was undetectable when cells were in G0 and did not rise to a detectable level until the cells reached late S phase. Peak levels of p170 topo II were observed when the cells were in the G2–M phase. The amount of p180 topo II remained constant throughout the cell cycle and was detectable at G0 (Woessner *et al.*, 1991).

Cells tend to be most sensitive to the antiproliferative effects of topo II antagonists such as the epipodophyllotoxin derivatives during log phase (Estey *et al.*, 1987a; Zwelling *et al.*, 1987)—the time when the levels of the p170 isozyme, which has greater drug sensitivity, is highest. Studies in NIH3T3 human fibroblasts showed that cells transformed with the *ras* oncogene had greater total topo II activity than normal NIH3T3 cells and that the proportion of the p170 enzyme was higher in the transformed cells. Both normal and *ras*-transformed NIH3T3 cells had similar levels of the p180 enzyme (Woessner *et al.*, 1990). As in the enzyme purified from A20 cells described earlier, p170 topo II from NIH3T3 cells was more sensitive to inhibition by VM-26. Consistent with this observation, *ras*-transformed NIH3T3 cells (which contain more of the p170 topo II) were more sensitive to the cytotoxic effects of VM-26 than normal NIH3T3 cells. Selectivity of topo II inhibitors for the p170 form of the enzyme may help explain why the drugs are most effective against rapidly growing tumours (Woessner *et al.*, 1990) and may be the molecular basis for the therapeutic index that allows topo II inhibitors to be employed successfully in the clinic.

Drug resistance due to qualitative alterations in drug–enzyme interactions

Levels of topo II activity may be similar in tumour cells sensitive to antagonists of the enzyme and cells which have been selected for resistance to these drugs. However, drug sensitivity of the topo II contained in each cell line may differ.

CHO cells were mutagenized with ethyl methanesulphonate and exposed to VP-16 once to select for drug-resistant cells. VpmR5 mutants were 20-fold resistant to the cytotoxic effects of VP-16 and they were also resistant to VP-16-induced DNA strand cleavage although there was no difference in cell associated VP-16 between parent CHO and VpmR5 (Glisson *et al.*, 1986a). VpmR5 cells were crossresistant to anthracyclines, amsacrine and mitoxantrone. Levels of daunorubicin and amsacrine were the same in wild type CHO and VpmR5 cells, but strand cleavage stimulated by Adriamycin, amsacrine, or mitoxantrone was reduced in the drug-resistant cells (Glisson *et al.*, 1986b). Nuclear extracts from both cell lines contained similar topo II decatenation activities and the catalytic activity of the enzyme in either extract was equally inhibited by VP-16. In contrast, VP-16-stimulated DNA cleavage activity differed between the two extracts as did DNA–protein crosslink formation. VP-16 induced cleavable complex formation by CHO nuclear extract but not by the extract derived from VpmR5 cells (Glisson *et al.*, 1986b). A somatic cell hybrid (M_1J_2-7) created by the fusion of the drug-resistant VpmR5 with the drug-sensitive CHO cell line EOT-3 was relatively sensitive to VP-16-induced cytotoxicity and DNA strand cleavage (Glisson *et al.*, 1986b). This suggests that the presence of drug-sensitive enzyme will render a cell sensitive even in the presence of a drug-resistant enzyme.

Immunoblotting showed comparable levels of topo II in nuclear extracts of wild-type and VpmR5 cells, but topo II purification revealed differences in the drug sensitivity of topo II from each cell line (Sullivan *et al.*, 1989). Formation of cleavable complexes was reduced in the presence of VP-16 or amsacrine when VpmR5 topo II was utilized when compared with drug effects on CHO topo II.

Another altered topo II has been characterized in HL60 human leukaemia cells selected for resistance to amsacrine. The HL60/AMSA cells were developed by repeated intermittent exposure to increasing concentrations of amsacrine and have a stable resistance phenotype (Odaimi *et al.*, 1986; Beran & Andersson, 1987). Although the cells are approximately 100-fold resistant to amsacrine, they are only two-fold resistant to VP-16 (Zwelling *et al.*, 1989).

Accumulation of amsacrine (Estey *et al.*, 1987b; Beran & Andersson, 1987) or VP-16 (Bakic *et al.*, 1987) in the HL60/AMSA cells was not less than in the parent cell line. Amsacrine-induced protein-associated DNA cleavage was markedly lower in HL60/AMSA than in HL60 cells or isolated nuclei exposed to equal concentrations of amsacrine. VP-16-induced cleavage was only minimally lower in HL60/AMSA. The magnitude of DNA cleavage in the cells correlated with amsacrine cytotoxicity (Bakic *et al.*, 1986). This indicated potential involvement of topo II in the drug resistance of these cells.

Nuclear extracts from HL60 and HL60/AMSA contained comparable decatenating activity, but differed in susceptibility to inhibition by amsacrine (Estey *et al.*, 1987b). Amsacrine stimulated more DNA cleavage in the presence of HL60 extract than in the presence of HL60/AMSA extract although cleavage stimulated by VP-16 was similar when either extract was present (Estey *et al.*, 1987b). The differences between the topo II in HL60 and HL60/AMSA cells were still present when studying purified enzyme from each cell line. Not only did topo II from HL60/AMSA resist stabilization in a complex with DNA in the presence of amsacrine, but HL60/AMSA topo II resisted stabilization induced by the anthracycline antibiotics, anthracenediones, and ellipticines which, like amsacrine, are DNA intercalators. VP-16, a non-intercalator, was able to stimulate DNA cleavage in the presence of topo II from either HL60 or HL60/AMSA (Zwelling *et al.*, 1989, 1991).

Study of topo II from HL60/AMSA may reveal differences in drug interaction with this enzyme between two classes of topo II inhibitors which can stimulate DNA cleavage—those which intercalate into DNA and those which do not. This suggests that these two drug classes interact with different sites on topo II.

The exact role of topo II in the drug resistance phenotype of CEM/ VM-1 cells is not easily defined. These cells were selected for resistance to VM-26 from the CCRF/CEM human leukaemia cell line by intermittent exposure to increasing concentrations of the drug. CEM/VM-1 was found to be crossresistant to VP-16, Adriamycin, mitoxantrone and amsacrine. CEM/VM-1 accumulated only 30% less VP-16 than parental CEM cells and HPLC analysis did not detect metabolites of the drug (Danks *et al.*, 1987). Although the cells were slightly resistant to the vinca alkaloids, the P-glycoprotein membrane transporter was not detected in CEM/VM-1 and verapamil (which can compete for this efflux pump, causing increases in intracellular concentration of other substrates) did not reverse this resistance (Beck *et al.*, 1987). Immunoblotting demonstrated that nuclear extracts from CEM parent, CEM/VM-1 and CEM/VM-1-5 (a cell line with even greater resistance to VM-26 than CEM/VM-1) cells contained similar amounts of topo II. Catalytic activity, however, was less sensitive to inhibition by VM-26 in extracts from the resistant cells, as was cleavable complex formation induced by VM-26 or amsacrine. Reduced sensitivity of the nuclear extracts from CEM/VM-1 and CEM/VM-1-5 was proportional to drug resistance in these cell lines (Danks *et al.*, 1988).

Hybrids of CEM and CEM/VM-1 cells were sensitive to the cytotoxic activities of VM-26. A nuclear extract from the hybrid was stimulated to form cleavable complexes with DNA in the presence of VM-26. Sensitivity was similar to the CEM cells, indicating that cells can be made sensitive to topo II inhibitors when a drug-sensitive enzyme is present (Wolverton *et al.*, 1989). Thus, hybrids containing sensitive and resistant enzymes will be drug sensitive such as the M_1J_2-7 cells mentioned previously (Glisson *et al.*, 1986b).

Subsequent studies in CEM, CEM/VM-1 and CEM/VM-1-5 have shown that nuclear extracts from the drug-resistant cell lines have an increased ATP requirement for DNA unknotting activity. Topo II from the drug-resistant cells seemed to have lower affinity for ATP. Novobiocin, which competetively inhibits the binding of ATP to topo II, increased the requirement for ATP during strand passage using extracts from CEM/ VM-1 and CEM/VM-1-5 cells to a greater extent than it did using CEM nuclear extract (Danks *et al.*, 1989). Although ATP is not required for cleavable-complex formation, it does stimulate formation of cleavable complexes. Danks *et al.*, (1989) postulated that ATP binding to topo II exposed more drug binding-sites on the enzyme. Therefore, decreased ATP binding exposed fewer sites for drug binding on the enzyme (Danks *et al.*, 1989). Topo II which has a lower affinity for ATP may not be as sensitive to drug interference as topo II which binds ATP more effectively.

Another observation made in CEM/VM-1 cells was that topo II in this cell line may be localized in these cells differently than in the parent CEM. The nuclear matrix is thought to be the site for DNA replication in the cell

(Pineta & Coffey, 1984). Topo II has been shown to be associated with this structure (Berrios *et al.*, 1985). In CEM cells, VP-16 and amsacrine inhibit DNA synthesis preferentially at the nuclear matrix, while they do not in CEM/VM-1 cells. Topo II was extracted from nuclear matrices of both cell lines. Topo II catalytic activity was lower in extract from the nuclear matrices of CEM/VM-1 cells than CEM extract and immunoblotting demonstrated that the amount of topo II was reduced in nuclear matrix from CEM/VM-1 cells, although non-matrix topo II levels were similar in both cell lines (Fernandes *et al.*, 1990). If matrix-associated topo II is that whose inhibition is most critical for drug cytotoxic activity, reduction in this pool of topo II would be expected to be associated with drug resistance.

Conclusion

Several investigators have shown that cell levels of topo II activity influence the response of the cell to drugs which target this enzyme. Drug resistance associated with low levels of topo II may be due to an alteration in the topo II gene which results in reduced synthesis of the enzyme as in the P388/ADR cells studied by Goldenberg *et al.* (1986) and the P388/amsacrine cells of Tan *et al.* (1989). Hypersensitivity of cells to topo II inhibitors has been linked to an increased enzyme activity in CHO-K-1 cells by Robson *et al.* (1987) and Davies *et al.* (1988). This phenomenon has also been observed in human Burkitt lymphoma cells that are nitrogen-mustard resistant apparently due to enhanced repair of DNA interstrand crosslinking. The cells have enhanced topo II activity compared to the sensitive parent lymphoma cells and are 4–11-fold more sensitive to topo II inhibitors such as VM-26, VP-16 and amsacrine (Tan *et al.*, 1987). Possibly patient tumours that responded initially to alkylating agents and have become resistant to these drugs could respond to treatment with a drug that targets topo II.

The interaction of topoisomerases I and II and how one enzyme may influence the other merits further study. Studies in DC3F/9-OHE cells by Pommier *et al.* (1986a,b) demonstrated that although purified cellular topo II may be drug sensitive, whole cells and nuclei may be resistant to cleavable-complex formation stimulated by inhibitors of this enzyme. This implies that cytoplasmic and nuclear factors (such as the topo I-like activity discovered by the Pommier group) may influence topo II cleavable-complex formation, thereby influencing drug sensitivity of the tumour cells. Other unknown modulators of cleavable-complex formation and/or cellular processing of the cleavable complex may exist in the cell. Identification of such factors and of means of controlling them could be useful in modulating tumour cell sensitivity to inhibitors of topo II.

Drake *et al.* (1989) have found that isozymes of topo II differ in their drug sensitivity as well as in their catalytic behaviour. Levels of these enzymes are not the same in drug-sensitive and drug-resistant cells. The p170 and p180 topo II isozymes are similar (but not identical) in amino acid sequence, yet are believed to be encoded by two separate topo II genes (Chung et al., 1989). Shifting topo II in normal cells away from the isozyme being targetted by drugs may improve the therapeutic index of the compound.

Studying mutant forms of topo II may help elucidate how drugs interact with the enzyme bound to DNA to cause formation of the cleavable complex. As the drug-binding site of topo II is elucidated, structural requirements of drug for optimal binding to the enzyme may be defined and could lead to the development of compounds which are more efficacious.

Mutant topo II in the HL60/AMSA cell line is resistant to cleavable complex formation stimulated by amsacrine, but not by VP-16 (Zwelling et al., 1989). Differential sensitivity of this enzyme to two classes of topo II antagonists (DNA intercalators versus non-intercalators) may provide insight on where drugs bind to the topo II/DNA complex and how mutations of the enzyme can influence the ability of certain drugs to inhibit topo II religation.

Lastly, the work of Danks and Beck et al. shows that different cofactor requirements (such as ATP) between topo II enzymes extracted from drug-sensitive parent cells and drug-resistant cells selected from the parent line may play a role in conferring drug resistance (Danks et al., 1989). In collaboration with Fernandes, this group of investigators has also found evidence that topo II may be localized differently in the CEM and CEM/VM-1 cell lines (Fernandes et al., 1990). Topo II activity was greater on the nuclear matrix (thought to be a primary site of DNA synthesis) in CEM cells than in CEM/VM-1, although non-matrix levels of topo II were similar in both cell lines. Further directions for this research may include assessing whether topo II not associated with the nuclear matrix is a target for inhibitors and what signals topo II to move onto or off the nuclear matrix if localization of topo II can be modulated within a cell.

A more complete understanding of topo II's normal function and regulation in the cell, its interaction with various classes of inhibitors, and what specific events following drug-stabilized cleavable-complex formation lead to cell death, may provide clues towards overcoming drug resistance associated with alteration of topo II in tumour cells.

Acknowledgements

Dr Zwelling is the recipient of a grant from the National Cancer Institute (CA40090) and American Cancer Society (CH-324D). We would also like to thank Diane Rivera for editing the manuscript and Michael Hinds for valuable criticisms.

References

Bakic, M., Beran, M., Andersson, B.S., Silberman, L., Estey, E. & Zwelling, L.A. (1986). The production of topoisomerase II-mediated DNA cleavage in human leukemia cells predicts their susceptibility to 4′-(9-acridinylamino)methanesulfon-*m*-anisidide (*m*-AMSA). *Biochemical and Biophysical Research Communications* **134**, 638–645.

Bakic, M., Chan, D., Andersson, B.S., Beran, M., Silberman, L., Estey, E., Ricketts, L. & Zwelling, L.A. (1987). Effect of 1-β-D-arabinofuranosylcytosine (ara-C) on nuclear topoisomerase II activity and on the DNA cleavage and cytoxicity produced by 4′-(9-acridinylamino) methanesulfon-*m*-anisidide (*m*-AMSA) and etoposide in *m*-AMSA-sensitive and -resistant human leukemia cells. *Biochemical Pharmacology* **36**, 4067–4077.

Beck, W.T., Cirtain, M.C., Danks, M.K., Felsted, R.L., Safa, A.R., Wolverton, J.S., Suttle, D.P. & Trent, J.M. (1987). Pharmacological, molecular, and cytogenetic analysis of 'atypical' multidrug-resistant human leukemia cells. *Cancer Research* **47**, 5455–5460.

Beran, M. & Andersson, B.S. (1987). Development and characterization of a human myelogenous leukemia cell line resistant to 4′-(9-acridinylamino)-3-methanesulfon-*m*-anisidide. *Cancer Research* **47**, 1897–1904.

Berrios, M., Osheroff, N. & Fisher, P.A. (1985). *In situ* localization of DNA topoisomerase II, a major polypeptide component of the *Drosophila* nuclear matrix fraction. *Proceedings of the National Academy of Sciences USA* **82**, 4124–4126.

Chung, T.D.Y., Drake, F.H., Tan, K.B., Per, S.R., Crooke, S.T. & Mirabelli, C.K. (1989). Characterization and immunological identification of cDNA clones encoding two human DNA topoisomerase II isozymes. *Proceedings of the National Academy of Sciences USA* **86**, 9431–9435.

Danks, M.K., Schmidt, C.A., Cirtain, M.C., Suttle, D.P. & Beck, W.T. (1988). Altered catalytic activity of and DNA cleavage by DNA topoisomerase II from human leukemic cells selected for resistance to VM-26. *Biochemistry* **27**, 8861–8869.

Danks, M.K., Schmidt, C.A., Deneka, D.A. & Beck, W.T. (1989). Increased ATP requirment for activity of and complex formation by DNA topoisomerase II from human leukemic CCRF-CEM cells selected for resistance to teniposide. *Cancer Communications* **1**, 101–109.

Danks, M.K., Yalowich, J.C. & Beck, W.T. (1987). Atypical multiple drug resistance in a human leukemia cell line selected for resistance to teniposide (VM-26). *Cancer Research* **47**, 1297–1301.

Davies, S.M., Robson, C.N., Davies, S.L. & Hickson, I.D. (1988). Nuclear topoisomerase II levels correlate with the sensitivity of mammalian cells to intercalating agents and epipodophyllotoxins. *Journal of Biological Chemistry* **263**, 17724–17729.

Deffie, A.M., Alam, T., Seneviratne, C., Beenken, S.W., Batra, J.K., Shea, T.C., Henner, W.D. & Goldenberg, G.J. (1988). Multifactorial resistance to Adriamycin: relationship of DNA repair, glutathione transferase activity, drug efflux, and P-glycoprotein in cloned cell lines of Adriamycin-sensitive and -resistant P388 leukemia. *Cancer Research* **48**, 3595–3602.

Deffie, A.M., Batra, J.K. & Goldenberg, G.J. (1989a). Direct correlation between DNA topoisomerase II activity and cytoxicity in Adriamycin-sensitive and -resistant P388 leukemia cell lines. *Cancer Research* **49**, 58–62.

Deffie, A.M., Bosman, D.J. & Goldenberg, G.J. (1989b). Evidence for a mutant allele of the gene for DNA topoisomerase II in Adriamycin-resistant P388 murine leukemia cells. *Cancer Research* **49**, 6879–6882.

de Jong, S., Zijlstra, J.G., de Vries, E.G.F. & Mulder, N.H. (1990). Reduced DNA topoisomerase II activity and drug-induced DNA cleavage activity in and Adriamycin-resistant human small cell lung carcinoma cell line. *Cancer Research* **50**, 304–309.

Drake, F.H., Hofman, G.A., Bartus, H.F., Mattern, M.R., Crooke, S.T. & Mirabelli, C.K. (1989). Biochemical and pharmacological properties of p170 and p180 forms of topoisomerase II. *Biochemistry* **28**, 8154–8160.

Drake, F.H., Zimmerman, J.P., McCabe, F.L., Bartus, H.F., Per, S.R., Sullivan, D.M., Ross, W.E., Mattern, M.R., Johnson, R.K., Crooke, S.T. & Mirabelli, C.K. (1987). Purification of topoisomerase II from amsacrine-resistant P388 leukemia cells. *Journal of Biological Chemistry* **262**, 16739–16747.

Estey, E., Adlakha, R.C., Hittleman, W.N. & Zwelling, L.A. (1987a). Cell cycle dependent variations in drug-induced topoisomerase II mediated DNA cleavage and cytotoxicity. *Biochemistry* **26**, 4338–4344.

Estey, E.H., Silberman, L., Beran, M., Andersson, B.S. & Zwelling, L.A. (1987b). The interaction between nuclear topoisomerase II activity from human leukemia cells, exogenous DNA, and 4'-(9-acridinylamino)methanesulfon-*m*-anside (*m*-AMSA) or 4-(4,6-*O*-ethylidene-*B*-*D*-glucopyranoside) (VP-16) indicates the sensitivity of the cells to the drugs. *Biochemical and Biophysical Research Communications* **144**, 787–793.

Ferguson, P.J., Fisher, M.H., Stephenson, J., Li, D., Zhou, B. & Cheng, Y. (1988). Combined modalities of resistance in etoposide-resistant human KB cell lines. *Cancer Research* **48**, 5956–5964.

Fernandes, D.J., Danks, M.K. & Beck, W.T. (1990). Decreased nuclear matrix DNA topoisomerase II in human leukemia cells resistant to VM-26 and *m*-AMSA. *Biochemistry* **29**, 4235–4241.

Gewirtz, D.A. (1991). Does bulk damage to DNA explain the cytostatic and cytotoxic effects of topoisomerase II inhibitors? *Biochemical Pharmacology* **42**, 2253–2258.

Glisson, B.S. & Ross, W.E. (1987). DNA topoisomerase II: a primer on the enzyme and its unique role as a multidrug target in cancer chemotherapy. *Pharmacological Therapeutics* **32**, 89–106.

Glisson, B., Gupta, R., Hodges, P. & Ross, W. (1986a). Cross-resistance to intercalating agents in an epipodophyllotoxin-resistant Chinese hamster ovary cell line: evidence for a common intracellular target. *Cancer Research* **46**, 1939–1942.

Glisson, B., Gupta, R., Smallwood-Kentro, S. & Ross, W. (1986b). Characterization of acquired epipodophyllotoxin resistance in a Chinese hamster ovary cell line: loss of drug-stimulated DNA cleavage activity. *Cancer Research* **46**, 1934–1938.

Goldenberg, G.J., Wang, H. & Blair, G.W. (1986). Resistance to Adriamycin: relationship of cytotoxicity to drug uptake and DNA single- and double-strand breakage in cloned cell lines of Adriamycin-sensitive and -resistant P388 leukemia. *Cancer Research* **46**, 2978–2983.

Liu, F. (1989). DNA topoisomerase poisons as antitumor drugs. *Annual Reviews in Biochemistry* **58**, 351–375.

Myers, C.E., Muinidi, J., Batist, G., Haim, N. & Sinha, B. (1985). Anthracyclines. In Pinedo, H.M. & Chabner, B.A. (eds) *Cancer Chemotherapy*, pp. 57–75. Scientific Publishers Ltd, Limerick.

Odaimi, M., Andersson, B.S., McCredie, K.B. & Beran, M. (1986). Drug sensitivity and cross-resistance of the 4'-(9-acridinylamino)methanesulfon-*m*-anisidide-resistant subline of HL-60 human leukemia. *Cancer Research* **46**, 3330–3333.

Osheroff, N. (1989). Effect of antineoplastic agents on the DNA cleavage/religation reaction of eukaryotic topoisomerase II: inhibition of DNA religation by etoposide. *Biochemistry* **28**, 6157–6160.

Per, S.R., Mattern, M.R., Mirabelli, C.K., Drake, F.H., Johnson, R.K. & Crooke, S.T. (1987). Characterization of a subline of P388 leukemia resistant to amsacrine: evidence of altered topoisomerase II function. *Molecular Pharmacology* **32**, 17–25.

Pineta, K.J. & Coffey, D.S. (1984). A structural analysis of the role of the nuclear matrix and DNA loops in the organization of the nucleus and chromosome. *Journal of Cell Sciences*, Suppl. 1, 123–235.

Pommier, Y., Kerrigan, D., Schwartz, R.E., Swack, J. & McCurdy, A. (1986a). Altered DNA topoisomerase II activity in Chinese hamster cells resistant to topoisomerase II inhibitors. *Cancer Research* **46**, 3075–3081.

Pommier, Y., Schwartz, R.E., Zwelling, L.A., Kerrigan, D., Mattern, M.R., Charcosset, J.Y., Jacquemin-Sablon, A. & Kohn, K.W. (1986b). Reduced formation of protein-associated DNA strand breaks in Chinese hamster cells resistant to topoisomerase II inhibitors. *Cancer Research* **46**, 611–616.

Robson, C.N., Hoban, P.R., Harris, A.L. & Hickson, I.D. (1987). Cross-sensitivity to topoisomerase II inhibitors in cytotoxic drug-hypersensitive Chinese hamster ovary cell lines. *Cancer Research* **47**, 1560–1565.

Salles, B., Charcosset, J.Y. & Jacquemin-Sablon, A. (1982). Isolation and properties of Chinese hamster lung cells resistant to ellipticine derivatives. *Cancer Treatment Reports* **66**, 327–338.

Seneviratne, C. & Goldenberg, G.J. (1989). Further characterization of drug-sensitivity and cross-resistance profiles of cloned cell lines of Adriamycin-sensitive and -resistant P388 leukemia. *Cancer Communications* **1**, 21–27.

Sullivan, D.M., Latham, M.D., Rowe, T.C. & Ross, W.E. (1989). Purification and characterization of an altered topoisomerase II from a drug-resistant Chinese hamster ovary cell line. *Biochemistry* **28**, 5680–5687.

Tan, K.B., Mattern, M.R., Boyce, R.A. & Schein, P.S. (1987). Elevated DNA topoisomerase II activity in nitrogen mustard-resistant human cells. *Proceedings of the National Academy of Sciences USA* **84**, 7668–7671.

Tan, K.B., Mattern, M.R., Eng, W.K., McCabe, F.L. & Johnson, R.K. (1989). Nonproductive rearrangement of DNA topoisomerase I and II genes: correlation with resistance to topoisomerase inhibitors. *Journal of the National Cancer Institute* **81**, 1732–1735.

Woessner, R.D., Chung, T.D.Y., Hofmann, G.A., Mattern, M.R., Mirabelli, C.K., Drake, F.H. & Johnson, R.K. (1990). Differences between normal and *ras*-transformed NIH-3T3 cells in expression of the 170 kD and 180 kD forms of topoisomerase II. *Cancer Research* **50**, 2901–2908.

Woessner, R.D., Mattern, M.R., Mirabelli, C.K., Johnson, R.K. & Drake, F.H. (1991). Proliferation- and cell cycle-dependent differences in expression of the 170 kilodalton and 180 kilodalton forms of topoisomerase II in NIH-3T3 cells. *Cell Growth and Differentiation* **2**, 209–214.

Wolverton, J.S., Danks, M.K., Schmidt, C.A. & Beck, W.T. (1989). Genetic characterization of the multidrug-resistant phenotype of VM-26 resistant human leukemic cells. *Cancer Research* **49**, 2422–2426.

Zijlstra, J.G., de Vries, E.G.E. & Mulder, N.H. (1987). Multifactorial drug resistance in an Adriamycin-resistant human small cell lung carcinoma cell line. *Cancer Research* **47**, 1780–1784.

Zwelling, L.A. (1985). DNA topoisomerase II as a target of antineoplastic drug therapy. *Cancer and Metastasis Reviews* **4**, 263–276.

Zwelling, L.A., Estey, E., Silberman, L., Doyle, S. & Hittleman, W. (1987). Effect of cell proliferation and chromatin conformation on intercalator-induced, protein-associated DNA cleavage in human brain tumor cells and human fibroblasts. *Cancer Research* **47**, 251–257.

Zwelling, L.A., Hinds, M., Chan, D., Mayes, J., Sie, K.L., Parker, E., Silberman, L., Radcliffe, A., Beran, M. & Blick, M. (1989). Characterization of an amsacrine-resistant line of human leukemia cells. *Journal of Biological Chemistry* **264**, 16411–16420.

Zwelling, L.A., Mayes, J., Hinds, M., Chan, D., Altschuler, E., Carroll, B., Parker, E., Diesseroth, K., Radcliffe, A., Seligman, M., Li, L. & Farquhar, D. (1991). Cross-resistance of an amsacrine-resistant human leukemia line to topoisomerase II reactive DNA intercalating agents. Evidence for two topoisomerase II directed drug actions. *Biochemistry* **30**, 4048–4055.

Chapter 9
Mammalian DNA topoisomerase I and its inhibitors
Yves Pommier and Akihiko Tanizawa

Introduction

DNA topoisomerase I has become an important target for chemotherapy since the discovery that camptothecin is a specific enzyme inhibitor, and that this effect is probably responsible for the potent antitumour activity of the drug. DNA topoisomerase I relaxes DNA supercoiling and is required for DNA synthesis, RNA transcription, and perhaps DNA repair and genetic rearrangements (for reviews see Wang, 1985, 1987, 1991; Champoux, 1990) (Fig. 9.1). Topoisomerase I catalyses DNA relaxation by making transient DNA single-strand breaks (Wang, 1985). Topo-isomerase I is concentrated in the nucleolus (Fleischmann *et al.*, 1984; Muller *et al.*, 1985; Garg *et al.*, 1987) and its activity seems tightly associ-ated with RNA polymerase I (Rose *et al.*, 1988).

Eukaryotic DNA topoisomerase I was first identified as the 'DNA untwisting enzyme' by Champoux and Dulbecco (Champoux & Dulbecco, 1972). In the following years, the enzyme has been purified from a variety of cell lines and tissues (Champoux, 1990), and is now commercially available (GIBCO-BRL, Gaithersburg, Maryland; Topogen, Columbus, Ohio). Its molecular mass is 100 kDa. Lower (68 kDa) and higher mole-cular mass (200 kDa) enzymes have also been isolated (Halligan *et al.*, 1985; Suzuki *et al.*, 1989; Pommier *et al.*, 1990). Although the 68-kDa form of the enzyme may be a proteolysis product of the 100-kDa enzyme

214

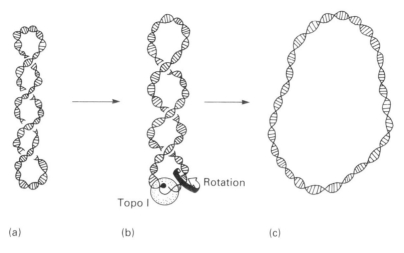

Fig. 9.1. DNA relaxation by topoisomerase I (topo I). Supercoiled DNA (a) is relaxed (c) by topo I in steps of one. (b) represents the first step of the reaction (one superturn being removed). The black dot in the middle panel indicates the covalent linkage between the enzyme (topo I) and the 3′–DNA terminus during the catalytic reaction. Topo I activity is processive under normal conditions.

(Halligan *et al.*, 1985), it is possible that both enzymes exist in cells. Indeed, antibodies raised against the 68-kDa form of topoisomerase I react with 68-kDa proteins in cell lysates and do not crossreact with the 100-kDa topoisomerase I (D. Kerrigan and Y. Pommier, unpublished observations). Thus, it is possible that several forms of topoisomerase I coexist in eukaryotic cells (Suzuki *et al.*, 1989; Pommier *et al.*, 1990; Wang, 1991). In addition, mitochondria contain a distinct topoisomerase I (Fairfield *et al.*, 1979; Brun *et al.*, 1981; Lazarus *et al.*, 1987). A 30-kDa DNA topoisomerase I is also encoded by vaccinia virus (Bauer *et al.*, 1977; Shuman & Moss, 1987, 1988).

Purified eukaryotic DNA topoisomerase I relaxes both negatively and positively supercoiled DNA plasmids and viruses (such as simian virus 40, SV40). This is in contrast to the prokaryotic DNA topoisomerase I (omega protein) which relaxes only negative supercoiling (Wang, 1985, 1987). Recent studies indicate, however, that prokaryotic DNA topoisomerase III encodes a protein homologous to eukaryotic DNA topoisomerase I (Wang, 1991). DNA relaxation by eukaryotic DNA topoisomerase I does not require nucleotide cofactor, unlike DNA topoisomerase II which hydrolyses 1 mol of adenosine triphosphate (ATP) per relaxation cycle (Osheroff *et al.*, 1983). Divalent cations are not required for topoisomerase I-mediated DNA relaxation, although their presence increases enzyme activity. This is also in contrast with prokaryotic topoisomerase I and eukaryotic DNA topoisomerase II which require divalent

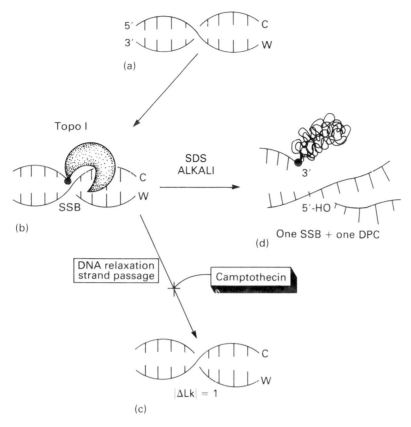

Fig. 9.2. Topoisomerase I-mediated DNA break. (a) One helical turn of duplex DNA is represented; the Watson strand (W) is above the Crick strand (C). (b) The intermediate represents topoisomerase I (topo I) covalently linked (black dot) to the 3′-terminus of the W strand; the covalent bond has been transferred by the enzyme from the phosphodiester DNA backbone to a tyrosine enzyme residue. Passage of the C strand through the DNA single-strand break (SSB) relaxes the DNA, and topo I reseals the break and dissociates from the DNA (c). The cleavage intermediate (b) can be detected after denaturation with sodium dodecylsulphate (SDS) and alkali ('cleavable complex') (d). Camptothecin stabilizes the intermediate (b). DPC, DNA–protein crosslink.

cations such as Mg^{2+} for activity. These different requirements are often used to differentiate topoisomerase I and II activities in crude nuclear extracts containing both enzymes (Pommier *et al.*, 1986).

DNA topoisomerase I catalyses DNA phosphodiester bond cleavage by transferring the covalent bond from the 3′-phosphate DNA terminus to the hydroxyl residue of a tyrosine (tyrosine 723 for human topo-isomerase I) (Champoux, 1977, 1978, 1981; Tse *et al.*, 1980; Wang, 1985, 1987; Lynn *et al.*, 1989). The 5′-DNA terminus at topoisomerase I cleavage sites is a 5′-OH-deoxyribose (Fig. 9.2). This intermediate cleavage complex is often referred to as a 'cleavable complex'. DNA relaxation may result either from free rotation of the DNA around the intact DNA phosphodiester bond opposite to the cleavage site or from passage of a duplex DNA segment through the gap formed by the cleavage site. The later model is less likely because single-stranded DNA fragments bearing a 5′-OH terminus can be exchanged with the strand 3′ to the cleavage site (Halligan *et al.*, 1982; McCoubrey & Champoux, 1986), indicating absence of strong binding of the 5′-OH DNA termini to the enzyme. The existence of such reactions is consistent with different observations showing that topoisomerase I may act as a recombination enzyme. There is good evidence that eukaryotic topoisomerase I is involved in the genomic excision of SV40 (Bullock *et al.*, 1985), and the integration of hepadnaviruses including hepatitis B virus DNA (Wang & Rogler, 1991). More recently, vaccinia virus topoisomerase I has been demonstrated to cause lambda prophage excision by an illegitimate recombination mechanism (Wang & Rogler, 1991). Thus, vaccinia topoisomerase I is capable of complementing *int* function *in vivo*. It is interesting to mention that the *int* protein is itself a topoisomerase I that can relax positive as well as negative supercoiling, and that the catalytic intermediate of this reaction is similar to a eukaryotic topoisomerase I-DNA cleavable complexes since the *int* protein nicks the DNA by making a covalent bond between tyrosine 342 and the 3′-DNA terminus (Kikuchi & Nash, 1979; Craig & Nash, 1983). These recent observations together with the recent report that camptothecin inhibits human immunodeficiency virus (HIV) replication (Priel *et al.*, 1991) suggest that topoisomerase I may be an important target for antiviral chemotherapy.

DNA cleavage and relaxation by eukaryotic topoisomerase I probably occur at many sequences, although most frequently at sites bearing a thymine at the 3′-DNA terminus of cleavage sites (Been *et al.*, 1984; Jaxel *et al.*, 1988, 1991a,b; Kjeldsen *et al.*, 1988b; Porter & Champoux, 1989a,b), and in bent DNA segments (Caserta *et al.*, 1989, 1990; Krogh *et al.*, 1991). This relatively limited DNA sequence selectivity is consistent with the functional role of the enzyme at many genomic sites during DNA metabolism (see below). DNA topoisomerase I cleavage occurs preferentially in double-stranded DNA (Been & Champoux, 1984; Jaxel *et al.*, 1991a). Also topoisomerase I binds preferentially to and cleaves supercoiled DNA (Muller, 1985; Caserta *et al.*, 1990; Camilloni *et al.*, 1989), as would be expected if it were involved in the relaxation of superhelical stress produced by the moving transcription or replication machinery. Single-stranded DNA is not cleaved unless its sequence is palindromic and can form duplex structures (Been & Champoux, 1984; Jaxel *et al.*, 1991a). Spontaneous cleavage at the site of a nick on a duplex DNA has also been demonstrated (McCoubry & Champoux, 1986). The occurrence of such a reaction may promote DNA recombination (see below).

DNA topoisomerase I is involved in many metabolic processes of DNA. Wang and Liu have clearly formulated in the 'twin supercoiled domain', that transcription generates supercoiling of the DNA template (Liu & Wang, 1987; Wu *et al.*, 1988; Ostrander *et al.*, 1990). As the transcription complex moves relative to the DNA template, positive supercoiling accumulates in front of the complex and negative supercoiling behind (Brill *et al.*, 1987; Brill & Sternglaz, 1988; Wu *et al.*, 1988). In prokaryotes, topoisomerase I probably acts as a swivel by relieving the negative supercoiling, while topoisomerase II (DNA gyrase) relieves positive supercoiling in front of the transcription complex (Wang, 1991). In eukaryotes, the relative roles of topoisomerases I and II is less clear since both enzymes can relax either positive or negative supercoiling. Nevertheless, several lines of evidence indicate that topoisomerase I is involved in transcription:

1 Yeast topoisomerase I mutants have reduced transcription rate (Thrash *et al.*, 1984; Brill *et al.*, 1987).

2 Topoisomerase I interacts preferentially with transcriptionally active region of the genome (Fleischmann *et al.*, 1984).

3 Topoisomerase I cleavage sites have been found within actively transcribing genes in diverse systems, including ribosomal DNA (Bonven *et al.*, 1985; Garg *et al.*, 1987; Culotta & Sollner-Webb, 1988; Rose *et al.*, 1988; Zhang *et al.*, 1988), the heat-shock genes (Fleischmann *et al.*, 1984; Gilmour & Elgin, 1987; Kroeger & Rowe, 1989), the tyrosine aminotransferase gene (Stewart & Schutz, 1987), and the c-*fos* gene (Stewart *et al.*, 1990).

4 Camptothecin is a potent RNA synthesis inhibitor (Horwitz *et al.*, 1971; Kann & Kohn, 1972; Zhang *et al.*, 1988; O'Connor *et al.*, 1991) which induces transcription blocks (Bendixen *et al.*, 1990; Stewart *et al.*, 1990).

5 Microinjection of antitopoisomerase I antibodies into cell nuclei leads to a blockage of transcription elongation.

6 Topoisomerase I and RNA polymerases may be associated within functional complexes (Rose *et al.*, 1988; Stewart *et al.*, 1990).

A role for topoisomerase I is also very likely during DNA replication which also generates supercoiling as a result of DNA unwinding by helicases and DNA replication fork progression (Brill *et al.*, 1987). Purified mammalian toposomerase I, in the absence of topoisomerase II, can support the complete replication of SV40 DNA in a cell-free replication system (Yang *et al.*, 1987). However, the product of DNA replication is a multiply interlocked molecule consisting of two replicated daughter SV40 DNA molecules (Yang *et al.*, 1987). In addition, treatment of SV40-infected cells with camptothecin yields abortive SV40 replication intermediates (Snapka, 1986; Yang *et al.*, 1987; Shin & Snapka, 1990a,b). Camptothecin also inhibits DNA synthesis rapidly but for a prolonged period of time in mammalian cells (Horwitz *et al.*, 1971; Duguet *et al.*, 1983; O'Connor *et al.*, 1991). Thus, topoisomerase I through its potent

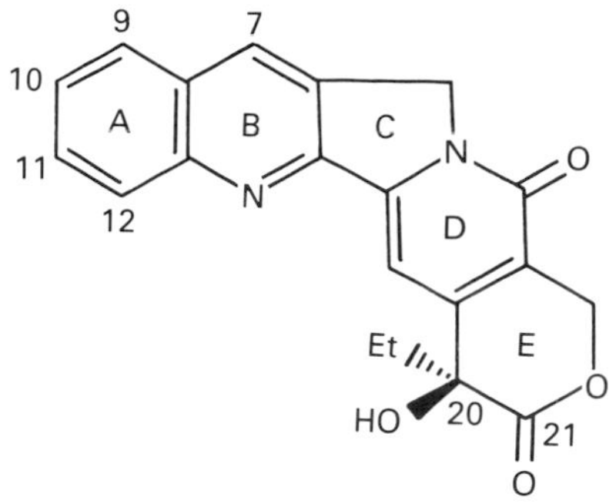

Fig. 9.3. Structure of natural camptothecin (20-S-camptothecin).

DNA relaxing activity probably acts as a key swivel for DNA metabolism, including replication, transcription, repair and recombinations.

Inhibition by camptothecin and its derivatives

Camptothecin (Fig. 9.3) was discovered by Monroe Wall *et al.* in the late 1960s as the alkaloid responsible for the potent antitumour activity of extracts from the Chinese tree, *Camptotheca acuminata* (Wall *et al.*, 1966; Wall, 1983). Soon after, camptothecin was found to cause rapid DNA fragmentation, associated with RNA and DNA synthesis inhibition in cultured cells (Bosmann, 1970; Horwitz & Horwitz, 1971, 1973; Horwitz *et al.*, 1971; Kessel, 1971; Kessel *et al.*, 1972). Clinical trials in the late 1970s showed that the compound was active against human tumours. However, severe side effects, including bladder, gastrointestinal and bone marrow toxicities led to the discontinuation of the clinical trials (Gottlieb *et al.*, 1970; Muggia *et al.*, 1972). A few years ago, camptothecin was tested against purified mammalian DNA topoisomerases and found to be a potent topoisomerase I inhibitor without affecting topoisomerase II (Hsiang *et al.*, 1985). More recently, four lines of evidence demonstrated that topoisomerase I is a major cellular target of camptothecin. Firstly, studies of a series of camptothecin derivatives showed a good correlation between topoisomerase I inhibition and antitumour activity (Jaxel *et al.*, 1989; Nicholas *et al.*, 1990). Secondly, the DNA fragmentation produced in camptothecin-treated cells corresponded to topoisomerase I-mediated DNA breaks (Mattern *et al.*, 1987; Hsiang & Liu, 1988; Covey *et al.*, 1989). Thirdly, cells made resistant to camptothecin failed to produce topoisomerase I-mediated DNA breaks, and their purified topoisomerase I was resistant to camptothecin (Andoh *et al.*, 1987; Kjeldsen *et al.*, 1988a; Tanizawa & Pommier, 1992). Finally, studies in yeast mutants showed that the cytotoxicity of campthotechin can be attributed to its action on topoisomerase I (Eng *et al.*, 1988; Nitiss & Wang, 1988; Bjornsti *et al.*, 1989).

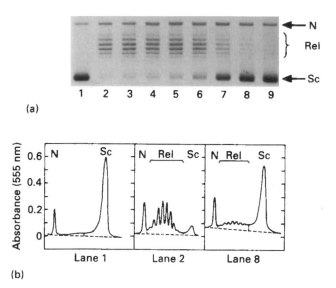

(a)

(b)

Fig. 9.4. Inhibition of DNA relaxation by camptothecin. (a) Native supercoiled simian virus 40 (SV40) DNA (0.2 μg) (Lane 1) was incubated for 10 min at 37°C with 1 unit topoisomerase I in the absence (Lane 2) or presence of *S*-camptothecin: 0.1, 0.3, 1, 3, 10, 30 and 100 μM in lanes 3–9, respectively. Reactions were stopped with 1% sodium dodecylsulphate, followed by digestion for 30 min with 0.5 mg/ml proteinase K. The DNA was analysed by agarose gel electrophoresis in the presence of chloroquine. N, nicked; Rel, relaxed; Sc, supercoiled. The gels were stained with ethidium and photographed. (b) The photographic negatives were densitometer scanned. Lane 1, DNA alone; lane 2, DNA plus enzyme; lane 8, DNA plus enzyme plus camptothecin (30 μM) (Jaxel *et al.*, 1989).

Effects of camptothecin upon purified DNA topoisomerase I

Camptothecin induces DNA single-strand breaks in the presence of DNA topoisomerase I. These breaks have the typical structure of topoisomerase I-mediated DNA breaks, with their 3′–DNA terminus covalently linked to the enzyme via a phosphotyrosine bond (Champoux, 1978; Hsiang & Liu, 1988) (see Fig. 9.2) The breaks are often referred to as 'protein-linked DNA breaks' (Covey *et al.*, 1989) or as 'cleavable complexes' (Hsiang *et al.*, 1985; Wang, 1991) because they are detectable after protein denaturation by sodium dodecylsulphate (SDS) (Champoux, 1976, 1977). Cleavable complexes can be detected either as DNA breaks, and/or as DNA–protein crosslinks. The breaks generate either nicked DNA molecules (form II) when supercoiled DNA is used as a substrate (Fig. 9.4), or single-stranded DNA fragments when linear end-labelled DNA is used, and reactions are run at alkaline pH in order to denature duplex DNA (Fig. 9.5) (Hsiang *et al.*, 1985; Thomsen *et al.*, 1987; Jaxel *et al.*, 1988; Porter & Champoux, 1989b). In the latter case, DNA labelling at the

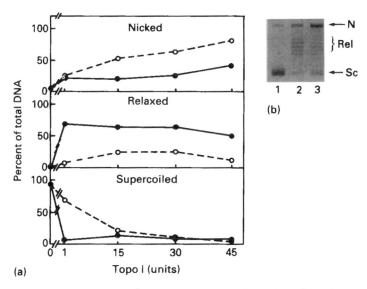

(a)   Topo I (units)

(b)

Fig. 9.5. Inhibition of supercoil relaxation and formation of topoisomerase I–DNA cleavage complexes by camptothecin; dependence on topoisomerase I (topo I) concentration. (a) Simian virus 40 (SV40) DNA (0.1 μg) was incubated with various concentrations of topo I in the presence (– – –o– – –) or absence (—●—) of 100 μM S-camptothecin and analysed by chloroquine agarose gel electrophoresis as in Fig. 9.4. (b) Part of the chloroquine gel. Lane 1, DNA only; lane 2, DNA and 0.75 unit/μl topo I (15 units); lane 3, same with 100 μM camptothecin. N, nicked; Rel, relaxed; Sc, supercoiled DNA (Jaxel et al., 1989).

3′–DNA terminus is preferable for DNA electrophoresis because camptothecin-induced DNA fragments that remain labelled after cleavage are not linked to the enzyme (see Fig. 9.2). While topoisomerase I alone is capable of generating breaks in the DNA, topoisomerase I in the presence of camptothecin exhibits differential cleavage (Fig. 9.5) (Thomsen et al., 1987; Jaxel et al., 1988, 1991b; Porter & Champoux, 1989a; Wassermann et al., 1990). Cleavable complexes can also be detected by SDS–KCl precipitation assay (Hsiang et al., 1985; Trask et al., 1984). In this case, camptothecin generates protein-linked DNA fragments that are labelled at their 5′ end and covalently linked to topoisomerase I at their 3′ end. Finally, cleavable complexes have also been measured by a filter binding assay using randomly labelled DNA as a substrate (Pommier et al., 1990).

Inhibition of topoisomerase I-mediated DNA relaxation by camptothecin is best detectable when limited amount of enzyme is used (Fig. 9.6) (Jaxel et al., 1989). Increasing topoisomerase I usually overcomes camptothecin inhibition (Fig. 9.4) (Jaxel et al., 1989). The most likely explanation of this effect is that camptothecin traps only a subset of the cleavable complexes (Fig. 9.5). Thus, when topoisomerase I is in excess, sites that are not sensitive to camptothecin are catalytically active.

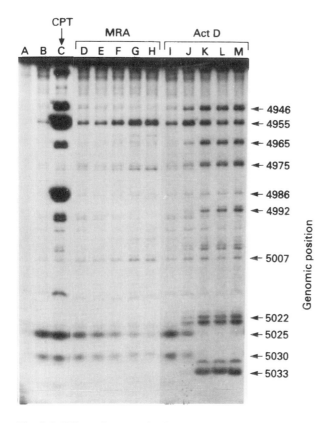

Fig. 9.6. Effect of camptothecin (CPT), morpholinyldoxorubicin (MRA), and actinomycin D (Act D) on sequence-specific cleavages of topoisomerase I (topo I). Reactions were performed with the 4912-5049 uniquely [^{32}P]-3'-end-labelled *Fok* I fragment (137 bp) (Jaxel *et al.*, 1988). The genomic positions of cleavage sites are marked to the right of the figure. Lane A shows the intact fragment. Topo I reactions are shown as follows: lane B, topo I alone; lane C, topo I in the presence of 10 μM CPT; lanes D–H, 0.1, 0.2, 0.5, 1 and 2 μM MRA; lanes I–M, 1, 2, 5, 10 and 20 μM Act D (Wassermann *et al.*, 1990).

Evidence for a camptothecin binding-site within topoisomerase I– DNA complexes

Previous studies indicate that camptothecin alone neither cleaves nor binds to purified DNA under physiological conditions (Li *et al.*, 1972; Fukada, 1985; Hsiang *et al.*, 1985; Kuwahara *et al.*, 1986). Camptothecin has a chiral centre at position 20 (Figs 9.3 & 9.7). Natural camptothecin is 20-S (e.g. the OH is above the plane and the ethyl below) (Fig. 9.7). Total synthesis yields a racemic mixture of 20-S and -R camptothecins. It is striking that the 20-R derivative (Fig. 9.7) is inactive against purified topoisomerase I and is devoid of antitumour activity (Jaxel *et al.*, 1989). Such a stereospecificity lets us hypothesize that camptothecin binds to a

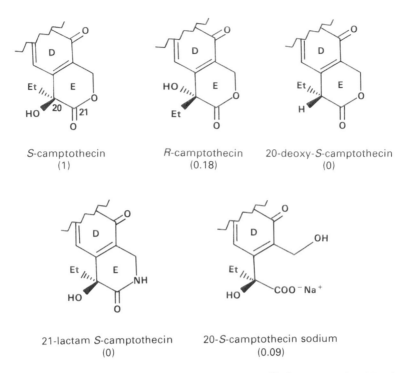

S-camptothecin
(1)

R-camptothecin
(0.18)

20-deoxy-S-camptothecin
(0)

21-lactam S-camptothecin
(0)

20-S-camptothecin sodium
(0.09)

Fig. 9.7. Structure of camptothecin derivatives modified on the E ring. Numbers in parentheses indicate the potency of the derivatives as inhibitors of purified topo-isomerase I, relative to that of camptothecin. No change can be made in the E ring without losing activity.

specific site. Studies with other camptothecin derivatives modified on the lactone ring (E ring, Fig. 9.7) indicate that in addition, opening of the keto–lactone bond is probably critical for activity. Indeed, 20-S camptothecin sodium which forms spontaneously within a few minutes at physiological pH is inactive (Hertzberg et al., 1980b; Hsiang et al., 1989b; Jaxel et al., 1989). The 20-S lactam and the 20-deoxy derivatives which do not undergo facile ring opening are inactive although their steric structure are almost superimposable to that of natural camptothecin (Hertzberg et al., 1989b; Jaxel et al., 1989). Therefore, the ring-opened drug may form a reversible covalent bond with the enzyme via an ester exchange reaction. This might be facilitated by hydrogen bonding of the 20-hydroxyl to an electronegative atom of the enzyme–DNA complex.

Camptothecin analogues modified on the A ring (Fig. 9.8) have also been synthesized (Kunimoto et al., 1987; Wani et al., 1987; Johnson et al., 1989; Kingsburg et al., 1991) and their study has provided important information supporting the hypothesis of a camptothecin receptor (Hertzberg et al., 1989a; Hsiang et al., 1989b; Jaxel et al., 1989). Substitutions at position 12, and to a lesser degree bulky substitutions at the 11 position

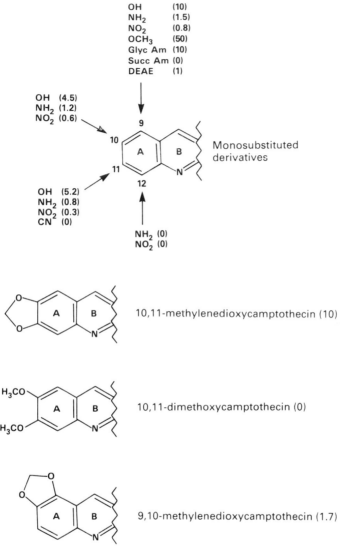

OH   (10)
NH$_2$ (1.5)
NO$_2$ (0.8)
OCH$_3$ (50)
Glyc Am (10)
Succ Am (0)
DEAE   (1)

OH (4.5)
NH$_2$ (1.2)
NO$_2$ (0.6)

9

10

A   B   Monosubstituted
derivatives

11

12

OH   (5.2)
NH$_2$ (0.8)
NO$_2$ (0.3)
CN   (0)

NH$_2$ (0)
NO$_2$ (0)

10,11-methylenedioxycamptothecin (10)

H$_3$CO
H$_3$CO
10,11-dimethoxycamptothecin (0)

9,10-methylenedioxycamptothecin (1.7)

Fig. 9.8. Structure of camptothecin derivatives modified on the A ring. Numbers in parentheses indicate the potency of the derivatives as inhibitors of purified topo-isomerase I, relative to those of the parent compound (20-*S*- or 20-*RS*-camptothecin for the semisynthetic and synthetic compounds, respectively). Substitutions around position 12 cannot be made without losing activity. Substitutions on the other positions can be used to synthesize active camptothecin derivatives.

abolish antitopoisomerase 1 and antitumour activities, indicating that substitutions in this region encroach upon a space that is in close proximity to the enzyme–DNA binding-site (Jaxel *et al.*, 1989). By contrast, substitutions at the 9 and 10 positions generally increase antitopo-

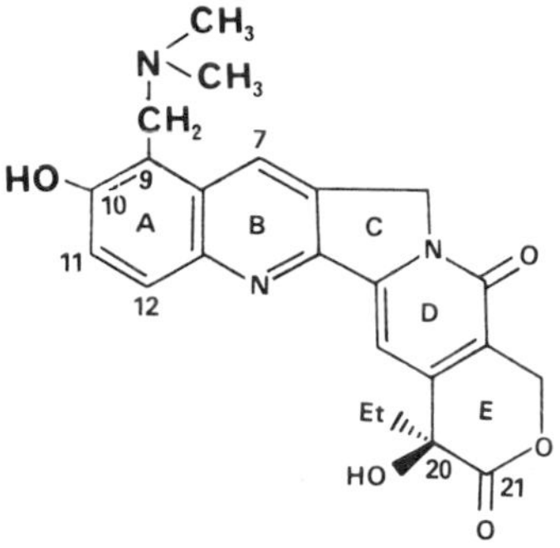

Topotecan (hycamptamine)
9-(dimethylamino)methyl-10-hydroxycamptothecin

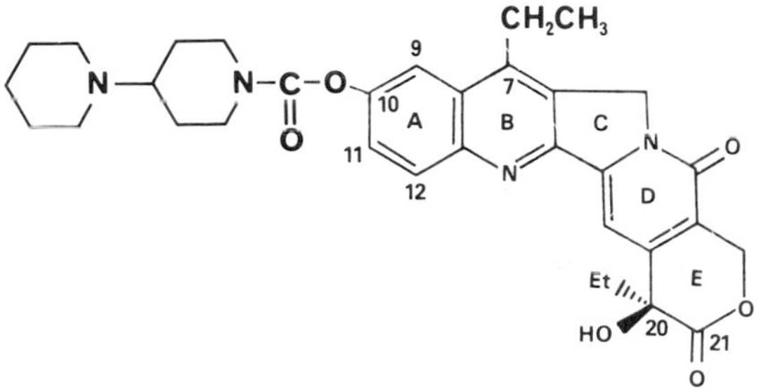

CPT-11 (camptothecin-11)
7-ethyl-10-[4-(1-piperidino)-1-piperidino]carbonyloxy-camptothecin

Fig. 9.9. Structure of topotecan and CPT-11.

isomerase I and antitumour activities (Hertzberg *et al.*, 1989b; Hsiang *et al.*, 1989b; Jaxel *et al.*, 1989). Among the 30 compounds that the authors have tested so far, 10,11-methylenedioxycamptothecin (Fig. 9.8) is one of the most active compounds, with a potency ratio close to 10 when compared to natural camptothecin (Jaxel *et al.*, 1989; O'Connor *et al.*, 1990, 1991; Pommier *et al.*, 1991b).

Drug binding studies with radiolabelled camptothecin and a derivative substituted with an alkylating group at the 9 position have provided further evidence for the existence of a binding site of camptothecin within topoisomerase I–DNA complexes. It was found that camptothecin does not bind to topoisomerase I or to DNA alone, but to the enzyme when in the presence of the DNA (Hertzberg *et al.*, 1990). The water-soluble derivatives that are currently in clinical trials are also semisynthetic camptothecin derivatives with A-ring substitutions. Topotecan (Hycamptamine) is 9-(dimethylamino)methyl-10-hydroxycamptothecin (Johnson *et al.*, 1989) and CPT-11 is 7-ethyl-10[4(1-piperidino)-1-piperidino]carbonyloxy-camptothecin (Kunimoto *et al.*, 1987) (Fig. 9.9). The latter is a prodrug for 7-ethyl-10-hydroxy-camptothecin (SN-38) which is more potent than camptothecin (Kaneda *et al.*, 1990; Kawato *et al.*, 1991).

Further clues for the nature of the drug binding-sites have been obtained by sequencing analysis of topoisomerase I cleavage sites induced in the absence and presence of camptothecin (Fig. 9.6). Camptothecin analogues differ in potency but produce a unique cleavage pattern (Jaxel *et al.*, 1989). This pattern is different from that of topoisomerase I in the absence of drug because only a subset of the enzyme cleavage sites are enhanced by camptothecins (Porter & Champoux, 1989a; Wasserman *et al.*, 1990; Jaxel *et al.*, 1991b). In other words, some topoisomerase I cleavage sites are not trapped by camptothecin and sometimes are even suppressed. Similar observations have been made by others in different genes (Kjeldsen *et al.*, 1988b). Thus, it is likely that camptothecin derivatives differ primarily by their binding constants to similar receptor sites. We have recently obtained evidence that these receptor sites involve the DNA base pairs immediately around the cleavage sites (Jaxel *et al.*, 1991a). Base preferences at camptothecin cleavage sites were analysed by first aligning the DNA sequences of all the cleavage sites in the 5′ to 3′ orientation with respect to the cleaved bond. The bases at the 3′- and at the 5′-termini of the breaks were numbered (-1) and $(+1)$, respectively (Fig. 9.10). At each position the number of occurrence of each base (A, G, T or C) was determined and the corresponding probability of random occurrence calculated (Fig. 9.10). By convention, probabilities of excessive base occurrence were plotted above the base line, and probabilities of defective base occurrence were plotted below the base line. Both in the absence of drug and in the presence of camptothecin, the strongest base preference was T at position (-1), e.g. at the 3′-terminus of the breaks where topoisomerase I is covalently linked to the DNA. By contrast, position $(+1)$ did not show significant preference in the absence of drug, while in the presence of camptothecin, G was strongly preferred (Fig. 9.10). The requirement for $G(+1)$ was further investigated in oligonucleotides containing the major SV40 DNA cleavage site (Jaxel *et al.*, 1988) in their centre. Mutations of the $(+1)$ base pair showed that topoisomerase I cleavage in the absence of drug was not affected by the nature of the $(+1)$ base, while in the presence of camptothecin, cleavage was maximal when a G was present, minimal when it was a T, and intermediate when it was either A or C (Jaxel *et al.*, 1991b). The simplest interpretation of these results is that camptothecin interacts with the base at the 5′-terminus of topoisomerase I-induced DNA breaks. Therefore, the current view is that the quasi-planar multiring system of camptothecin binds by stacking with the G at the 5′-terminus of the breaks $((+1)$ positions) (Fig. 9.11). Such a model is attractive because it is consistent with the one that the authors have recently developed for topoisomerase II inhibitors (Capranico *et al.*, 1990b; Pommier *et al.*, 1991a).

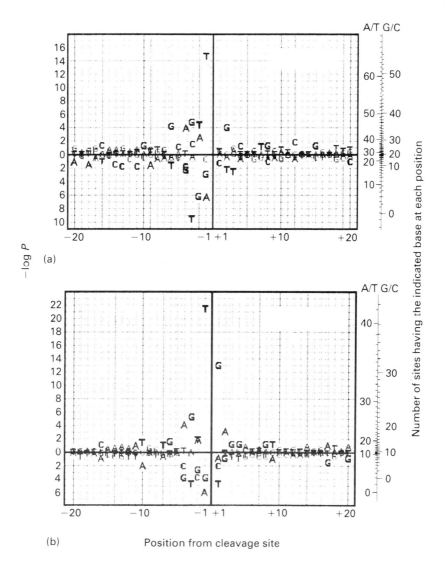

Fig. 9.10. Probability of base occurrence at topoisomerase I cleavage sites induced in the absence (a, 91 sites) or presence of camptothecin (b, 41 sites). In the ordinate, P is the probabilities of the observed base frequency deviations from expectation at each position, either as excess (above base-line) or deficiency (below base-line) relative to the expected frequency for each individual base. The expected frequencies are based on the overall base frequency of simian virus 40 (SV40) DNA. The number of occurrences of each base (A/T or G/C) corresponding to the log P scale are given on separate scales on the right (Jaxel *et al.*, 1991a).

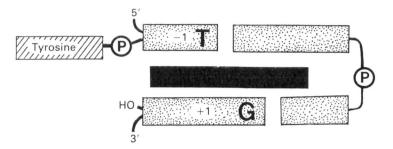

Fig. 9.11. Model for camptothecin binding to topoisomerase I–DNA complexes. Schematic representation of a ternary complex between camptothecin (black rectangle), DNA and topoisomerase I (topo I) (tyrosine residue). Camptothecin binds reversibly between the -1 and $+1$ base pairs, and stabilizes the covalent topo I cleavage intermediate preferentially at $+1$ G sites.

Camptothecin-induced DNA damage in cells

Camptothecin-induced DNA breaks were first detected by alkaline sucrose sedimentation (Horwitz & Horwitz, 1971). Presently, the two methods of choice are measurement of cleavable complexes by alkaline elution (Mattern *et al.*, 1987; Covey *et al.*, 1989; Hsiang *et al.*, 1989b) and SDS-KCl precipitation assays (Hsiang & Liu, 1988). Alkaline elution measures DNA single- and double-strand breaks and DNA–protein cross-links, while SDS-KCl precipitation measures only DNA–protein complexes. By using alkaline elution, we have shown that camptothecin produces equal frequencies of DNA single-strand breaks and DNA–protein crosslinks in Chinese hamster and human colon carcinoma cells and in their isolated nuclei (Covey *et al.*, 1989; Holm *et al.*, 1989; O'Connor *et al.*, 1990, 1991). The 1:1 stoichiometry between the two types of lesion is expected for topoisomerase I-mediated DNA breaks. In addition, the breaks are 'protein-linked' since they are not detectable under non-deproteinizing conditions. Three important technical comments must be made regarding the detection of camptothecin-induced DNA damage by alkaline elution (for more details see Covey *et al.*, 1989). Firstly, the detergent used for cell lysis is critical since two-fold more breaks and DNA–protein crosslinks are detectable with SDS than with sarkosyl (LS-10 lysis solution). This property is inherent to topoisomerase I–DNA cleavable complexes since similar results are obtained with purified topoisomerase I (Covey *et al.*, 1989). Secondly, camptothecin must be kept in the culture medium until cell lysis because camptothecin-induced DNA breaks reverse within minutes after drug removal even if the drug is removed from cells at 0°C. Thirdly, internal standard cells must be added immediately before lysis. Otherwise the presence of camptothecin in the medium induces DNA breaks in the internal standard cells even if these cells are added to the test cells at 0°C. The fact that camptothecin-induced DNA damage forms and reverses at 0°C is also observed with purified topoisomerase I (Covey *et al.*, 1989). This is different from topoisomerase II-induced cleavable complexes which fail to form or to reverse after drug removal at 0°C (Zwelling *et al.*, 1981).

DNA double-strand breaks have recently been detected by pulse-field gel electrophoresis (Ryan *et al.*, 1991). In contrast to the protein-linked single-strand breaks described above, they persist for several hours following drug removal. It is likely that these breaks are analogous to the double-stranded breaks that arise in replicating SV40 DNA (Yang *et al.*, 1987; Avemann *et al.*, 1988; Shin & Snapka, 1990a,b), and that they correspond to damaged replication forks (see below).

Other topoisomerase I inhibitors

DNA intercalators inhibit topoisomerase I activity at drug concentrations that produce detectable DNA unwinding (Pommier *et al.*, 1987). This effect is not associated with the formation of cleavable complexes and is detectable with limited amount of enzyme (Pommier *et al.*, 1987). It is not specific since it can be observed with a variety of intercalators, including ethidium bromide, acridine derivatives, anthracyclines and ellipticines (Pommier *et al.*, 1987). The most likely explanation for this effect is that DNA intercalators bind directly at topoisomerase I catalytic sites and/or alter DNA structure and topoisomerase I binding.

The DNA minor groove binder, distamycin; also inhibits catalytic activity at high-affinity topoisomerase I binding sequences (Mortensen *et al.*, 1990) and in bent DNA from kinetoplast (Caserta *et al.*, 1989). In contrast to camptothecin, and by analogy with DNA intercalators, this inhibition is not associated with cleavable complex formation. Inhibition of catalytic activity is probably due to distamycin binding directly at enzyme cleavage sites, since distamycin inhibits topoisomerase I-mediated DNA cleavage at drug binding-sites. Also, distamycin and other DNA minor groove binders decrease camptothecin-induced DNA damage in isolated nuclei (McHugh *et al.*, 1990). Thus, inhibition of both DNA topoisomerases I and II by distamycin are comparable (Fesen & Pommier, 1989). Both in the case of DNA intercalators and distamycin, the most likely explanation for topoisomerase I inhibition is that drug binding to the DNA at topoisomerase I binding sequences prevent catalytic activity.

Three intercalators, actinomycin D (Trask & Muller, 1988; Wassermann *et al.*, 1990), morpholinyldoxorubicin (Trask & Muller, 1988) and saintopin (Yamashita *et al.*, 1991) can also induce topoisomerase I cleavable complexes (Trask & Muller, 1988; Wassermann *et al.*, 1990). It is quite remarkable that for each drug, cleavable complexes have a specific sequence selectivity (Fig. 9.6) (Wassermann *et al.*, 1990; Yamashita *et al.*, 1991). In the case of actinomycin D, which also induces topoisomerase II

cleavable complexes, there is no obvious relationship between topoisomerase I cleavage sites and preferential intercalation sequences (Wassermann *et al.*, 1990). Therefore, DNA intercalation is probably not
sufficient for poisoning of topoisomerase I and II complexes. Saintopin
inhibits both topoisomerase I and II (Yamashita *et al.*, 1991). Topoisomerase I inhibition by morpholinyldoxorubicin appears more specific
since morpholinyldoxorubicin does not induce topoisomerase II cleavable
complexes, while doxorubicin induces only topoisomerase II but not topoisomerase I cleavable complexes. Nevertheless, these findings suggest
topoisomerase I and II inhibition may share common mechanisms.

Topoisomerase I gene(s)

A partial human topoisomerase I cDNA clone has been isolated and
sequenced (D'Arpa *et al.*, 1988). It encodes 765 amino acids and its active
tyrosine, presumably Tyr^{723} (Lynn *et al.*, 1989), is located in the carboxyl
terminus of the protein. The Genbank data base accession number of this
topoisomerase I sequence is J03250 (Huang, 1990). By using this probe, a
single copy gene has been identified on chromosone 20q (D'Arpa *et al.*,
1988; Juan *et al.*, 1988). Two additional truncated topoisomerase I genes
have also been mapped on human chromosome 1 q23-24, and 22 q11.2–
13.1 (Kunze *et al.*, 1990; Yang *et al.*, 1990). These pseudogenes harbour
sequences corresponding to the 3′ half of the coding sequence of the active
topoisomerase I gene. The apparent discrepancy between chromosomal
locations might depend on the hybridization probes. D'Arpa *et al.* used
the whole topoisomerase I cDNA to search for the gene, while Juan *et al.*
used a 5′ section of the gene, and Kunze *et al.* the 3′ terminal portion.
Zhou *et al.* (1989) characterized the 3′ region of topoisomerase I gene(s)
from six human cell lines and also suggested the existence of pseudogenes
which appeared to be hypomethylated. A three allele Taq I polymorphism
at the active topoisomerase I gene has also been reported (Sunde *et al.*,
1990). At the present time, it is unknown whether the different pseudogenes encode active enzymes.

   In addition to the above studies on human topoisomerase I, extensive
genetic analyses have been performed in yeast (Thrash *et al.*, 1985;
Uemura *et al.*, 1987), and in vaccinia virus which encodes a 33 kDa
topoisomerase I (Shuman & Moss, 1987), and more recently in Shope
fibroma virus (Upton *et al.*, 1990). Amino acid sequence homology
between human and yeast topoisomerase I (*Saccharomyces cerevisiae*) is
42% (D'Arpa *et al.*, 1988), while there is no significant sequence similarity
between human and *Escherichia coli* topoisomerases I. By using site-
directed mutagenesis and peptide sequencing of covalent enzyme–DNA
adducts, the amino acid covalently linked to the cleaved 3′-DNA terminus
has been mapped at tyr-771 for *S. pombe* and tyr-727 for *S. cerevisiae* (Eng

et al., 1989; Lynn *et al.*, 1989). Covalent linkage at a tyrosine residue is also the case for *E. coli* (tyr-319; Lynn *et al.*, 1989) and vaccinia virus topoisomerases I (tyr-274; Shuman *et al.*, 1989). By amino acid sequence analogy, tyr-723 has been deduced as the active tyrosine of human topoisomerase I. A motif, Ser-Lys-Xaa-Xaa-Tyr, is proposed to be common to the active site of viral and cellular topoisomerases I (Shuman *et al.*, 1989). In addition to the active tyr site, several reports indicate that other regions are also important for topoisomease I activity. In *E. coli* topoisomerase I, Beran-Steed and Tse-Dinh (1989) found that the carboxyl terminal domain confers higher affinity to DNA when compared to a truncated topoisomerase I which lacks C-terminal domain. Interestingly vaccinia topoisomerase I is resistant to the effect of camptothecin (Shuman & Moss, 1988). Since vaccinia virus topoisomerase I is smaller than its human counterpart, it is possible that the vaccinia enzyme lacks the camptothecin binding-site(s). Comparison of the amino acids immediately around the active tyrosine shows that the vaccinia enzyme lacks the three amino acid residues immediately towards the C-terminus end of the enzyme (Asp-Prol-Arg), indicating that these amino acids may be involved in the formation of the camptothecin binding-site. Further studies using site-directed mutagenesis are underway in order to test this observation.

Regulation of topoisomerase I

Understanding the regulation of topoisomerase I may provide important insights for improving the chemotherapeutic efficiency of topoisomerase I inhibitors alone or in combination with other anticancer agents.

Cell cycle regulation

While topoisomerase II activity appears to be tightly linked to cell proliferation, increasing sharply during S phase before dropping to low level G1 phase, topoisomerase I activity is more constant during cell cycle and is present in non-dividing cells. However, the data are not consistent. Some reports indicate that topoisomerase I activity, as measured by the DNA relaxing activity of nuclear extracts, increases during or just prior to S phase (Rosenberg *et al.*, 1976; Poccia *et al.*, 1978; Taudou *et al.*, 1984; Tricoli *et al.*, 1985), while others find very little fluctuations in enzymatic activity (Duguet *et al.*, 1983). In addition, immunoblotting with topoisomerase I antibodies shows that the enzyme does not significantly fluctuate in content or stability across the cell cycle in normal and transformed chicken cell lines (Heck *et al.*, 1988), and increases two-fold in serum-stimulated fibroblasts while its specific activity remains constant (Romig & Richter, 1990a). The quantitative discrepancies above may depend on cell types and/or topoisomerase I extraction and assay procedures (Tricoli *et al.*, 1985). Nevertheless, topoisomerase I activity appears to fluctuate less than that of topoisomerase II as a function of cell cycle. This point may be of considerable interest with respect to chemotherapy since a large fraction of tumour cells divide very slowly, and therefore could be targetted with topoisomerase I inhibitors..

Gene regulation

Increased transcription (five- to 10-fold *m*RNA increase) has been reported in serum-stimulated fibroblasts (Romig & Richter, 1990a) and after treatment with phorbol 12-myristate 13-acetate (PMA) (Hwong *et al.*, 1989), as well as in HeLa cells infected with adenovirus 5 (Romig & Richter, 1990b). This three- to five-fold increase is due to a transactivation of the topoisomerase I gene by the E1A protein, which is an early adenovirus protein coded by the E1A region. However, in this case the amount of topoisomerase I protein and its activity remain constant. These results suggest that topoisomerase I activity is regulated both at the transcriptional and at the translational and post-translational levels. More recently, the 5′ region of the topoisomerase I gene has been cloned and several regulatory binding sequences have been identified, including a retinoic acid binding-site (A. Harris, personal communication). By using the same approach, Kunze *et al.* (1990) found that the gene contains neither a 'TATA' nor a 'CAAT' box, but several motifs which are known as binding sites for transcription factors (Oct1, Sp1, Ap2). This type of study coupled with the use of reporter genes will probably provide important information for the regulation mechanisms involved in topoisomerase I expression.

Topoisomerase I phosphorylation

Several reports demonstrated that active topoisomerase I is a phosphoprotein since dephosphorylation by alkaline phosphatase abolishes catalytic activity and camptothecin sensitivity (Durban *et al.*, 1983; Tse-Dinh *et al.*, 1984; Kaiserman *et al.*, 1988; Samuel *et al.*, 1989; Coderoni *et al.*, 1990; Pommier *et al.*, 1990). The observations that: (i) topoisomerase I phosphorylation by purified protein kinase C restores catalytic activity and camptothecin sensitivity; (ii) protein kinase C copurifies with topoisomerase I; and (iii) certain forms of protein kinase C have been identified in isolated nuclei (Girard *et al.*, 1985; Capitani *et al.*, 1987; Kraft *et al.*, 1987; Misra & Sahyoun, 1987; Masmoudi *et al.*, 1989; Pommier *et al.*, 1990), suggest that topoisomerase I may be regulated by signal transduction pathways. This hypothesis is supported by the findings that treatment of cells with hormones and growth factors (Nambi *et al.*, 1989, 1990), as well as leukotriene D_4 (Mattern *et al.*, 1990) and phorbol esters rapidly stimulate topoisomerase I catalytic activity and camptothecin-induced DNA breaks (D. Kerrigan & Y. Pommier, unpublished results). Other protein kinases may also act upon topoisomerase I (Durban *et al.*, 1983). While casein kinase II which phosphorylates serine and threonine residues, activates topoisomerase II (Ackerman *et al.*, 1985, 1988), its role in regulating topoisomerase I has not been established. Tyrosine phosphorylation by P60^{src} has been shown to inactivate purified topoisomerases *in vitro* (Tse-Dinh *et al.*, 1984), but there is no evidence of such a role in cells.

Poly(adenosine diphosphoribosylation)

Purified topoisomerase I is a major acceptor of poly(ADP-ribose) and the activity of the topoisomerase I associated with poly(ADP-ribose) is diminished three- to five-fold (Ferro *et al.*, 1983, 1984a,b; Jongstra-Bilen *et al.*, 1983; Ferro & Olivera, 1984; Darby *et al.*, 1985; Krupita & Cerutti, 1989). Consistent with these data is the finding that the camptothecin-induced DNA breaks are reduced in cells pretreated with the poly(ADP-ribose) inhibitor, 3-aminobenzamide (Mattern *et al.*, 1987). Other, post-transcriptional modifications, such as interactions with acidic phospholipids (Tamura *et al.*, 1990) and heparin (Ishii *et al.*, 1987) may also down-regulate catalytic activity.

Chromatin structure

At the DNA level, topoisomerase I-binding can be influenced by chromatin structure. Comparison of camptothecin-induced DNA breaks in SV40 DNA and in minichromosomes, demonstrate that nucleosome formation abolishes topoisomerase I cleavage (Capranico *et al.*, 1990a; Jaxel *et al.*, 1991b). By contrast, histone H1 and high mobility group (HMG) proteins have been shown to stimulate catalytic activity *in vitro* and to form tight complexes with topoisomerase I (Javaherian & Liu, 1983). Thus, it is likely that specific DNA binding proteins, including transcription factors, regulate enzyme binding and catalytic activity. In addition, natural polyamines, such as spermine and spermidine also modulate enzyme activity with stimulation at low concentrations and inhibition at millimolar concentrations (Srivenugopal & Morris, 1985).

Cytotoxicity of camptothecin

Camptothecin-induced cell killing is different from topoisomerase II inhibitor-induced cell killing. This is best exemplified by the observation that 30-min treatments of exponentially growing cells with various camptothecin concentrations yields limited toxicity (Fig. 9.12a), while in the

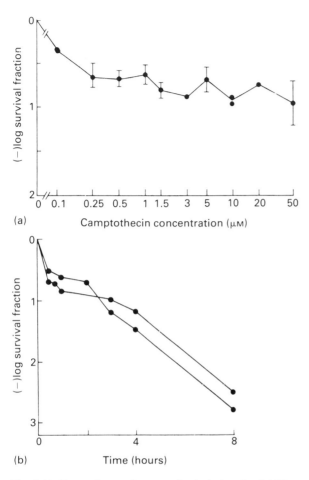

Fig. 9.12. Dependence of camptothecin-induced cell killing upon drug concentration and exposure time in Chinese hamster DC3F cells (Holm *et al.*, 1989). (a) Concentration-dependence of 30-min treatments at 37°C. Error bars denote standard deviation of at least three independent experiments. (b) Time-dependence of camptothecin-induced cytotoxicity. Cells were treated with 0.25 μM camptothecin for the indicated time periods. Two independent experiments are shown.

case of topoisomerase II inhibitors cytotoxicity is almost a linear function of the drug concentration logarithm (Holm *et al.*, 1989). With camptothecin, maximum cytotoxicity is obtained at low drug concentrations (between 0.1 and 0.5 μM) and is not increased further by increasing drug concentration 100-fold. Thus, 10–20% of exponentially growing cells are naturally resistant to camptothecin. The finding that resistance can be overcome by increasing drug exposure time (Fig. 9.12b), suggests that camptothecin is only active against a subpopulation of proliferating cells. This is in agreement with early studies demonstrating that S and G2-phase cells are more sensitive than G1 phase cells, although DNA breaks are

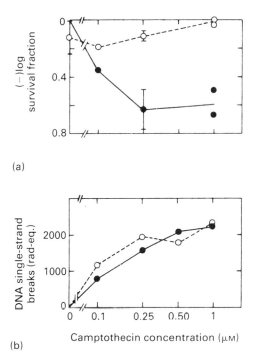

(a)

(b)

Camptothecin concentration (μM)

Fig. 9.13. Effects of aphidicolin on camptothecin-induced cytotoxicity (a) and DNA single-strand breaks (b) in DC3F cells. Cells were either treated with camptothecin alone (●) or camptothecin and aphidicolin (○). Aphidicolin treatments (10 μM) were started 5 min before the addition of camptothecin and continued throughout the 30-min camptothecin treatments. DNA breaks were assayed by alkaline elution immediately at the end of drug treatments; a typical experiment is shown in (b). Error bars denote standard deviations of at least three independent cloning experiments (Holm *et al.*, 1989).

detectable in both populations (Kessel *et al.*, 1972; Li *et al.*, 1972; Horwitz & Horwitz, 1973). The finding of similar DNA breaks in both cell populations is consistent with the above-mentioned fact that topoisomerase I is present throughout the cell cycle.

This key observation has been explored further in order to demonstrate the role of active replication in the cytoxicity of camptothecin. Short pretreatment of cells with the DNA synthesis inhibitors, aphidicolin or hydroxyurea abolish the cytotoxicity of camptothecin (Fig. 9.13) (Holm *et al.*, 1989; Hsiang *et al.*, 1989a). However, under these conditions, the frequency of camptothecin-induced DNA breaks is not altered by DNA synthesis inhibition (Fig. 9.13). By contrast, similar pretreatments inhibit only partially the cytotoxicity of topoisomerase II inhibitors (Holm *et al.*, 1989). These observations demonstrate that the occurrence of topoisomerase I-mediated DNA breaks is not sufficient for cell killing by camptothecin. Rather, collision of active replication forks with

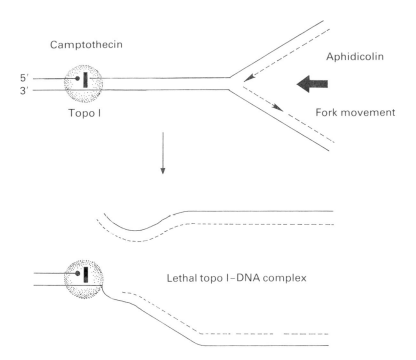

Fig. 9.14. Model for camptothecin-induced cytotoxicity (replication forks).

camptothecin-trapped topoisomerase I–DNA cleavage complexes must occur for lethality. This model implies that only those few camptothecin-induced DNA breaks occurring within replicating genes may be lethal. The exact alterations of the replication complexes that 'collide' into the topoisomerase I–DNA complexes remain poorly defined. It is possible that DNA polymerase dissociates from the DNA at the 5′-OH termini of the topoisomerase I-mediated DNA breaks, and that this process generates DNA double-strand breaks in newly replicated DNA (Fig. 9.14). This type of DNA lesion may be difficult to repair for the cell. Such lesions have been identified in genomic DNA by pulse-field gel electrophoresis (Ryan *et al.*, 1991), and in replicating SV40 DNA (Fleischmann *et al.*, 1987; Yang *et al.*, 1987; Avemann *et al.*, 1988; Shin & Snapka, 1990a). A corollary of these observations is that topoisomerase I plays an active role in DNA replication. The enzyme may relax the torsional tension that accumulates on both the leading and the lagging strands upstream and downstream of replication bubbles (Shin & Snapka, 1990a). This may explain why DNA replication inhibition is only partially reversible after camptothecin removal, while topoisomerase I-induced DNA breaks reverse very quickly (Horwitz *et al.*, 1971; Kessel *et al.*, 1972; Covey *et al.*, 1989; Holm *et al.*, 1989; O'Connor *et al.*, 1991).

We have shown recently that calcium is an important cofactor of camptothecin-induced cytoxicity. Calcium-depleted cells are resistant to camptothecin although DNA synthesis and topoisomerase I-mediated DNA breaks still occur (Bertrand *et al.*, 1991). Calcium is an important cofactor of protein kinases and cell signalling pathways. Therefore, cell death may involve the active participation of such processes that in turn induce active cell death. In HL-60 cells, indeed, camptothecin can induce DNA fragmentation by apoptosis (Kaufmann, 1989).

Finally, independent investigators have demonstrated that association of camptothecin with topoisomerase II inhibitors produces antagonistic effect (D'Arpa *et al.*, 1990; Kaufmann, 1991; Bertrand *et al.*, 1992). The protective effect of simultaneous camptothecin and VP-16 exposure is not due to reduced formation or alterations in the rates of cleavable complex formation and reversal since protection persists for a considerably longer period of time than DNA strand breaks (Bertrand *et al.*, 1992). Rather, protection correlates with the kinetics of DNA and RNA synthesis inhibition produced by either drug (see above). Remarkably, full cytotoxic protection could be afforded by one drug over the other, in the presence of only partial inhibition of DNA or RNA synthesis (50–60%).

Resistance to camptothecin

Drug-resistant cell lines are useful for understanding not only the mechanism of drug-induced cell killing but also the molecular interactions between the drugs and their target enzymes or substrates. Since camptothecin has not been used routinely in the clinical field yet, there is no available camptothecin-resistant cell line isolated from cancer patients and no available data to explain how camptothecin-resistance develops in malignant cells following clinical chemotherapy. However, several camptothecin- or CPT-11-resistant cell lines have been established *in vitro* and two cell lines have been developed from P388 cells *in vivo* (Andoh *et al.*, 1987; Gupta *et al.*, 1988; Eng *et al.*, 1990; Kanzawa *et al.*, 1990; Sugimoto *et al.*, 1990). Two different approaches have been used to isolate camptothecin-resistant cell lines. In one procedure, parental cells are first treated with alkylating agent such as ethylmethanesulphonate (EMS) to mutagenize and then selected for camptothecin resistance. In the other, cells are continuously cultured in the presence of camptothecin at concentrations that are gradually increased. Based on the mechanism for camptothecin resistance, these cell lines can be categorized into two groups. In one group, resistant cells have reduced amounts of camptothecin-sensitive topoisomerase I protein. In the other, camptothecin-resistant enzyme is presumably responsible for drug resistance, regardless of the amount of topoisomerase I present.

Quantitative reduction of topoisomerase I is a common mechanism of drug-induced resistance. Sugimoto *et al.* (1990) found a reduction of cellular topoisomerase I content in three out of four camptothecin-resistant cell lines, with purified topoisomerase I from one of these cell lines showing similar relaxation activity compared to the parental line. The authors concluded that the most frequently occurring event in the development of camptothecin resistance was the quantitative reduction of topoisomerase I. Three other camptothecin-resistant cell lines were also found to have decreased enzyme levels: camptothecin-resistant CHO cells (Gupta et al., 1988), P388 cells (Eng et al., 1990) and human lung cancer cells (Kanzawa et al., 1990). In the P388 resistant cells, down-regulation of topoisomerase I was postulated as secondary to rearrangement and hypermethylation of the topoisomerase I gene (Eng et al., 1990).

Qualitative alterations of topoisomerase I have been identified in a variety of camptothecin-resistant cell lines (Andoh et al., 1987; Gupta et al., 1988; Kanzawa et al., 1990; Tanizawa & Pommier, 1992). These cell lines have been isolated by two different procedures: either by continuous and stepwise exposure to camptothecin or CPT-11 (Andoh et al., 1987 and Kanzawa et al., 1990, respectively), or by selection of mutagenized cells (with EMS) with camptothecin (Gupta et al., 1988; Tanizawa & Pommier, 1992). Topoisomerase I alterations have been well characterized in the cell line described by Andoh et al. Its mutant topoisomerase I cleaves an enzyme recognition sequence with two-fold higher efficiency than the wild-type enzyme and forms more stable cleavable complexes (Kjeldsen et al., 1988a). Resistance has been attributed to the presence of two mutations which cause amino acid changes from aspartic acid to glycine (Tamura et al., 1990). These mutations may confer resistance by altering the camptothecin binding-sites. However the two mutations are not in a vicinity of active tyrosine, suggesting some protein folding in order for these amino acids to be in close proximity to the DNA cleavage site where camptothecin probably binds (Jaxel et al., 1991a).

Camptothecin uptake or metabolism may also be subject to regulation. In CPT-11-resistant cells, intracellular formation of SN-38, an active metabolite of CPT-11 (Kaneda et al., 1990), is two-fold less than in parental cells (Kanzawa et al., 1990). At the present time, there is no resistant cell line that exhibits reduced intracellular camptothecin accumulation as a primary mechanism for resistance. Furthermore, camptothecin does not inhibit [^{3}H]vincristine binding to plasma membrane of Adriamycin-resistant K562 cells (Naito et al., 1988) and CPT-11 is active against pleiotropic drug-resistant tumours, such as vincristine-resistant and Adriamycin-resistant P388 cell lines (Tsuruo et al., 1988). These observations indicate that camptothecin and CPT-11 are not substrates for multidrug-resistant drug efflux systems and suggest some camptothecin derivatives may be useful in overcoming human tumour multidrug resistance.

Mutant cell lines exhibiting either collateral hypersensitivity or cross-resistance to camptothecin may be interesting for understanding the biochemical function of topoisomerase I and the cellular effects of camptothecin. Chatterjee *et al.* (1989) reported that a poly(ADP-ribose) polymerase-deficient Chinese hamster cell line was hypersensitive to camptothecin. In these cells, camptothecin-induced DNA single-strand breaks were similar to those of parental cells, indicating that defective DNA repair may increase the cytotoxicity of camptothecin. Consistent with this hypothesis is the finding that the X ray-senstive CHO-K1 cell line, which was first selected for hypersensitivity to topoisomerase II inhibitors, is defective in DNA double-strand break repair and is five-fold crossresistant to camptothecin (Hickson *et al.*, 1990).

It is also interesting that several camptothecin-resistant cell lines show collateral hypersensitivity to topoisomerase II inhibitors (Gupta *et al.*, 1988; Sugimoto *et al.*, 1990). Sugimoto *et al.* (1990) demonstrated increase of cellular content of topoisomerase II protein and *m*RNA in camptothecin-resistant cell lines. In yeast, topoisomerase I is not essential for viability and topoisomerase II can substitute for topoisomerase I (Thrash *et al.*, 1985).

Conclusion

Topoisomerase I has become an important target for cancer chemotherapy since camptothecin has been shown to be a specific enzyme inhibitor and a potent antitumour agent in animal model systems (Giovanella *et al.*, 1989). Clinical trials of water soluble camptothecin are underway and will determine the anticancer activity of this type of drugs. New camptothecin analogues are also being considered for development. The availability of purified topoisomerase I has facilitated screening procedures. It will be interesting to find new families of topoisomerase I inhibitors and to investigate their molecular interactions with purified topoisomerase I.

We are presently learning a lot about topoisomerase I, its gene(s), and its cellular regulation. This will enable a rational approach to the application of topoisomerase I inhibitors to both sensitive and resistant tumours. The cytotoxic mechanisms of camptothecin are better understood than those of topoisomerase II inhibitors. It is clear that topoisomerase I inhibition is a prerequisite for drug activity. However, the formation of cleavable complexes is not sufficient for cell death and DNA replication and protein kinases are probably key determinants of drug activity.

The molecular interactions between camptothecin and topoisomerase I–DNA complexes remain to be determined. Although structure–activity studies suggest that camptothecin binds with stereospecificity to a specific binding or even receptor site, the structure of its binding site remains to be determined. Determination of the molecular structure of this binding site may provide enormous possibilities for the rational design of new topoisomerase I inhibitors.

Acknowledgements

We wish to thank Ms Donna Kerrigan and Dr Mark Fesen for critical reading of the manuscript and valuable suggestions. Thanks to Dr K.W. Kohn for his support during the course of our studies with topoisomerase inhibitors.

References

Ackerman, P., Glover, C.V. & Osheroff, N. (1985). Phosphorylation of DNA topoisomerase II by casein kinase II: modulation of eukaryotic topoisomerase II activity *in vitro*. *Proceedings of the National Academy of Sciences USA* **82**, 3164–3168.

Ackerman, P., Glover, C.V. & Osheroff, N. (1988). Phosphorylation of DNA topoisomerase II *in vivo* and in total homogenates of *Drosophila* Kc cells. The role of casein kinase II. *Journal of Biological Chemistry* **263**, 12653–12660.

Andoh, T., Ishii, K., Suzuki, Y., Ikegami, Y., Kusunoki, Y., Takemoto, Y. & Okada, K. (1987). Characterization of a mammalian mutant with a camptothecin-resistant DNA topoisomerase I. *Proceedings of the National Academy of Sciences USA* **84**, 5565–5569.

Avemann, K., Knippers, R., Koller, T. & Sogo, J.M. (1988). Camptothecin, a specific inhibitor of type I DNA topoisomerase, induces DNA breakage at replication forks. *Molecular and Cellular Biology* **8**, 3026–3034.

Bauer, W.R., Ressner, E.C., Kates, J. & Patzke, J.V. (1977). A DNA nicking-closing enzyme encapsidated in vaccinia viurs: partial purification and properties. *Proceedings of the National Academy of Sciences USA* **74**, 1841–1845.

Been, M.D., Burgess, R.R. & Champoux, J.J. (1984). Nucleotide sequence preference at rat liver and wheat germ type 1 DNA topoisomerase breakage sites in duplex SV40 DNA. *Nucleic Acids Research* **12**, 3097–3114.

Been, M.D. & Champoux, J.J. (1984). Breakage of single-stranded DNA by eukaryotic type 1 topoisomerase occurs only at regions with the potential for base-pairing. *Journal of Molecular Biology* **180**, 515–531.

Bendixen, C., Thomsen, B., Alsner, J. & Westergaard, O. (1990). Camptothecin-stabilized topoisomerase I-DNA adducts cause premature termination of transcription. *Biochemistry* **29**, 5613–5619.

Beran-Steed, R.K. & Tse-Dinh, Y. (1989). The carboxyl terminal domain of *Escherichia coli* DNA topoisomerase I confers higher affinity to DNA. *Proteins, Structure, Function and Genetics* **6**, 249–258.

Bertrand, R., Kerrigan, D., Sarang, M. & Pommier, Y. (1991). Cell death induced by topoisomerase inhibitors: role of calcium in mammalian cells. *Biochemical Pharmacology* **42**, 77–85.

Bertrand, R. O'Connor, P.M., Kerrigan, D. & Pommier, Y. (1992). Sequential administration of camptothecin and etoposide circumvents the antagonistic cytotoxicity of simultaneous drug administration in slowly growing human colon carcinoma, HT-29 cells. *European Journal of Cancer*, **28A**, 743–748.

Bjornsti, M.-A., Beneditti, P., Viglianti, G.A. & Wang, J.C. (1989). Expression of human DNA topoisomerase I in yeast cells lacking yeast DNA topoisomerase I: restoration of sensitivity of the cells to the antitumor drug camptothecin. *Cancer Research* **49**, 6318–6323.

Bonven, B.J., Gocke, E. & Westergaard, O. (1985). A high affinity topoisomerase I binding sequence is clustered at DNAase I hypersensitive sites in tetrahymena R-chromatin. *Cell* **41**, 541–551.

Bosmann, H.B. (1970). Camptothecin inhibits macromolecular synthesis in mammalian cells but not in isolated mitochondria or *E. coli. Biochemical and Biophysical Research Communications* **41**, 1412–1420.

Brill, S.J. & Sternglanz, R. (1988). Transcription-dependent DNA supercoiling in yeast DNA topoisomerase mutants. *Cell* **54**, 403–411.

Brill, S.J., DiNardo, S., Voelkel-Meiman, K. & Sternglanz, R. (1987). Need for DNA topoisomerase activity as a swivel for DNA replication for transcription of ribosomal RNA [published erratum appears in *Nature* 1987 Apr 23–29; **326**(6115):812]. *Nature* **326**, 414–416.

Brun, G., Vannier, P., Scovassi, I. & Callen, J.-C. (1981). DNA topoisomerase I from mitochondria of *Xenopus laevis* oocytes. *European Journal of Biochemistry* **118**, 407–415.

Bullock, P., Champoux, J.J. & Botchan, M. (1985). Association of crossover points with topoisomerase I cleavage sites: a model for nonhomologous recombination. *Science* **230**, 954–958.

Camilloni, G., Di Martino, E., Di Mauro, E. & Caserta, M. (1989). Regulation of the function of eukaryotic topoisomerase I: topological conditions for inactivity. *Proceedings of the National Academy of Sciences USA* **86**, 3080–3084.

Capitani, S., Girard, P.R., Mazzei, G.J., Kuo, J.R., Berezney, R. & Manzoli, F.A. (1987). Immunochemical characterization of protein kinase C in rat liver nuclei and subnuclear fractions. *Biochemical and Biophysical Research Communications* **142**, 367–375.

Capranico, G., Jaxel, C., Roberge, M., Kohn, K.W. & Pommier, Y. (1990a). Nucleosome positioning as a critical determinant for the DNA cleavage sites of mammalian DNA topoisomerase II in reconstituted Simian virus 40 chromatin. *Nucleic Acids Research* **18**, 4553–4559.

Capranico, G., Kohn, K.W. & Pommier, Y. (1990b). Local sequence requirements for DNA cleavage by mammalian topoisomease II in the presence of doxorubicin. *Nucleic Acids Research* **18**, 6611–6619.

Caserta, M., Amadei, A., Camilloni, G. & Di Mauro, E. (1990). Regulation of the function of eukaryotic DNA topoisomerase I: analysis of the binding step and of the catalytic constants of topoisomerization as a function of DNA topology. *Biochemistry* **29**, 8152–8157.

Caserta, M., Amadei, A., Di Mauro E. & Camilloni, G. (1989). *In vitro* preferential topoisomerization of bent DNA. *Nucleic Acids Research* **17**, 8463–8474.

Champoux, J.J. (1976). Evidence for an intermediate with a single-strand break in the reaction catalyzed by the DNA untwisting enzyme. *Proceedings of the National Academy of Sciences USA* **73**, 3488–3491.

Champoux, J.J. (1977). Strand breakage by the DNA untwisting enzyme results in covalent attachment of the enzyme to DNA. *Proceedings of the National Academy of Sciences USA* **74**, 3800–3804.

Champoux, J.J. (1978). Mechanism of the reaction catalyzed by the DNA untwisting enzyme: attachment of the enzyme to 3′-terminus of the nicked DNA. *Journal of Molecular Biology* **118**, 441–446.

Champoux, J.J. (1981). DNA is linked to the rat liver DNA nicking-closing enzyme by a phosphodiester bond to tyrosine. *Journal of Biological Chemistry* **256**, 4805–4809.

Champoux, J.J. (1990). Mechanistic aspects of type-I topoisomerases. In Cozzarelli, N.R. & Wang, J.C. (eds) *DNA Topology and its Biological Effects*, pp. 217–242. Cold Spring Harbor Laboratory Press, Cold Spring Harbor.

Champoux, J.J. & Dulbecco, R. (1972). An activity from mammalian cells that untwists superhelical DNA—a possible swivel for DNA replication (polyoma-ethidium bromide-mouse-embryo cells-dye binding assay). *Proceedings of the National Academy of Sciences USA* **69**, 143–146.

Chatterjee, S., Cheng, M.-F., Trivedi, D., Petzold, S.J. & Berger, N.A. (1989). Camptothecin hypersensitivity in poly(adenosine diphosphate-ribose) polymerase-deficient cell lines. *Cancer Communications* **1**, 389–394.

Coderoni, S., Paparelli, M., Luigi, G. & Gianfranceschi, G.L. (1990). Phosphorylation sites for type N II protein kinase in DNA-topoisomerase I from calf thymus. *International Journal of Biochemistry* **22**, 737–746.

Covey, J.M., Jaxel, C., Kohn, K.W. & Pommier, Y. (1989). Protein-linked DNA strand breaks induced im mammalian cells by camptothecin, an inhibitor of topoisomerase I. *Cancer Research* **49**, 5016–5022.

Craig, N.L. & Nash, H.A. (1983). The mechanism of phage lambda site-specific recombination: site-specific breakage of DNA by *int* topoisomerase. *Cell* **35**, 795–803.

Culotta, V. & Sollner-Webb, B. (1988). Sites of topoisomerase I action on *X. laevis* ribosomal chromatin: transcriptionally active rDNA has an ~200 bp repeating structure. *Cell* **52**, 585–597.

Darby, M.K., Schmitt, B., Jongstra-Bilen, J. & Vosberg, H.P. (1985). Inhibition of calf thymus type II DNA topoisomerase by poly(ADP-ribosylation). *EMBO Journal* **4**, 2129–2134.

D'Arpa, P., Beardmore, C. & Liu, L.F. (1990). Involvement of nucleic acid synthesis in cell killing mechanisms of topoisomerase poisons. *Cancer Research* **50**, 6919–6924.

D'Arpa, P., Machlin, P.S., Ratrie, H., Rothfield, N.F., Cleveland, D.W. & Earnshaw, W.C. (1988). cDNA cloning of human DNA topoisomerase I: catalytic activity of a 67.7-kDa carboxyl-terminal fragment. *Proceedings of the National Academy of Sciences USA* **85**, 2543–2547.

Duguet, M., Lavenot, C., Harper, F., Mirambeau, G. & De Recondo, A.M. (1983) DNA topoisomerases from rat liver: physiological variations. *Nucleic Acids Research* **11**, 1059–1075.

Durban, E., Goodenough, M., Mills, J. & Busch, H. (1985). Topoisomerase I phosphorylation *in vitro* and in rapidly growing Novikoff hepatoma cells. *EMBO Journal* **4**, 2921–2926.

Durban, E., Mills, J.S., Roll, D. & Busch, H. (1983). Phosphorylation of purified Novikoff hepatoma topoisomerase I. *Biochemical and Biophysical Research Communications* **111**, 897–905.

Eng, W.K., Faucette, L., Johnson, R.K. & Sternglanz, R. (1988). Evidence that DNA topoisomerase I is necessary for the cytotoxic effects of camptothecin. *Molecular Pharmacology* **34**, 755–760.

Eng, W.K., McCabe, F.L., Tan, K.B., Mattern, M.R., Hofmann, G.A., Woessner, R.D., Hertzberg, R.P. & Johnson, R.K. (1990). Development of a stable camptothecin-resistant subline of P388 leukemia with reduced topoisomerase I content. *Molecular Pharmacology* **38**, 471–480.

Eng, W.K., Pandit, S.D. & Sternglanz, R. (1989). Mapping of the active site tyrosine of eukaryotic DNA topoisomerase I. *Journal of Biological Chemistry* **264**, 13373–13376.

Fairfield, F.R., Bauer, W.R. & Simpson, M.Y. (1979). Mitochondria contain a distinct DNA topoisomerase. *Journal of Biological Chemistry* **259**, 9352–9354.

Ferro, A.M. & Olivera, B.M. (1984). Poly(ADP-ribosylation) of DNA topoisomerase I from calf thymus. *Journal of Biological Chemistry* **259**, 547–554.

Ferro, A.M., Higgins, N.P. & Olivera, B.M. (1983). Poly (ADP-ribosylation) of a DNA topoisomerase. *Journal of Biological Chemistry* **258**, 6000–6003.

Ferro, A.M., McElwain, M.C. & Olivera, B.M. (1984a). Poly (ADP-ribosylation) of DNA topoisomerase I: a nuclear response to DNA-strand interruptions. *Cold Spring Harbour Symposium of Quantitative Biology* **49**, 683–690.

Ferro, A.M., Thompson, L.H. & Olivera, B.M. (1984b). Poly (ADP-ribosylation) and DNA topoisomerase I in different cell lines. *Advances in Experimental and Medical Biology* **179**, 441–447.

Fesen, M. & Pommier, Y. (1989). Mammalian topoisomerase II activity is modulated by the DNA minor groove binder distamycin in simian virus 40 DNA. *Journal of Biological Chemistry* **264**, 11354–11359.

Fleischmann, G., Filipski, R. & Elgin, S.C. (1987). Isolation and distribution of a *Drosophila* protein preferentially associated with inactive regions of the genome. *Chromosoma* **96**, 83–90.

Fleischmann, G., Pflugfelder, G., Steiner, E.K., Javaherian, K., Howard, G.C., Wang, J.C. & Elgin, S.C. (1984). *Drosophila* DNA topoisomerase I is associated with transcriptionally active regions of the genome. *Proceedings of the National Academy of Sciences USA* **81**, 6958–6962.

Fukada, M. (1985). Action of camptothecin and its derivatives on deoxyribonucleic acid. *Biochemical Pharmacology* **34**, 1225–1230.

Garg, L.C., DiAngelo, S. & Jacob, S.T. (1987). Role of DNA topoisomerase I in the transcription of supercoiled rDNA gene. *Proceedings of the National Academy of Sciences USA* **84**, 3185–3188.

Gilmour, D.S. & Elgin, S.C. (1987). Localization of specific topoisomerase I interactions within the transcribed region of active heat shock genes by using the inhibitor camptothecin. *Molecular and Cellular Biology* **7**, 141–148.

Giovanella, B.C., Stehlin, J.S., Wall, M.E., Wani, M.C., Nicholas, A.W., Liu, L.F., Silber, R. & Potmesil, M. (1989). DNA topoisomerase I-targeted chemotherapy of human colon cancer in xenografts. *Science* **246**, 1046–1048.

Girard, P.R., Mazzei, G.J., Wood, J.G. & Kuo, J.F. (1985). Polyclonal antibodies to phospholipid/Ca^{2+}-dependent protein kinase and immunocytochemical localization of the enzyme in rat brain. *Proceedings of the National Academy of Sciences USA* **82**, 3030–3034.

Gottlieb, J.A., Guarino, A.M., Call, J.B., Olivero, V.T. & Block, J.B. (1970). Preliminary pharmacologic and clinical evaluation of camptothecin sodium (NSC-100880). *Cancer Chemotherapy Reports* **54**, 461–470.

Gupta, R.S., Gupta, R., Eng, B., Lock, R.B., Ross, W.E., Hertzberg, R.P., Caranfa, M.J. & Johnson, R.K. (1988). Camptothecin-resistant mutants of Chinese hamster ovary cells containing a resistant form of topoisomerase I. *Cancer Research* **48**, 6404–6410.

Halligan, B.D., Davis, J.L., Edwards, K.A. & Liu, L.F. (1982). Intra- and intermolecular strand transfer by HeLa DNA topoisomerase I. *Journal of Biological Chemistry* **257**, 3995–4000.

Halligan, B.D., Edwards, K.A. & Liu, L.F. (1985). Purification and characterization of a type II DNA topoisomerase from bovine calf thymus. *Journal of Biological Chemistry* **260**, 2475–2482.

Heck, M.M., Hittelman, W.N. & Earnshaw, W.C. (1988). Differential expression of DNA topoisomerases I and II during the eukaryotic cell cycle. *Proceedings of the National Academy of Sciences USA* **85**, 1086–1090.

Hertzberg, R.P., Busby, R.W., Caranfa, M.J., Holden, K.G., Johnson, R.K., Hecht, S.M. & Kingsbury, W.D. (1990). Irreversible trapping of the DNA–topoisomerase I covalent complex. *Journal of Biological Chemistry* **265**, 19287–19295.

Hertzberg, R.P., Caranfa, M.J. & Hecht, S.M. (1989a). On the mechanism of topoisomerase I inhibition by camptothecin: Evidence for binding to an enzyme-DNA complex. *Biochemistry* **28**, 4629–4638.

Hertzberg, R.P., Caranfa, M.J., Holden, K.G., Jakas, D.R., Gallagher, H., Mattern,

M.R., Mong, S.M., Bartus, J.O., Johnson, R.K. & Kingsbury, W.D. (1989b). Modification of the hydroxy lactone ring of camptothecin: inhibition of mammalian topoisomerase I and biological activity. *Journal of Medicinal Chemistry* **32**, 715–720.

Hickson, I.D., Davies, S.L., Davies, S.M. & Robson, C.N. (1990). DNA repair in radiation sensitive mutants of mammalian cells: possible involvement of DNA topoisomerases. *International Journal of Radiation and Biology* **58**, 561–568.

Holm, C., Covey, J.M., Kerrigan, D. & Pommier, Y. (1989). Differential requirement of DNA replication for the cytoxicity of DNA topoisomerase I and II inhibitors in Chinese hamster DC3F cells. *Cancer Research* **49**, 6365–6368.

Horwitz, M.S. & Horwitz, S.B. (1971). Intracellular degradation of HeLa and adenovirus type 2 DNA induced by camptothecin. *Biochemical and Biophysical Research Communications* **45**, 723–727.

Horwitz, S.B. & Horwitz, M.S. (1973). Effects of camptothecin on the breakage and repair of DNA during the cell cycle. *Cancer Research* **33**, 2834–2836.

Horwitz, S.B., Chang, C.K. & Grollman, A.P. (1971). Studies on camptothecin. I. Effects of nucleic acid and protein synthesis. *Molecular Pharmacology* **7**, 632–644.

Hsiang, Y.H. & Liu, L.F. (1988). Identification of mammalian DNA topoisomerase I as an intracellular target of the anticancer drug camptothecin. *Cancer Research* **48**, 1722–1726.

Hsiang, Y.H., Hertzberg, R., Hecht, S. & Liu, L.F. (1985). Camptothecin induces protein-linked DNA breaks via mammalian DNA topoisomerase I. *Journal of Biological Chemistry* **260**, 14873–14878.

Hsiang, Y.-H., Lihou, M.G. & Liu L.F. (1989a). Arrest of DNA replication by drug-stabilized topoisomerase I-DNA cleavable complexes as a mechanism of cell killing by camptothecin. *Cancer Research* **49**, 5077–5082.

Hsiang, Y.-H., Liu, L.F., Wall, M.E., Wani, M.C., Nicholas, A.W., Manikumar, G., Kirschenbaum, S., Silber, R. & Potmesil, M. (1989b). DNA topoisomerase I-mediated DNA cleavage and cytotoxicity of camptothecin analogs. *Cancer Research* **49**, 4385–4389.

Huang, W.M. (1990). Nucleotide sequences and the encoded amino acids of DNA topoisomerase genes. In Cozzarelli, N.R. & Wang, J.C. (eds) *DNA Topology and its Biological Effects*, pp. 409–457. Cold Spring Harbor Laboratory Press, Cold Spring Harbor.

Hwong, C.-L., Chen, M.-S. & Hwang, J. (1989). Phorbol ester transiently increases topoisomerase I mRNA levels in human skin fibroblasts. *Journal of Biological Chemistry* **264**, 14923–14926.

Ishii, K., Katase, A., Andoh, T. & Seno, N. (1987). Inhibition of topoisomerase I by heparine. *Biochemical and Biophysical Research Communications* **104**, 541–547.

Javaherian, K. & Liu, L.F. (1983). Association of eukaryotic DNA topoisomerase I with nucleosomes and chromosomal proteins. *Nucleic Acids Research* **11**, 461–472.

Jaxel, C., Capranico, G., Kerrigan, D., Kohn, K.W. & Pommier, Y. (1991a). Effect of local DNA sequence on topoisomerase I cleavage in the presence or absence of camptothecin. *Journal of Biological Chemistry* **266**, 20418–20423.

Jaxel, C., Capranico, G., Wasserman, K., Kerrigan, D., Kohn, K.W. & Pommier, Y. (1991b). DNA sequence at sites of topoisomerase I cleavage induced by camptothecin in SV40 DNA. In Potmesil. M. & Kohn, K.W. (eds.) *DNA Topoisomerases in Cancer*, pp. 182–195. Oxford University Press, New York.

Jaxel, C., Kohn, K.W. & Pommier, Y. (1988). Topoisomerase I interaction with SV40 DNA in the presence and absence of camptothecin. *Nucleic Acids Research* **16**, 11157–11170.

Jaxel, C., Kohn, K.W., Wani, M.C., Wall, M.E. & Pommier, Y. (1989). Structure-activity study of the actions of camptothecin derivatives on mammalian topoisomerase I: evidence for a specific receptor site and a relation to antitumor activity. *Cancer Research* **49**, 1465–1469.

Johnson, R.K., McCabe, F.L., Faucette, L.F., Hertzberg, R.P., Kingsbury, W.D., Boehm, J.C., Caranfa, M.J. & Holden, K.G. (1989). SK&F 10864, a water-soluble analog of camptothecin with broad-spectrum activity in preclinical tumor models. *Proceedings of the American Accociation of Cancer Research* **30**, 623.

Jongstra-Bilen, J., Ittel, M.E., Niedergang, C., Vosberg, H.P. & Mandel, P. (1983). DNA topoisomease I from calf thymus is inhibited *in vitro* by poly(ADP-ribosylation). *European Journal of Biochemistry* **136**, 391–396.

Juan, C.C., Hwang, J.L., Liu, A.A., Whang-Peng, J., Knutsen, T., Huebner, K., Croce, C.M., Zhang, H., Wang, J.C. & Liu, L.F. (1988). Human DNA topoisomerase I is encoded by a single-copy gene that maps to chromosome region 20q12-13.2. *Proceedings of the National Academy of Sciences USA* **85**, 8910–8913.

Kaiserman, H.B., Ingebritsen, T.S. & Benbow, R.M. (1988). Regulation of *Xenopus laevis* DNA topoisomerase I activity by phosphorylation *in vitro*. *Biochemistry* **27**, 3216–3222.

Kaneda, N., Nagata, H., Furuta, T. & Yokokura, T. (1990). Metabolism and pharmacokinetics of the camptothecin analogue CPT-11 in the mouse. *Cancer Research* **50**, 1715–1720.

Kann, H.E. Jr & Kohn, K.W. (1972). Effects of deoxyribonucleic acid-reactive drugs on ribonucleic acid synthesis in leukemia L1210 cells. *Molecular Pharmacology* **8**, 551–560.

Kanzawa, F., Sugimoto, Y., Minato, K., Kasahara, K., Bungo, M., Nakagawa, K., Fujiwara, Y., Liu, L.F. & Saijo, N. (1990). Establishment of a camptothecin analogue (CPT-11)-resistant cell line of human non-small cell lung cancer: characterization and mechanism of resistance. *Cancer Research* **50**, 5919–5924.

Kasid, U.N., Halligan, B., Liu, L.F., Dritschilo, A. & Smulson, M. (1989). Poly(ADP-ribose)-mediated post-translational modification of chromatin-associated human topoisomerase I. Inhibitory effects on catalytic activity. *Journal of Biological Chemistry* **264**, 18687–18692.

Kaufmann, S.H. (1989). Induction of endonucleolytic DNA cleavage in human acute myelogenous leukemia cells by etoposide, camptothecin, and other cytotoxic anticancer drugs: a cautionary note. *Cancer Research* **49**, 5870–5878.

Kaufmann, S.H. (1991). Antagonism between camptothecin and topoisomerase II-directed chemotherapeutic agents in a human leukemia cell line. *Cancer Research* **51**, 1129–1136.

Kawato, Y., Aonuma, M., Hirota, Y., Kuga, H. & Sato, K. (1991). Intracellular roles of SN-38, a metabolite of the camptothecin derivative CPT-11, in the antitumor effect of CPT-11. *Cancer Research* **51**, 4187–4191.

Kessel, D. (1971). Effects of camptothecin on RNA synthesis in leukemia cells. *Biochimica Biophysica Acta* **246**, 225–232.

Kessel, D., Bosmann, H.B. & Lohr, K. (1972). Camptothecin effects on DNA synthesis in murine leukemia cells. *Biochimica Biophysica Acta* **269**, 210–216.

Kikuchi, Y. & Nash, H.A. (1979). Nicking-closing activity associated with bacteriophage lambda *Int* gene product. *Proceedings of the National Academy of Sciences USA* **76**, 3760–3764.

Kingsbury, W.D., Boehm, J.C., Jakas, D.R., Holden, K.G., Hecht, S.M., Gallagher, G., Caranfa, M.J., McCabe, F., Faucette, L.F., Johnson, R.K. & Hertzberg, R.P. (1991). Synthesis of water-soluble (aminoalkyl)camptothecin analogues: inhibition of topoisomerase I and antitumour activity. *Journal of Medicinal Chemistry* **34**, 98–107.

Kjeldsen, E., Bonven, B.J., Andoh, T., Ishii, K., Okada, K., Bolund, L. & Westergaard, O. (1988a). Characterization of a camptothecin-resistant human DNA topoisomerase I. *Journal of Biological Chemistry* **263**, 3912–3916.

Kjeldsen, E., Mollerup, S., Thomsen, B., Bonven, B.J., Bolund, L. & Westergaard, O. (1988b). Sequence-dependent effect of camptothecin on human topoisomerase I DNA cleavage. *Journal of Molecular Biology* **202**, 333–342.

Kraft, A.S., Appling, C. & Berkow, R.L. (1987). Specific binding of phorbol esters to nuclei of human promyelocytic leukemia cells. *Biochemical and Biophysical Research Communications* **144**, 393–401.

Kroeger, P.E. & Rowe, T.C. (1989). Interaction of topoisomerase I with the transcribed region of the *Drosophila* HSP 70 heat shock gene. *Nucleic Acids Research* **17**, 8495–8509.

Krogh, S., Mortensen, U.H., Westergaard, O. & Bonven, B.J. (1991). Eurkaryotic topoisomerase I–DNA interaction is stabilized by helix curvature. *Nucleic Acids Research* **19**, 1235–1241.

Krupita, G. & Cerutti, P. (1989). ADP-ribosylation of ADPR-transferase and topoisomerase I in intact mouse epidermal cell JB6. *Biochemistry* **28**, 2034–2040.

Kunimoto, T., Nitta, K., Tanaka, T., Uehara, N., Baba, H., Takeuchi, M., Yokokura, T., Sawada, S., Miyasaka, T. & Mutai, M. (1987). Antitumor activity of 7-ethyl-10-[4-(1-piperidino)-1-piperidino]carbonyloxy-camptothecin, a novel water-soluble derivative of camptothecin, against murine tumors. *Cancer Research* **47**, 5944–5947.

Kunze, N., Klein, M., Richter, A. & Knippers, R. (1990). Structural characterization of the human DNA topoisomerase I gene promoter. *European Journal of Biochemistry* **194**, 323–330.

Kuwahara, J., Suzuki, T., Funakoshi, K. & Sugiura, Y. (1986). Photosensitive DNA cleavage and phage inactivation by copper(II)-camptothecin. *Biochemistry* **25**, 1216–1221.

Lazarus, G.M., Henrich, J.P., Kelly, W.G., Schmitz, S.A. & Castora, F.J. (1987). Purification and characterization of a type I DNA topoisomerase from calf thymus mitochondria. *Biochemistry* **26**, 6195–6203.

Li, L.H., Fraser, T.J., Olin, E.J. & Bhuyan, B.K. (1972). Action of camptothecin on mammalian cells in culture. *Cancer Research* **32**, 2643–2650.

Liu, L.F. & Wang, J.C. (1987). Supercoiling of the DNA template during transcription. *Proceedings of the National Academy of Sciences USA* **84**, 7024–7027.

Lynn, R.M., Bjornsti, M.A., Caron, P.R. & Wang, J.C. (1989). Peptide sequencing and site-directed mutagenesis identify tyrosine-727 as the active site tyrosine of *Saccharomyces cerevisiae* DNA topoisomerase I. *Proceedings of the National Academy of Sciences USA* **86**, 3559–3563.

McCoubrey, W.K. Jr & Champoux, J.J. (1986). The role of single-strand breaks in the catenation reaction catalyzed by the rat type I topoisomerase. *Journal of Biological Chemistry* **261**, 5130–5137.

McHugh, M.M., Sigmund, R.D. & Beerman, T.A. (1990). Effects of minor groove binding drugs on camptothecin-induced DNA lesions in L1210 nuclei. *Biochemical Pharmacology* **39**, 707–714.

Masmoudi, A., Labourdette, G., Mersel, M., Huang, F.L., Huang, K.-P., Vincendon, G. & Malviya, A.N. (1989). Protein kinase C located in rat liver nuclei. *Journal of Biological Chemistry* **264**, 1172–1179.

Mattern, M.R., Mong, S.M., Bartus, H.F., Mirabelli, C.K., Crooke, S.T. & Johnson, R.K. (1987). Relationship between the intracellular effects of camptothecin and the inhibition of DNA topoisomerase I in cultured L1210 cells. *Cancer Research* **47**, 1793–1798.

Mattern, M.R., Mong, S., Mong, S.-M., Bartus, J., Sarau, H.M., Clark, M.A., Foley, J.J. & Crooke, S.T. (1990). Transient activation of topoisomerase I in leukotriene D4 signal transduction in human cells. *Biochemical Journal* **265**, 101–107.

Misra, U.K. & Sahyoun, N. (1987). Protein kinase C binding to isolated nuclei and its activation by a Ca^{2+}/phospholipid-independent mechanism. *Biochemical and Biophysical Research Communications* **142**, 367–375.

Mortensen, U.H., Stevnsner, T., Krogh, S., Olesen, K., Westergaard, O. & Bonven, B.J. (1990). Distamycin inhibition of topoisomerase I-DNA interaction: a mechanistic analysis. *Nucleic Acids Research* **18**, 1983–1989.

Muggia, F.M., Creaven, P.J., Hansen, H.H., Cohen, M.H. & Selawry, O.S. (1972). Phase I clinical trial of weekly and daily treatment with camptothecin (NSC-100800): correlation with preclinical studies. *Biochemistry* **56**, 515–521.

Muller, M.T. (1985). Quantitation of eukaryotic topiosomerase I reactivity with DNA. Preferential cleavage of supercoiled DNA. *Biochimica Biophysica Acta* **824**, 263–267.

Muller, M.T., Pfund, W.P., Mehta, V.B. & Trask, D.K. (1985). Eukaryotic type I topoisomerase is enriched in the nucleolus and catalytically active on ribosomal DNA. *EMBO Journal* **4**, 1237–1243.

Naito, M., Hamada, H. & Tsuruo, T. (1988). ATP/Mg^{2+}-dependent binding of vincristine to the plasma membrane of multidrug-resistant K562 cells. *Journal of Biological Chemistry* **263**, 11887–11891.

Nambi, P., Mattern, M., Bartus, J.O.L., Aiyar, N. & Crooke, S.T. (1989). Stimulation of intracellular topoisomerase I activity by vasopressin and thrombin. *Biochemical Journal* **262**, 485–489.

Nambi, P., Wu, H.-L., Woessner, R.D. & Mattern, M.R. (1990). Inhibition of endothelium-mediated topoisomerase I activation by pertussis toxin. *FEBS Letters* **276**, 17–20.

Nicholas, A.W., Wani, M.C., Manikumar, G., Wall, M.E., Kohn, K.W. & Pommier, Y. (1990). Plant antitumor agents. 29. Synthesis and biological activity of ring D and ring E modified analogues of camptothecin. *Journal of Medicinal Chemistry* **33**, 972–978.

Nitiss, J. & Wang, J.C. (1988). DNA topoisomerase-targeting antitumor drugs can be studied in yeast. *Proceedings of the National Academy of Sciences USA* **85**, 7501–7505.

O'Connor, P.M., Kerrigan, D., Bertrand, R., Kohn, K.W. & Pommier, Y. (1990). 10,11-methylenedioxycamptothecin, a topoisomerase I inhibitor of increased potency: DNA damage and correlation to cytotoxicity in human colon carcinoma (HT-29) cells. *Cancer Communications* **2**, 395–400.

O'Connor, P.M., Nieves-Neira, W., Kerrigan, D., Bertrand, R., Goldman, J., Kohn, K.W. & Pommier, Y. (1991). S-phase population analysis does not correlate with the cytoxicity of camptothecin and 10,11-methylenedioxycamptothecin in human colon carcinoma HT-29 cells. *Cancer Communications* **3**, 233–240.

Osheroff, N., Shelton, E.R. & Brutlag, D.L. (1983). DNA topoisomerase II from *Drosophila* melanogaster. Relaxation of supercoiled DNA. *Journal of Biological Chemistry* **258**, 9536–9543

Ostrander, E.A., Benedetti, P. & Wang, J.C. (1990). Template supercoiling by a chimera of yeast GAL4 protein and phage T7 RNA polymerase. *Science* **249**, 1261–1265.

Poccia, D.L., LeVine, D. & Wang, J.C. (1978). Activity of a DNA topoisomerase (nicking-closing enzyme) during sea urchin development and the cell cycle. *Developmental Biology* **64**, 273–283.

Pommier, Y., Capranico, G. & Kohn, K.W. (1991a). Local DNA sequence requirements for topoisomerase II-induced DNA cleavage produced by amsacrine and teniposide. *Proceedings of the American Association for Cancer Research* **32**, 335.

Pommier, Y., Covey, J.M., Kerrigan, D., Markovits, J. & Pham, R. (1987). DNA unwinding and inhibition of mouse leukemia L1210 DNA topoisomerase I by intercalators. *Nucleic Acids Research* **15**, 6713–6731.

Pommier, Y., Kerrigan, D., Hartmann, K.D. & Glazer, R.I. (1990). Phosphorylation of mammalian DNA topoisomerase I and activation by protein kinase C. *Journal of Biological Chemistry* **265**, 9418–9422.

Pommier, Y., Kerrigan, D., Schwartz, R.E., Swack, J.A. & McCurdy, A. (1986). Altered DNA topoisomerase II activity in Chinese hamster cells resistant to topoisomerase II inhibitors. *Cancer Research* **46**, 3075–3081.

Pommier, Y., Jaxel, C., Kerrigan, D. & Kohn, K.W. (1991b). Structure–activity relationship of topoisomerase I inhibition by camptothecin derivatives: evidence for the existence of a ternary complex. In Potmesil, M. & Kohn, K.W. (eds.) *DNA Topoisomerases in Cancer*, pp. 121–132. Oxford University Press, New York.

Porter, S.E. & Champoux, J.J. (1989a). The basis for camptothecin enhancement of DNA breakage by eukaryotic topoisomerase I. *Nucleic Acids Research* **17**, 8521–8532.

Porter, S.E. & Champoux, J.J. (1989b). Mapping *in vivo* topoisomerase I sites on simian virus 40 DNA: asymmetric distribution of sites on replicating molecules. *Molecular and Cellular Biology* **9**, 541–550.

Priel, E., Showalter, S.D. & Blair, D.G. (1991). Inhibition of human immunodeficiency virus (HIV-1) replication *in vitro* by noncytotoxic doses of camptothecin, a topoisomerase I inhibitor. *AIDS Research and Human Retroviruses* **7**, 65–72.

Romig, H. & Richter, A. (1990a). Expression of the topoisomerase I gene in serum stimulated human fibroblasts. *Biochimica Biophysica Acta* **1048**, 274–280.

Romig, H. & Richter, A. (1990b). Expression of the type I DNA topoisomerase gene in adenovirus-5 infected human cells. *Nucleic Acids Research* **18**, 801–808.

Rose, K.M., Szopa, J., Han, F.S., Cheng, Y.C., Richter, A. & Scheer, U. (1988). Association of DNA topoisomerase I and RNA polymerase I: a possible role for topoisomerase I in ribosomal gene transcription. *Chromosoma* **96**, 411–416.

Rosenberg, B.H., Ungers, G. & Deutsch, J.F. (1976). Variation in DNA swivel enzyme activity during the mammalian cell cycle. *Nucleic Acids Research* **3**, 3305–3311.

Ryan, A.J., Squires, S., Strutt, H.L. & Johnson, R.T. (1991). Camptothecin cytotoxicity in mammalian cells is associated with the induction of persistent double strand breaks in replicating DNA. *Nucleic Acids Research* **19**, 3295–3300.

Samuel, D.S., Shimizu, Y. & Shimizu, N. (1989). Protein kinase C phosphorylates DNA topoisomerase I. *FEBS Letters* **259**, 57–60.

Shin, C.-G. & Snapka, R.M. (1990a). Exposure to camptothecin breaks leading and lagging strand simian virus 40 DNA replication forks. *Biochemical and Biophysical Research Communications* **168**, 135–140.

Shin, C.-G. & Snapka, R.M. (1990b). Patterns of strongly protein-associated simian virus 40 DNA replication intermediates resulting from exposures to specific topoisomerase poisons. *Biochemistry* **29**, 10934–10939.

Shuman, S., Kane, E.M. & Morham, S.G. (1989). Mapping of the active-site tyrosine of vaccinia virus DNA topoisomerase I. *Proceedings of the National Academy of Sciences USA* **86**, 9793–9797

Shuman, S. & Moss, B. (1987). Identification of a vaccinia virus gene encoding a type I DNA topoisomerase. *Proceedings of the National Academy of Sciences USA* **84**, 7478–7482.

Shuman, S. & Moss, B. (1988). Characterization of vaccina virus DNA topoisomerase I expressed in *Escherichia coli*. *Journal of Biological Chemistry* **263**, 16401–16407.

Snapka, R.M. (1986). Topoisomerase inhibitors can selectively interfere with different stages of simian virus 40 DNA replication. *Molecular and Cellular Biology* **6**, 4221–4227.

Srivenugopal, K.S. & Morris, D.R. (1985). Differential modulation by spermidine of reactions catalyzed by type 1 prokaryotic and eukaryotic topoisomerases. *Biochemistry* **24**, 4766–4771.

Stewart, A.F. & Schütz, G. (1987). Camptothecin-induced *in vivo* topoisomerase I cleavages in the transcriptionally active tyrosine aminotransferase gene. *Cell* **50**, 1109–1117.

Stewart, A.F., Herrera, R.E. & Nordheim, A. (1990). Rapid induction of c-*fos* transcription reveals quantitive linkage of RNA polymerase II and DNA topoisomerase I enzyme activities. *Cell* **60**, 141–146.

Sugimoto, Y., Tsukahara, S., Oh-hara, T., Liu, L.F. & Tsuruo, T. (1990). Elevated expression of DNA topoisomerase II in camptothecin-resistant human tumour cell lines. *Cancer Research* **50**, 7962–7965.

Sunde, L., Kjeldsen, E., Andoh, T., Keene, J. & Bolund, L. (1990). A three allele Taq1 polymorphism at TOP1 gene. *Nucleic Acids Research* **18**, 5919.

Suzuki, M., Takagi, E., Kojima, K., Izuta, S. & Yoshida, S. (1989). Rapid purification and structural study of DNA topoisomerase I from human Burkitt lymphoma Raji cells. *Journal of Biochemistry* **106**, 742–744.

Tamura, H., Ikegami, Y., Ono, K., Sekimizu, K. & Andoh, T. (1990). Acidic phospholipids directly inhibit DNA binding of mammalian DNA topoisomerase I. *FEBS Letters* **261**, 151–154.

Tanizawa, A. & Pommier, Y. (1992). Topoisomerase I alteration in a camptothecin-resistant cell line derived from Chinese hamster DC3F cells in culture. *Cancer Research* **52**, 1848–1854.

Taudou, G., Mirambeau, G., Lavenot, C., Dergarabedian, A., Vermeersch, J. & Duguet, M. (1984). DNA topoisomerase activities in concanavalin A-stimulated lymphocytes. *FEBS Letters* **176**, 431–435.

Thomsen, B., Mollerup, S., Bonven, B.J., Frank, R., Blöcker, H., Nielsen, O.F. & Westergaard, O. (1987). Sequence specificity of DNA topoisomerase I in the presence and absence of camptothecin. *EMBO Journal* **6**, 1817–1823.

Thrash, C., Bankier, A.T., Barrell, B.G. & Sternglanz, R. (1985). Cloning, characterization, and sequence of the yeast DNA topoisomerase I gene. *Proceedings of the National Academy of Sciences USA* **82**, 4374–4378.

Thrash, C., Voelkel, K., DiNardo, S. & Sternglanz, R. (1984). Identification of *Saccharomyces cerevisiae* mutants deficient in DNA topoisimerase I activity. *Journal of Biological Chemistry* **259**, 1375–1377.

Trask, D.K. & Muller, M.T. (1988). Stabilization of type I topoisomerase–DNA covalent complexes by actinomycin D. *Proceedings of the National Academy of Sciences USA* **85**, 1417–1421.

Trask, D.K., DiDonato, J.A. & Muller, M.T. (1984). Rapid detection and isolation of covalent DNA/protein complexes: application to topoisomerase I and II. *EMBO Journal* **3**, 671–676.

Tricoli, J.V., Sahai, B.M., McCormick, P.J., Jarlinski, S.J., Bertram, J.S. & Kowalski, D. (1985). DNA topoisomerase I and II activities during cell proliferation and the cell cycle in cultured mouse embryo fibroblasts (C3H 10T1/2) cells. *Experimental Cell Research* **158**, 1–14.

Tse, Y.-C., Kirkegaard, K. & Wang, J.C. (1980). Covalent bonds between protein and DNA. Formation of phosphotyrosine linkage between certain DNA topoisomerases and DNA. *Journal of Biological Chemistry* **255**, 5560–5565.

Tse-Dinh, Y.C., Wong, T.W. & Goldberg, A.R. (1984). Virus- and cell-encoded tyrosine protein kinases inactivate DNA topoisomerases *in vitro*. *Nature* **312**, 785–786.

Tsuruo, T., Matsuzaki, T., Matsushita, M., Saito, H. & Yokokura, T. (1988). Antitumor effect of CPT-11, a new derivative of camptothecin, against pleiotropic drug-resistant tumours *in vitro* and *in vivo*. *Cancer Chemotherapy and Pharmacology* **21**, 71–74.

Uemura, T., Morino, K., Uzawa, S., Shiozaki, K. & Yanagida, M. (1987). Cloning and sequencing of *Schizosaccharomyces pombe* DNA topoisomerase I gene, and effect of gene disruption. *Nucleic Acids Research* **15**, 9727–9739.

Upton, C., Opgenorth, A., Traktman, P. & McFadden, G. (1990). Identification and DNA sequence of the Shope fibroma virus DNA topoisomerase I gene. *Virology* **176**, 439–447.

Wall, M.E. (1983). A new look at older drugs in cancer treatment: natural products. *Bioscience Reports* **11**, 480A–489A.

Wall, M.E., Wani, M.C., Cooke, C.E., Palmer, K.H., McPhail, A.T. & Slim, G.A. (1966). The isolation and structure of camptothecin, a novel alkaloidal leukemia and tumor inhibitor from *Camptotheca acuminata*. *Journal of the Americal Chemical Society* **88**, 3888–3890.

Wang, H.-P. & Rogler, C.E. (1991). Topoisomerase I-mediated integration of hepadnavirus DNA *in vitro*. *Journal of Virology* **65**, 2381–2392.

Wang, J.C. (1985). DNA topoisomerases. *Annual Reviews of Biochemistry* **54**, 665–697.

Wang, J.C. (1987). Recent studies of DNA topoisomerases. *Biochemica Biophysica Acta* **990**, 1–9.

Wang, J.C. (1991). DNA topoisomerases: why so many? *Journal of Biological Chemistry* **266**, 6659–6662.

Wani, M.C., Nicholas, A.W., Manikumar, G. & Wall, M.E. (1987). Plant antitumor agents. 25. Total synthesis and antileukemic activity of ring A substituted camptothecin analogues. Structure–activity correlations. *Journal of Medicinal Chemistry* **30**, 1774–1779.

Wassermann, K., Markovits, J., Jaxel, C., Capranico, G., Kohn, K.W. & Pommier, Y. (1990). Effects of morpholinyl doxorubicins, doxorubicin, and actinomycin D on mammalian DNA topoisomerases I and II. *Molecular Pharmacology* **38**, 38–45.

Wu, H.Y., Shyy, S.H., Wang, J.C. & Liu, L.F. (1988). Transcription generates positively and negatively supercoiled domains in the template. *Cell* **53**, 433–440.

Yamashita, Y., Kawada, S.-Z., Fujii, N. & Nakano, H. (1991). Induction of mammalian topoisomerase I and II mediated DNA cleavage by saintopin, a new antitumor agent from fungus. *Biochemistry* **30**, 5838–5845.

Yang, G., Kunze, N., Baumgartner, B., Jiang, Z., Sapp, M., Knipper, R. & Richter, A. (1990). Molecular structure of human DNA topoisomerase I retrosequences. *Gene* **91**, 247–253.

Yang, L., Wold, M.S., Li, J.J., Kelly, T.J. & Liu, L.F. (1987). Roles of DNA topoisomerases in simian virus 40 DNA replication *in vitro*. *Proceedings of the National Academy of Sciences USA* **84**, 950–954.

Zhang, H., Wang, J.C. & Liu, L.F. (1988). Involvement of DNA topoisomerase I in transcription of human ribosomal RNA genes. *Proceedings of the National Academy of Sciences USA* 1060–1064.

Zhou, B.-Z., Bastow, K.F. & Cheng, Y.-C. (1989). Characterization of the 3′ region of the human DNA topoisomerase I gene. *Cancer Research* **49**, 3922–3927.

Zwelling, L.A., Michaels, S., Erickson, L.C., Ungerleider, R.S., Nichols, M. & Kohn, K.W. (1981). Protein-associated deoxyribonucleic acid strand breaks in L1210 cells treated with the deoxyribonucleic acid intercalating agents 4′-(9-acridinylamino) methanesulfon-*m*-anisidide and adriamycin. *Biochemistry* **20**, 6553–6563.

Chapter 10
DNA-sequence specificity of anticancer agents

John A. Hartley and Robert L. Souhami

Introduction

The interaction of chemical and physical agents with DNA appears to be the basis of a wide range of biological phenomena. Examples of carcinogens, mutagens, antiviral agents, antitumour drugs, metal ions, antibiotics, as well as many proteins, can interact with DNA and induce changes of potential biological significance. Not surprisingly, there is considerable effort directed towards understanding the exact nature of these interactions with the hope that it may provide clues to the way in which specific modifications of DNA could have specific biological effects.

Many agents that possess antitumour activity have been shown to bind to DNA. Several aspects of the binding of such agents could contribute to their biological activity, such as their mode of binding, the kinetics of the binding interaction, and the selectivity of the drug for particular base sites (base-pair specificity) or sequences of bases (base-sequence specificity). The modes of binding to DNA are diverse. Simple bifunctional alkylating agents can bind covalently to and crosslink the bases of DNA. Metal derivatives such as cisplatin can also crosslink DNA through the formation of coordination complexes. Other agents bind non-covalently to DNA either by intercalating between the base pairs (e.g. the anthracyclines), or by non-intercalative groove binding (particularly in the minor groove, e.g. distamycin A) employing a combination of hydrophobic, electrostatic, hydrogen-bonding and dipolar forces. Indeed some agents may employ more than one mode, an example being the extensively studied, potent antitumour antibiotic CC1065 which binds strongly and reversibly in the minor groove of DNA specifically at stretches of AT base pairs, and bonds covalently to the N3 position on adenine.

It is becoming increasingly clear that a crucial aspect in the understanding of antitumour drug–DNA interactions is an appreciation of the precise structure of DNA itself. There have been significant advances in our understanding of the way in which the nucleotide sequence and various external factors can effect DNA conformation. Right-handed, double helical B-DNA is generally assumed to be the most relevant DNA structure *in vivo* (Wing *et al.*, 1980). Sequences containing runs of contiguous guanines, however, have a tendency to adopt an A conformation (Wang *et al.*, 1982). Similarly, the left-handed Z-DNA helix is favoured by alternative G-C sequences (Wang *et al.*, 1979), the conversion from Z to B-DNA being influenced by metal ions, ionic stength, supercoiling and various DNA binding proteins (Rich *et al.*, 1984; Wells & Harvey, 1987). DNA sequence can also cause bending, particularly in $(dA)_n$ sequences ($n = 4$–6) when they are appropriately and repeatedly spaced along the DNA (Koo *et al.*, 1986). Recently, other alternative DNA structures have received much attention, such as the triple-stranded helix containing both Watson–Crick and Hoogsteen base pairing which can form with homo-purine–homopyrimidine sequences (Le Doan *et al.*, 1987; Moser & Dervan, 1987). Clearly a full appreciation of the conformational polymorphism of DNA is crucial to any understanding of the binding mechanisms of anticancer drugs.

In addition to diverse modes of binding to DNA, antitumour agents can have quite distinct base-pair specificities. For example, most simple alkylating agents are guanine specific, binding primarily to the guanine-N7 position in the major groove of DNA (Hemminki & Ludlum, 1984). Other guanine-specific agents include the natural products anthramycin and mitomycin C, but in these cases binding is primarily to the N2 position in the minor groove of DNA (Hurley & Thurston, 1984; Tomasz *et al.*, 1987). In contrast, agents like CC1065 bind primarily to adenine bases in the minor groove (Reynolds *et al.*, 1985). Coupled to this, following the development of more sophisticated methodologies, it is now apparent that many, if not all the antitumour agents that bind to DNA, do so with some degree of base-sequence specificity. This can vary from agents which show a limited discrimination between the target base in different sequence contexts, to those which show a high degree of selectivity to certain unique sequences, with the corresponding avoidance of others. It is this primary base-sequence specificity that this chapter will address. It is by no means intended as an exhaustive review of this rapidly expanding area, but rather to illustrate how even relatively simple molecules can interact with DNA in quite specific and predictable ways, to discuss what relevance this may have to the mechanism of action of these drugs, and how this knowledge could aid in the future rational design of more sequence-specific agents.

Methods for determining DNA base-sequence specificity

The base specificity for a number of antitumour agents has been known for many years as the result of, for example, spectroscopic methods, DNA homopolymer studies, and from the analysis of modified base products by high pressure liquid chromatography, but is is only in recent years that it has become possible to examine the precise DNA primary base-sequence specificity of such agents. Undoubtedly the major advances in this area have been the result of modifications of DNA sequencing-based techniques in which a fragment of DNA of known sequence is used to pinpoint the precise position of drug binding.

The principles of four of the main sequencing-based methods are shown in Fig. 10.1. A number of strategies are available for those agents which can bind covalently to DNA. For example for those compounds which can cause strand cleavage directly, or whose binding can be converted into a strand break by an appropriate reaction, the sites of binding are determined relatively easily (Fig. 10.1a). Two examples of the latter reactions which have been used extensively are the quantitative conversion of alkylations at the guanine-N7 position to strand breaks by treatment with hot piperidine (Mattes et al., 1986b) and the thermal cleavage at sites of adenine-N3 alkylation (Reynolds et al., 1985).

Where strand cleavage is not possible, sites of covalent modification can be determined as blocks to the function of enzymes such as exonucleases (Fig. 10.1c), or DNA polymerases (Fig. 10.1d). For example, various kinds of damage block the 3' to 5' exonuclease action of enzymes such as Escherichia coli exonuclease III (Royer-Pokora et al., 1981) or the 5' to 3' exonuclease action of lambda exonuclease, the latter enzyme appearing to be particularly sensitive to obstructions in the minor groove of DNA, and not to alkylations at the guanine-N7 position in the major groove (Mattes, 1990). Similarly, a number of drugs, including bifunctional alkylating agents and platinum analogues, can impede the progress of E. coli DNA polymerase (Gralla et al., 1987) and the thermostable Taq DNA polymerase (Ponti et al., 1991a), the latter assay having the advantage that sensitivity can be increased by using many cycles of polymerization.

These methods are only applicable to agents which can bind covalently to DNA. The determination of the base-sequence specificity of non-covalently or equilibrium binding drugs requires a different approach, that of 'footprinting' (Fig. 10.1b). This powerful technique was originally developed to investigate protein–DNA interactions and relies on the ability of ligands bound to DNA to protect the DNA from cleavage by enzymes such as DNase I (Drew, 1984), or radical-producing chemicals such as methidiumpropyl-Fe-EDTA (Dervan, 1986). This technique is now used extensively to reveal both the position and length of drug

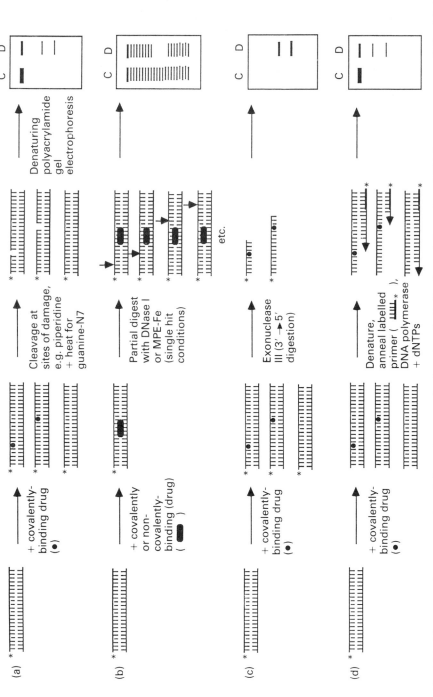

Fig. 10.1. Diagrammatic representation of the main sequencing-based methods for determining a drug–DNA base-sequence specificity: (a) strand cleavage at the site of drug binding, e.g. piperidine cleavage and thermal cleavage assays; (b) footprinting; (c) exonuclease stop assay; and (d) polymerase stop assay. Site of radioactive labelling is indicated by *. In each case drug doses are used that give at most one drug molecule bound per DNA fragment (so-called single hit kinetics). Under these conditions the intensity of a band produced in assays (a), (c) and (d) is related to the

binding-sites and has recently been reviewed (Portugal, 1989). The method has also been refined recently by Dabrowiak *et al.* to enable binding constants for drugs at specific sites within a DNA sequence to be obtained (Dabrowiak & Goodisman, 1989).

The sequencing-based techniques can give information on the precise location of drug binding-sites on relatively large (up to several hundred base pair) fragments of DNA, but gives little information about the type and dynamics of the interaction and the functional groups involved. The ability to produce large quantities of oligonucleotides of known sequence for drug binding studies is now enabling such information to be obtained. The application of two-dimensional nuclear magnetic resonance (NMR) methods to the study of oligonucleotide–drug complexes is beginning to provide high resolution data on the conformation of both drug and nucleic acid at the binding site, and can identify the structural basis of sequence specificity in drug binding from analysis of the complexes formed with oligonucleotides of differing sequence. This approach in solution is paralleled by recent advances in the X-ray crystallographic analysis of similar complexes. Despite the inherent problems of 'end-effects' when using short oligonucleotides, these techniques are proving to be invaluable in the study of ligand–DNA interactions, and the application of each method to the study of antitumour-drug complexes has recently been reviewed (Leupin, 1990; Wang *et al.*, 1990). The two techniques yield complimentary information and such data; in conjunction with computational methods, can generate three-dimensional models of ligand–DNA complexes (e.g. Neidle *et al.*, 1987). A number of theoretical methods have also been applied to the problem of the base-sequence selectivity of antitumour drugs. This area has been reviewed extensively by Pullman (1989). An example relevant to studies to be described later is the calculation of the molecular electrostatic potential which has become, in recent years, a useful index in the description of the properties of biological macromolecules such as DNA with a direct bearing on their chemical and biochemical reactivity towards charged attacking species (Pullman & Pullman, 1981).

Examples of DNA sequence-specific reactions by antitumour agents

In this section the diversity of the sequence specificity of DNA binding antitumour agents is illustrated by some of the more widely studied examples of major groove alkylators, minor groove alkylators, intercalators and non-intercalative groove binders. The major points are summarized in Table 10.1. See Chapter 11 for a discussion of agents which can cleave DNA.

Table 10.1. A summary of the diverse modes of binding and sequence specificities for a number of synthetic and naturally occurring antitumour agents

Drug	Mode of binding	Sequence preference	Remarks	Reference
Mechlorethamine	Covalent, guanine-N7 in major groove	$(G)_n$*	Preference is for internal guanines	Mattes et al., 1986a
		5'-GNC	Interstrand crosslink preference	Millard et al., 1990
Chloroethylnitrosoureas	Covalent, guanine-N7 in major groove	$(G)_n$*	Preference is for internal guanines	Hartley et al., 1986
Uracil mustard	Covalent, guanine-N7 in major groove	5'PyGC	–	Kohn et al., 1987
Quinacrine mustard	Intercalation, covalent guanine-N7	5'GGPu, 5'GTPu	Preference is for alkylation event	Kohn et al., 1987
DZQ	Covalent, guanine-N7 in major groove	$(G)_n$*	Quinone form of drug	Hartley et al., 1991a
		5'-GC (particularly TGC)	Hydroquinone form of drug	
Cisplatin	Coordination, guanine-N7	5'GC	Interstrand crosslink preference	Hopkins et al., 1991
Mitomycin C	Covalent, guanine-N2 in minor groove	5'CG	Interstrand crosslink preference	Teng et al., 1989 Weidner et al., 1990 Borowy-Borowski et al., 1990a,b

Anthramycin	Covalent, guanine-N2 in minor groove	PuGPu	—	Hertzberg et al., 1986 Hurley et al., 1988
CC-1065	Covalent, adenine-N3 in minor groove	5'-AAAAA and 5'-PuNTTA	—	Reynolds et al., 1985
Doxorubicin	Intercalation	5'(A/T)CG, 5'(A/T)GC 5'-CA, (particularly 5'-TCA)	From footprint data From in vitro transcription assay	Chaires et al., 1990 Phillips et al., 1990
Actinomycin D	Intercalation	5'GC (particularly 5'-(T/C)GC)	—	Rehfuss et al., 1990
Echinomycin	Bis-intercalation	5'-CG	—	Low et al., van Dyke & Dervan, 1984
Netropsin	Non-covalent, minor groove	$(A/T)_4$	—	Zimmer & Wahnert, 1986
Distamycin A	Non-covalent minor groove	$(A/T)_5$	—	Zimmer & Wahnert, 1986

* $n = \geqslant 3$.
DZQ, 3,6-diaziridinyl-1,4-benzoquinone.

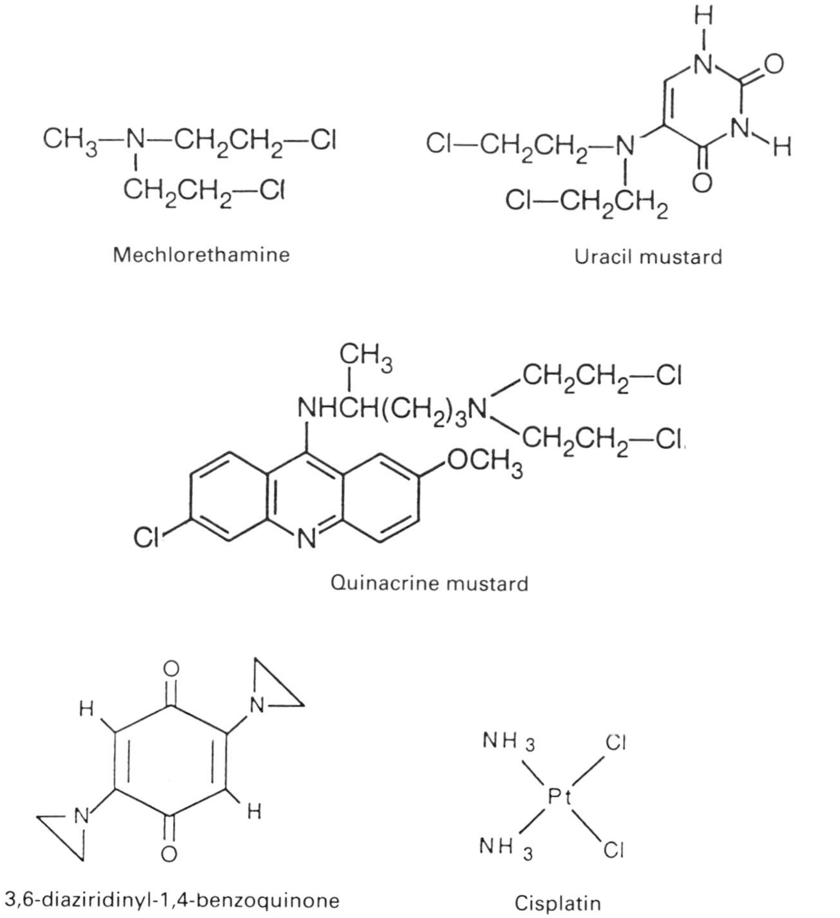

Mechlorethamine   Uracil mustard

Quinacrine mustard

3,6-diaziridinyl-1,4-benzoquinone   Cisplatin

Fig. 10.2. Structures of the DNA major groove alkylating drugs described in the text.

Major groove alkylators

Mechlorethamine (Fig. 10.2) was the first clinically effective anticancer agent, and other nitrogen mustard derivatives such as melphalan, cyclophosphamide and chlorambucil, are still among the most useful clinical agents despite their apparently non-specific chemical reaction mechanism. Covalent binding may occur at many nucleophilic sites within nucleic acids and proteins, but DNA is probably the most important target with reaction predominantly at the N7 position of guanine in the major groove. The cytotoxic lesion produced by these agents is generally assumed to be a DNA interstrand crosslink between two guanine N7 positions.

Simple highly reactive agents of this type would not generally be considered candidates for any degree of sequence-specific reaction with

DNA. Recent results, however, indicate that agents of this type do react with a predictable sequence specificity. Using a sequencing-based technique, a direct examination of the guanine-N7 reaction by this type of alkylating agent at the individual base level was possible. Large variations in alkylation were found to exist among guanines in a DNA sequence following treatment with, for example, nitrogen mustards (Fig. 10.3) (Mattes *et al.*, 1986a; Kohn *et al.*, 1987, Hartley *et al.*, 1990) and chloroethylnitrosoureas (Hartley *et al.*, 1986). The most striking finding was that most agents reacted preferentially within runs of contiguous guanines, the degree of preference being much greater than would be expected from the number of guanines alone. This may be due to a number of factors, including an increased accessibility of the guanine-N7 in such sequences but in general reaction by those agents that can produce a positively charged alkylating intermediate (such as the aziridinium ion produced in aqueous solution from nitrogen mustards) correlates well with the calculated molecular electrostatic potential at the reactive site. The molecular electrostatic potential is sequence dependent and strongly influenced by its nearest neighbour base pairs (Pullman & Pullman, 1981). Correspondingly, the lack of any distinct sequence selectivity for agents such as busulphan is consistent with its inability to form a charged or partially charged intermediate (Ponti *et al.*, 1991b).

It is, therefore, clear that for these relatively simple agents the sequence specificity of reaction is imposed directly by the DNA. In addition, however, the substituent attached to the reactive group can introduce a distinct sequence preference for reaction, as clearly demonstrated in the case of uracil and quinacrine mustards (Figs 10.2 and 10.3) (Kohn *et al.*, 1987). The preference of uracil mustard for 5′-Py*G*C sequences (which are some of the weakest sites for other mustards) was proposed to be due to a specific favourable interaction between the uracil-04 position on the drug and the 3′-cytosine amino group facilitating reaction at the 5′-guanine. In the case of quinacrine mustard a rapid initial non-covalent (intercalative) binding is indicated by the high reactivity of this compound. The observed distinct sequence preference for alkylation relies on the two bases 3′ to the reactive guanine which must be GPu or TPu. Intercalation occurs between these two base pairs and the reacting side chain can stretch over the intervening guanine or thymine (but not an adenine or cytosine because of unfavourably placed amino groups) and alkylate the guanine-N7. These two examples clearly demonstrate how changing the non-alkylating portion of even a simple molecule can introduce specific base-sequence preferences for the drug.

Another example that has recently emerged clearly demonstrates how even the same drug under different conditions can react with a different DNA sequence specificity. 3,6-diaziridinyl-1,4-benzoquinone (DZQ, Fig. 10.2) reacts with all guanine-N7 positions with a selectivity similar to other

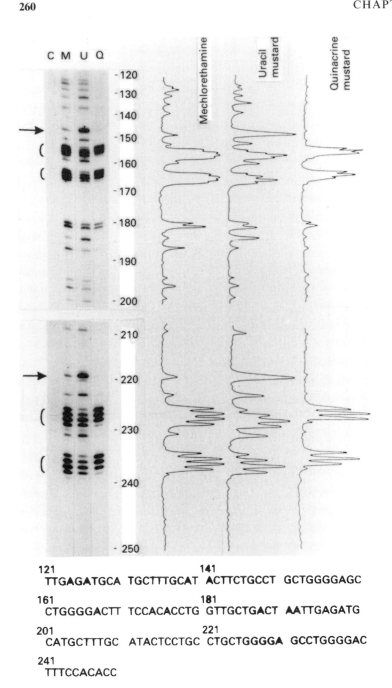

121   141
TTGAGATGCA TGCTTTGCAT ACTTCTGCCT GCTGGGGAGC
161   181
CTGGGGACTT TCCACACCTG GTTGCTGACT AATTGAGATG
201   221
CATGCTTTGC ATACTCCTGC CTGCTGGGGA GCCTGGGGAC
241
TTTCCACACC

Fig. 10.3. Sites of guanine-N7 alkylation produced in a fragment of simian virus 40 (SV40) DNA following treatment with mechlorethamine (M), uracil mustard (U) or quinacrine mustard (Q). C is control unalkylated DNA. The dose of drug was chosen to give approximately the same level of overall alkylation in each case. Brackets indicate the runs of contiguous guanines, and the arrows sites of preferred alkylation by uracil mustard. The corresponding densitometric scans are shown aligned with the gel, and the appropriate base sequence is given.

alkylating agents. However, upon reduction of the drug to the hydroquinone form (either chemically or enzymatically) this agent not only becomes more reactive overall, but now only alkylates guanines in a 5'-GC sequence (and particularly 5'-TGC sequences) (Hartley *et al.*, 1991a). A model to explain this unique reaction has been proposed in which the drug can intercalate between the base pairs in the 5'-GC sequence and as the hydroquinone can produce hydrogen bonding to the cytosine amino group and cytosine O2 position, orienting the drug in an ideal position to alkylate the guanine-N7 position in this sequence.

The above sequence specificities are for the initial monoalkylation event of these bifunctional agents. It has been assumed for many years from measurements on static B-DNA that the interstrand crosslink produced by nitrogen mustards would be between the two guanine-N7 positions in the sequence 5'-GC. Recent experimental evidence however, from the laboratory of Hopkins (Millard *et al.*, 1990), and confirmed in our own laboratory (Berardini *et al.*, 1991), suggests that crosslinking by mechlorethamine occurs preferentially in the sequence 5'-GNC (where N = any base). This clearly shows that care must be taken in extrapolating directly from calculations on static non-distorted DNA to the situation in solution. The preference for 5'-GNC sequences also appears to hold for the longer crosslinking aziridinylbenzoquinones (Berardini *et al.*, 1991), although DZQ is an exception in that upon reduction it crosslinks preferentially in a 5'-GC sequence (Berardini *et al.*, 1992) consistent with the altered sequence selectivity for the hydroquinone form of this drug, and the model proposed for its interaction with DNA (see above). Cisplatin (Fig. 10.2), another agent which can link two guanines through their guanine-N7 positions was, however, found to produce crosslinks preferentially in the sequence 5'-GC (Hopkins *et al.*, 1991). In the case of the nitrogen mustards, although the substituent attached to the reactive group can influence the sequence specificity of monoalkylation (see above) and the rate of interstrand crosslink formation (Hartley *et al.*, 1991b), it remains to be seen to what extent it can influence the base-sequence specificity of the crosslink.

Minor groove alkylators

Mitomycin C (Fig. 10.4) is a potent antitumour antibiotic that is used in clinical treatment. Under physiological conditions it is unreactive towards DNA, but upon reduction of the quinone function gives rise to a reactive form which can bind covalently to DNA and produce interstrand crosslinks, the latter lesion assumed to be the cytotoxic lesion. The alkylation event is specific for the N2 position of guanine in the minor groove (Tomasz *et al.*, 1987). Evidence that the site of crosslinking is preferentially in 5'-CG sequences has been derived from a number of techniques

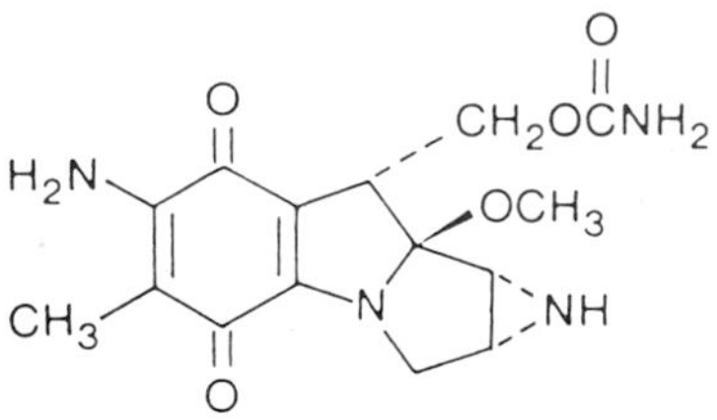

Mitomycin C 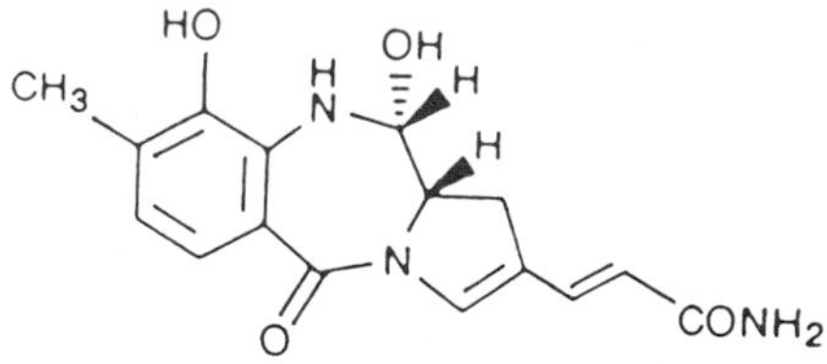   Anthramycin

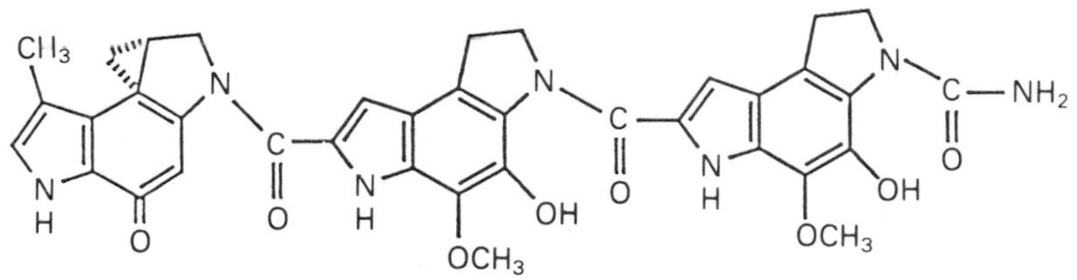

CC-1065

Fig. 10.4. Structures of the DNA minor groove alkylating drugs described in the text.

utilizing synthetic DNA oligomers and electrophoresis (Teng *et al.*, 1989), chemical cleavage (Weidner *et al.*, 1990), and high pressure liquid chromatographic separation of digests (Borowy-Borowski *et al.*, 1990a,b). It has been suggested that the base selectivity stems solely from the crosslinking event (Teng *et al.*, 1989). Other recent studies, however, suggest that a base-sequence preference exists for the mitomycin C monoalkylation step and the specificity for 5'-CG sequences is reinforced by the second, crosslinking event (Borowy-Borowski *et al.*, 1990b; Li & Kohn, 1991) although the mechanisms proposed to account for this differ.

Anthramycin (Fig. 10.4) is a member of the pyrrolo[1,4] benzodiazepine class of antitumour antibiotics which can also bind covalently to the guanine-N2 position but this agent does not produce crosslinks (Thurston & Hurley, 1983; Hurley & Thurston, 1984). The resultant drug adducts lie snugly in the minor groove, following the curvature of the double helix. Footprinting and exonuclease III digestion experiments have shown that the bound drug spans three base pairs with the attacked GC base pair in the centre, and exhibits a preference for purine–guanine–purine sequences (Hertzberg *et al.*, 1986; Hurley *et al.*, 1988). In a series of natural and synthetic analogues a good correlation was found between the extent of DNA alkylation and *in vitro* and *in vivo* potency (Hurley *et al.*, 1988), although recent evidence suggests that non-covalent binding may contribute to biological activity in some cases (Jones et al., 1990).

CC-1065 (Fig. 10.4) is a potent antitumour antibiotic produced by Streptomyces zenensis (Reynolds et al., 1985). Although never clinically evaluated because of its delayed and irreversible toxicity in rodents at therapeutic doses, the mechanism of action of this agent has been the subject of extensive investigation (Warpehoski & Hurley, 1988; Warpehoski et al., 1990). It lies within the minor groove of DNA and covalently binds through the N3 position of adenine (Hurley et al., 1984). The drug covalently binds preferentially to two consensus sequences, 5'-AAAAA* and 5'-PuNTTA*, where (*) indicates the covalently modified base and N represents any base (Reynolds et al., 1985). The most stringent sequence specificity lies at the 3' end of the sequences at AAA* and TTA* (Hurley et al., 1990). There are several interesting features of the binding of the drug. For example, the primary molecular basis for the sequence selectivity of this agent is postulated to be determined not by sequence-specific non-covalent binding, but by the sequence requirement inherent in the covalent bonding step itself (Warpehoski & Hurley, 1988). This can be envisioned as either a sequence-dependent catalytic activation of the drug, or a sequence-dependent conformational flexibility of the DNA, or possibly a combination of the two.

The CC-1065 molecule consists of three repeating pyrroloindole subunits, one of which contains a DNA-reactive cyclopropyl function. This subunit alone contains sufficient structural information to mediate both the sequence specificity, DNA bending and antitumour efficacy of the drug (Warpehoski et al., 1990; Lee et al., 1991). The other two subunits can fine-tune the sequence specificity of subunit A (Warpehoski & Hurley, 1988). Bonding of CC-1065 bends the DNA in towards the minor groove by about 15° and winds DNA by about the equivalent of one base pair per drug (Lee et al., 1991).

Intercalating drugs

Anthracycline antibiotics, daunomycin and Adriamycin (Fig. 10.5), are among the most potent compounds in current clinical use in cancer chemotherapy. While the intercalative mode of binding of these drugs to DNA is well established (Quigley et al., 1980), the assessment of the base-sequence preference has been the subject of numerous experimental studies with conflicting results (reviewed in Pullman, 1989). In this case theoretical studies by Pullman et al. were useful in suggesting that daunomycin binds preferentially to a triplet sequence consisting of contiguous GC base pairs flanked by an AT base pair (Chen et al., 1985, 1986). Recent footprinting titration experiments are consistent with this prediction with the triplet sequences 5'-(A/T)CG and 5'-(A/T)GC sequences identified as

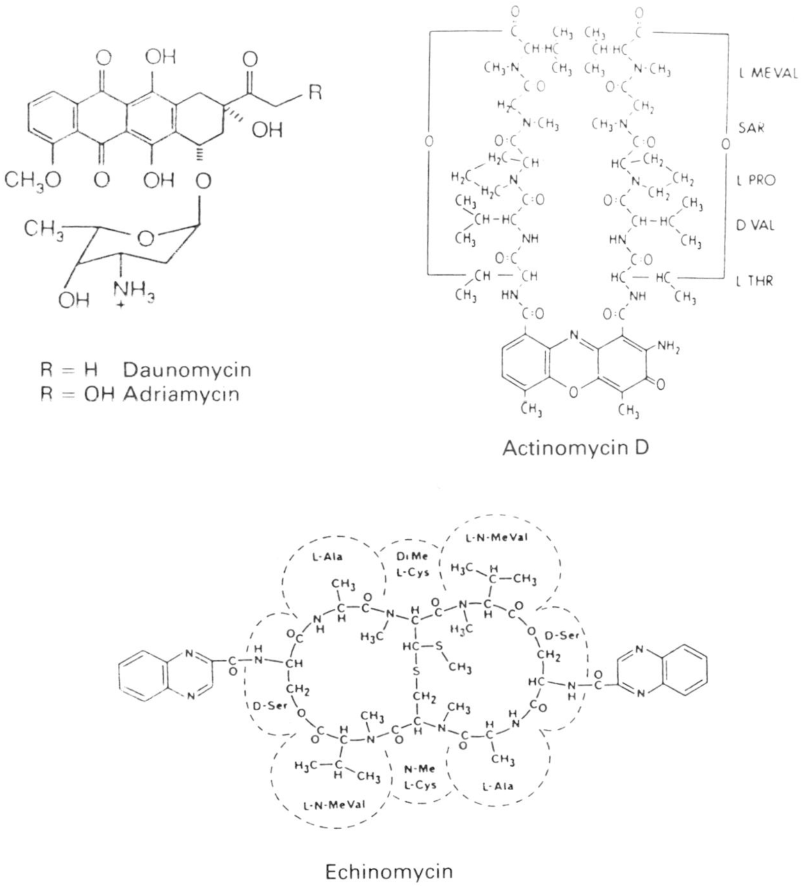

R = H   Daunomycin
R = OH Adriamycin

Actinomycin D

Echinomycin

Fig. 10.5. Structures of the DNA intercalating drugs described in the text.

most preferred daunomycin binding-sites (Chaires *et al.*, 1990). Other recent results, however, using an *in vitro* transcription assay, indicate that the preferred intercalative binding-site for daunomycin and Adriamycin is at 5′-CA sequences (and particularly 5′-TCA sites) and, furthermore, that irreversible adducts produced by Adriamycin were found at 5′-GC sequences (reviewed in Phillips *et al.*, 1990). High-resolution X-ray crystallographic studies have provided the structure of daunomycin bound to the oligonucleotides 5′-d(CGATCG)$_2$ and 5′-d(CGTACG)$_2$ (Wang *et al.*, 1987; Moore *et al.*, 1989; Frederick *et al.*, 1990). In these cases daunomycin molecules are intercalated in the CG sequences at both ends of the distorted B helix and these high-resolution structures provide some explanations for the DNA base triplet specificity derived from the solution and theoretical studies.

The sequence specificity of other intercalating drugs has been easier to determine. Actinomycin D (Fig. 10.5) is used in the treatment of Wilm's tumour. The drug binds to DNA via the minor groove at GC-rich sites. The ring system of the drug intercalates between the base pairs of DNA, while the amide carbonyl groups of the drugs threonine moieties hydrogen bond to the 2-amino group of guanine in the minor groove (Scott *et al.*, 1988). This agent was one of the first to be studied by footprinting methods which suggested a preference for the sequence 5'-GC (van Dyke *et al.*, 1982; Lane *et al.*, 1983). This has recently been refined by a quantitative footprinting analysis to show the sites of highest binding constant for the drug being in 5'-TGC and 5'-CGC sequences (Rehfuss *et al.*, 1990).

Echinomycin (Fig. 10.5) is one member of a family of quinoxaline antitumour antibiotics which react with DNA from the minor groove so as to form a *bis*-intercalated complex in which two GC base pairs are sandwiched between the quinoxaline chromophores. The binding to DNA has been studied extensively by solution studies, footprinting, NMR and crystallography and recently reviewed in detail (Waring, 1990). Footprinting revealed a clear preference for strong binding to a 5'-CG sequence although the actual binding site size is at least four base pairs (Low *et al.*, 1984; van Dyke & Dervan, 1984). The origins of the sequence selectivity of echinomycin and a related compound triostin A were revealed in the crystal structures of their complexes with oligonucleotides (Quigley *et al.*, 1986). The alanine residues of the peptide ring are crucial determinants in the observed specificity, their CO and NH groups forming hydrogen bonds to the 2-amino groups and N3 atoms respectively of the sandwiched guanines.

The most unusual structural feature of these complexes is that the bases flanking the sandwiched dinucleotides are Hoogsteen paired. However, recent studies of longer stretches of DNA in solution have concluded that the bulk of the structural changes induced by the binding of echinomycin to DNA do not involve Hoogsteen and non-Watson–Crick base pairing, but are due to sequence-specific unwinding of the helix in a manner which is strongly dependent on the nature of the surrounding nucleotide sequence (McLean & Waring, 1988; McLean *et al.*, 1989).

Non-intercalative minor groove-binding drugs

A number of natural and synthetic compounds are known to bind to DNA in a non-intercalative and non-covalent manner. Perhaps the best known compounds of this type are the antitumour antibiotics netropsin and distamycin (Fig. 10.6). It is clear that these compounds bind in the minor groove of DNA, preferentially at AT-rich sequences with a binding site size of four and five base pairs respectively (Zimmer & Wahnert, 1986). Several studies, including footprinting and affinity cleaving studies [in which distamycin is tagged with an EDTA(Fe) moiety which generates

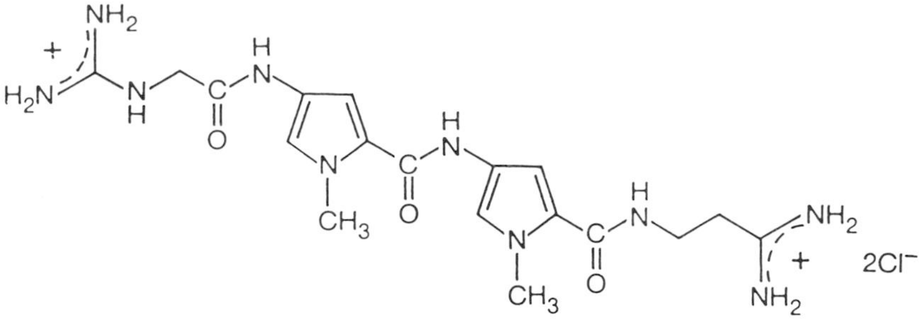

Netropsin

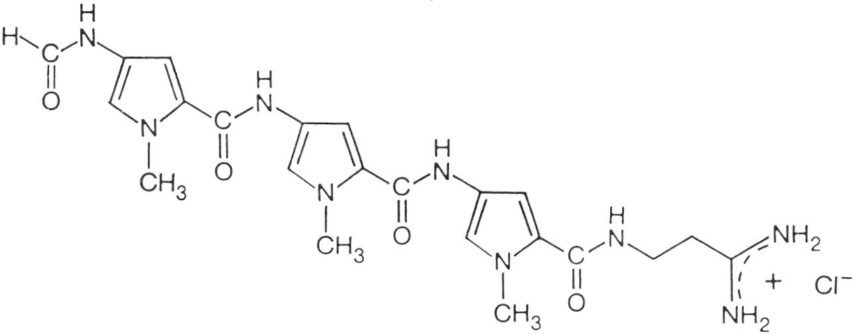

Distamycin A

Fig. 10.6. Structures of the DNA non-intercalative minor groove binding drugs described in the text.

radicals at binding sites and leads to local cleavage of the DNA], indicate that there is discrimination among different AT-rich sequences (Schultz & Dervan, 1984; Zimmer & Wahnert, 1986). The molecular basis of their interaction with DNA has become better understood as a result of several X-ray diffraction analyses, using DNA oligomers containing binding sites of AATT (Kopka *et al.*, 1985), ATAT (Coll *et al.*, 1989) and AAATTT (Coll *et al.*, 1987), and from several NMR studies (e.g. Pelton & Wemmer, 1989, 1990). It is clear that binding in the narrow minor groove of B-DNA by these agents uses a complex combination of interactions including hydrogen bonds, ionic charge interactions and van der Waal's interactions, and that it is a highly dynamic binding process reflecting the fluidity of the DNA molecule.

Development of novel DNA sequence-specific agents

There is considerable interest in the development of more highly sequence-specific agents. One guiding principle behind such efforts is that increased sequence specificity will lead to increased biological effect with hopefully less toxic side effects. Related to this is the hope that it may be possible ultimately to selectively suppress the transcription of particular gene sequences. Approaches towards this latter goal include the targeting of single-strand sequences with β-oligonucleotides or their modified counterparts (the so-called 'antisense strategy', Dolnick, 1991) and the targeting of double-stranded sequences to form triplex structures (the so-called 'anti-gene strategy', Maher et al., 1989). Another approach utilizes the knowledge gained from the sequence-specific interactions of natural products to develop novel structures which can recognize unique sequences in double-stranded DNA. One elegant example which will be used to describe such an approach is based on netropsin and distamycin, leading to the development of 'lexitropsins' or information-reading oligopeptides (Lown, 1988, 1990).

Netropsin and distamycin contain, respectively, two and three pyrrole units joined by peptide linkages. A close examination of the structural requirements for the molecular recognition of the drugs to their AT-rich sequences led to the suggestion that replacement of one or more of the pyrrole units, with a heterocycle capable of accepting a hydrogen bond from guanine-(2)NH_2 such as imidazole, should alter the preference to allow the recognition of GC base pairs in a predictable fashion (Kopka et al., 1985: Lown et al., 1986). Compounds of this type containing imidazole instead of pyrrole units were synthesized and shown by footprinting experiments to recognize some GC-containing sites whilst retaining a memory for AT sequences (Lown et al., 1986).

The memory for AT sequences was overcome by producing a second generation of lexitropsins in which one of the two positive charges was removed. This was found to overcome the natural bias of dicationic compounds for AT-rich sequences in which the site of greatest negative potential occurs in the minor groove (Lavery et al., 1982). These monocationic compounds were shown by footprinting to target cleanly for GC sites (Kissinger et al., 1987) such that a compound containing two imidazole units showed a preference for the sequence CCGT. It was deduced from NMR analysis of a complex of this compound with d[CATG-GCCATG]$_2$ that the dominant factor which determines the reading of the 3'-terminal AT base pair is the van der Waal's interaction between the methylenes at the carboxyl terminus of the lexitropsin and the DNA (Lee et al., 1988a). These methylenes would enter into steric contact with the guanine-NH_2 of a GC base pair thereby forcing the recognition of an AT base pair. To test this, a third generation 'truncated' lexitropsin was designed and synthesized with only one methylene at the C terminus. A detailed NMR analysis has revealed that on binding to d[CGCAATTGCG]$_2$, whereas the parent pyrrole containing compound binds to the central AATT, the 'truncated' molecule is displaced to read the sequence ATTG (Lee et al., 1988b). Thus it became possible to predictably alter the structure of an AT-recognizing minor groove ligand

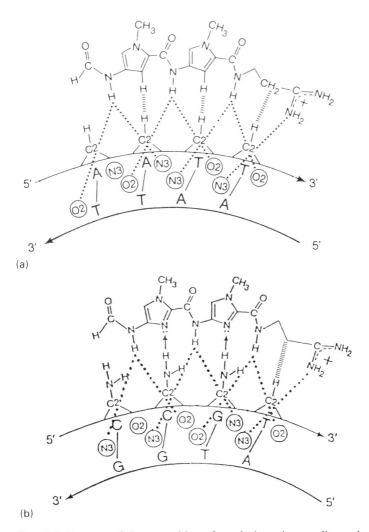

Fig. 10.7. Features of the recognition of two lexitropsins on oligonucleotide sequences as determined by high-field ¹H-NMR (nuclear magnetic resonance). (a) a singly charged compound related to netropsin binding to its preferred AATT sequence. (b) a GC-recognizing compound in which pyrrole groups are replaced by imidazole groups capable of accepting hydrogen bonds from guanine-(2) amino groups. The preferred binding site of this drug is now CCGT. In both cases dotted lines indicate hydrogen bonding and dashed lines represent intermolecular van der Waals interactions.

to produce GC-specific compounds. The features of the recognition of an AT-recognizing versus a GC-recognizing lexitropsin, as deduced from high field ¹H-NMR of oligonucleotide–drug complexes, are shown in Fig. 10.7.

Each refinement of the lexitropsin model gave information of specific contacts and, in turn, suggested future avenues for development. The properties of hydrogen bond accepting heterocycles other than imidazole have been examined. For example, monocationic *bis*-furan compounds confer GC recognition but, whereas the *bis*-imidazole counterpart reads 5'-CCAT in the oligomer d[CATGGCCATG]$_2$, this compound recognizes 5'-GCCA (Lee *et al.*, 1988a, 1989). Conversely, lexitropsins containing thiazole units in which the sulphur is directed towards the floor of the minor groove exhibit very strict preferences for AT sequences, and are even more sequence discriminating than distamycin (Rao *et al.*, 1990).

Because the lexitropsins are made up of units linked together, targetting for longer sequences should be possible by adding further heterocyclic units. However, it may not be a coincidence that the longest natural compounds of this type (distamycin and anthelvencin) contain only three pyrrole units. Longer molecules may get 'out of phase' with the corresponding DNA sequence. This problem is being approached by connecting netropsin moieties with both flexible and rigid linkers of variable length and assessing their DNA-binding properties (Lown *et al.*, 1989; Lown, 1990).

Many of the lexitropsins synthesized have been shown to have cytostatic activity against human and murine cell lines, and are often superior to netropsin and distamycin (Lown *et al.*, 1989). In addition, the attachment of an alkylating function to netropsin and distamycin significantly increases their antitumour activity (Krowicki *et al.*, 1988; Broggini *et al.*, 1991), although antiviral activity is not significantly altered (Krowicki *et al.*, 1988). A distamycin derivative containing a nitrogen mustard group at one end is a potent agent presently under investigation (Broggini *et al.*, 1991). DNA binding is directed by the distamycin portion of the molecule, and alkylation only occurs at a very few adenine-N3 sites in the minor groove with no detectable guanine-N7 alkylation in the major groove, or crosslinking, detected. Thus although this molecule now recognizes the same number of bases, similar sequences, and can alkylate at the same base position as CC-1065, their mechanisms are quite distinct. A number of GC-recognizing lexitropsins containing alkylating groups have also been synthesized recently. It will be interesting to compare their binding, bonding and antitumour properties with their AT-recognizing counterparts.

Other groove binding agents are being used as models for rational structural modification to produce altered sequence specificity, including anthramycins (Thurston *et al.*, 1990) and the Hoechst dye 33258 (Bathini *et al.*, 1990). CC-1065 has also been the object of considerable analogue design including the production of dimers capable of crosslinking DNA, some of which are five- to 10-fold more potent than the already highly potent CC-1065 itself (Mitchell *et al.*, 1989). A rationally designed, highly efficient sequence-specific DNA interstrand crosslinking agent based on the pyrrolobenzodiazepine ring system has recently been synthesized (Bose *et al.*, 1992). This agent spans six base pairs, crosslinking guanine-N2 positions in a central 5′-GATC sequence, and is remarkably cytotoxic *in vitro*. Clues to the further rational design of sequence-specific drugs will emerge as the intricate mechanisms involved in the recognition of DNA by proteins and small molecules are unravelled.

Conclusion and future directions

Little is understood of the basis for the wide differences in sensitivity to cytotoxic drugs shown by tumours of different pathological types. Many mechanisms are likely to be involved. One possible contributing factor might be that sensitive tumour cells are maintained in growth by the action of certain genes whose DNA contains sequences which are unusually susceptible to damage by DNA-binding cytotoxic drugs. The previous description indicates that, even with simple chemical structures, base-sequence specificity is a feature of drug–DNA interaction and that we may now be in a position to modify drugs so that they can be made selective for defined base sequences. Alternatively, or additionally, susceptibility to DNA damage may reside in less effective repair when damage occurs at certain regions of susceptible genes. Testing of these hypotheses will involve a combination of chemical and molecular biological techniques.

The data from reactions on isolated DNA suggests that GC-rich regions in genes could be preferred sites of damage to alkylating agents such as nitrogen mustards. The production of interstrand and intrastrand crosslinks would be especially favoured. The human genome contains regions of unexpectedly high GC content ($> 80\%$) which accounts for approximately 1.3% of the genome and includes regions in a number of oncogenes (Zerial *et al.*, 1986). The 5′ flank of the c-*Ha-ras* oncogene is particularly GC-rich and these sequences do indeed serve as preferred sites of alkylation *in vitro* by nitrogen mustards and chloroethylnitrosoureas (Mattes *et al.*, 1988).

A functional role of GC-rich sequences is suggested by their frequent occurrence in genes associated with proliferation. Certainly for some genes these runs are part of sequences known to be involved in the control of gene expression (e.g. SP1 transcription factor binding-sites in the preferentially alkylated regions of the c-*Ha-ras* gene). A search of the Genbank DNA data base, as well as revealing a significant number of oncogenes (Mattes *et al.*, 1988), also included a number of viral sequences, including the Epstein–Barr virus (EBV). In EBV large regions of extraordinary GC-richness are located within the 3-kb repeats beginning about 3 kb from the replication origin and have features suggesting an important control function (Karlin, 1986). It is interesting to note that the nuclei of tumour cells from the endemic African form of Burkitt's lymphoma contain multiple copies of the EBV genome, and this form of lymphoma is extraordinarily sensitive to chemotherapy: one or two doses of nitrogen mustard (cyclophosphamide) can produce dramatic regression of the tumour (Ziegler, 1981).

The definition of which lesions produced by a given drug are biologically the most important requires new methods of analysis. The most frequent sites of binding may not be the most biologically significant. Critical experiments to determine especially vulnerable target sequences will require model systems in which the specificity of drug binding to base sequences of a known gene can be measured and the biological effect assessed by the resulting effect on protein synthesis. It has been shown (Futscher & Erickson, 1990) that alkylating agents produce changes in expression of oncogene mRNA (causing elevation then depression of the level of transcripts), but the regions of the gene which are critical for the changes are not known. The analysis of the detailed pattern of binding to these and other early growth response genes will be of great interest.

In cell-free systems, DNA-binding drugs can be shown to interfere specifically with a number of biochemical functions. For example, alkylating agents and platinum analogues can block at specific base sites the progress of both DNA polymerases (Gralla $et\ al.$, 1987; Ponti $et\ al.$, 1991a) and RNA polymerases (Pieper $et\ al.$, 1989; Pieper & Erickson, 1990). Distamycins can specifically inhibit the binding of DNA transcription factors which contain $(A/T)_4$ within their recognition sequence (Broggini $et\ al.$, 1989) by either shielding the protein recognition site, or changing the DNA conformation at these sites. In some cases drug binding can augment a protein–DNA interaction, for example, in the formation of stable ternary complexes with topoisomerases and several intercalating drugs. Again, there is evidence of sequence specificity here (Capranico $et\ al.$, 1990). In these, and other examples, the direct relationship between the basic observations in simple model systems and the biochemical and biological consequences of such drug binding in cells remains largely undetermined.

One of the major limitations of current methodology has been that the detailed analysis of base sequence specificity has been performed on isolated DNA fragments, or synthetic oligonucleotides. The question of whether the preferential reactivity is preserved in intact cells is therefore critical. Using the highly reiterated α-sequence of human DNA as a target it has now been shown (Hartley $et\ al.$, 1991c) that the particular base-sequence specificities of mechlorethamine, uracil mustard and quinacrine mustard are maintained when α-DNA is extracted, and sequenced, from drug-treated cells. Although very encouraging this result is only a first step since the analysis (using piperidine cleavage) is limited to drugs which bind at guanine-N7, excluding many important drug–DNA interactions. Furthermore, α-DNA is not the desired target.

We need to be able to determine the base-sequence specificity of DNA binding and repair in defined gene sequences in drug-treated intact cells, both for drugs which bind covalently and those which do not. A possible technical advance is the use of *Taq* DNA polymerase, referred to earlier (Ponti *et al.*, 1991a), which is impeded by a number of covalently binding drugs when bound to isolated DNA. This method might be applicable to defined gene sequences in drug-treated intact cells if the resulting products can be sufficiently amplified. It is likely, however, that this method will be restricted to drugs which bind covalently to DNA.

When designing new sequence-specific agents how many bases should we target? A drug which recognized a unique base sequence of 15 base pairs would be able to bind to only one site in the genome. Such precision can hardly be the aim for treating cancer (but might be for treating viral diseases). As new sequence-selective agents are synthesized it will be necessary to determine the *biological* benefit which comes from increasing selectivity and complexity of structure. It is entirely possible that even small gains in specificity of base binding might lead to considerable increases in biological effect. Conversely, as the complexity of drug structure increases there may be additional pharmacological problems of drug metabolism, distribution and penetration, which limit the degree of selectivity which can be achieved.

How important is covalent binding? Although it may not be important in the case of intercalating agents [although mechanisms have been proposed for the production of covalent binding for agents such as Adriamycin following chemical and enzymatic reduction (Myers *et al.*, 1988)] in general, agents that can covalently attach are more biologically potent. For example, the synthetic modification of Adriamycin to its cyanomorpholinyl analogue which can covalently bind (and crosslink) DNA increases potency by 1000-fold. Similarly, as already discussed, the attachment of an alkylating function to netropsin and distamycin also significantly increases their antitumour activity, and although distamycin and CC-1065 both recognize similar sequences and the same number of bases in the minor groove, the covalent binder CC-1065 shows some six orders of magnitude greater cytotoxicity.

This section so far has dealt with the selectivity of drug binding and the consequences of specific binding. Of equal importance may be the specificity of repair of this binding which would depend on the type of lesion, the primary base sequence containing the lesion, or the genomic location of the damage. There is now clear evidence that repair of DNA damage differs in transcriptionally active and inactive genes. Madhani *et al.* (1986) showed that the pyrimidine dimers induced in DNA by ultraviolet (u.v.) light were equally frequent in the c-*abl* gene (which was expressed in 3T3 fibroblasts) and in the inactive c-*mos* gene. The overall repair of these lesions at 24 h was considerably greater in the transcriptionally active gene. Damage by u.v. light differs from that induced by chemicals in that it is uniform in different genomic locations. Psoralen, a furocoumarin, intercalates into DNA binding covalently to pyrimidine bases after activation with u.v. light. Both monoadducts and interstrand crosslinks can be formed. Vos and Hanawalt (1987) showed that repair of psoralens adducts could be measured in the actively transcribed, amplified, gene dihydrofolate reductase and that monoadducts were repaired more slowly than crosslinks. Thus repair proficiency was shown to be related to the type of chemical lesion. Bohr *et al.* (1987) have pointed out that many chemical agents react preferentially with regions of chromatin which are transcriptionally active and might thus be more 'accessible' to repair enzymes. Bohr and Hanawalt (1987) later showed that u.v. sensitive Chinese hamster ovary (CHO) cells did not repair u.v. damage but repair was restored by transfection with the denV gene (which repairs pyrimidine dimers). The human repair gene ERCC-1 repaired the actively transcribing DHFR gene more efficiently than non-transcribing sequences (Bohr *et al.*, 1988).

Wasserman *et al.* (1990) have now shown that nitrogen mustard mono-adducts are repaired preferentially when a gene is transcriptionally active and, within a gene, the coding region is repaired more efficiently than the non-coding. This was not the case after dimethylsulphate damage implying heterogeneity of repair not only within a gene but between alkylating agents. Furthermore, the adducts were preferentially located in specific genomic regions compared with the genome as a whole.

Another approach towards an analysis at the gene level has been taken by Govan *et al.* (1990) who have shown using *Taq* polymerase that there were different rates of overall repair in small segments (< 500 base pairs) of three different genes after exposure to u.v. light. In similar experiments using 4-nitroquinoline-1-oxide, which produces bulky adducts on purine bases, the chosen regions of the three genes showed varying time courses of adduct removal.

There is therefore good reason to believe that in addition to base-sequence specificity of adduct formation, there are important differences in removal of adducts depending on genomic site and transcriptional activity. The methods to date, however, measure the *overall* repair in particular gene sequences in cells. Techniques that will enable us to examine damage and repair at *individual base sites* within genes will therefore be extremely important in the future.

References

Bathini, Y., Rao, K.E., Shea, R.G. & Lown, J.W. (1990). Molecular recognition between ligands and nucleic acids: novel pyridine- and benzoxazole-containing agents related to Hoechst 33258 that exhibit altered DNA sequence specificity deduced from footprinting analysis and spectroscopic studies. *Chemical Research and Toxicology* **3**, 268–280.

Berardini, M.D., Lee, C.S., Hartley, J.A. & Gibson, N.W. (1992). Nucleotide preferences for DNA interstrand crosslinking by 3,6-diaziridinyl-1,4-benzoquinone (DZQ) and 2,5-dimethylDZQ (MeDZQ) upon reduction by DT-diaphorase (DTD). *Proceedings of the American Association of Cancer Research* **33**, 403.

Berardini, M.D., Souhami, R.L. & Hartley, J.A. (1991). DNA interstrand crosslinking specificity of bifunctional alkylating agents. *British Journal of Cancer* **63** (Suppl. XIII), 46.

Bohr, V.A. & Hanawalt, P.C. (1987). Enhanced repair of pyrimidine dimers in coding and non-coding genomic sequences in CHO cells expressing a prokaryotic DNA repair gene. *Carcinogenesis* **8**, 1333–1336.

Bohr, V.A., Chu, E.H.Y., van Duin, M., Hanawalt, P.C. & Okomoto, D.S. (1988). Human repair gene restores normal pattern of preferential DNA repair in repair defective CHO cells. *Nucleic Acids Research* **16**, 7397–7403.

Bohr, V.A., Phillips, D.H. & Hanawalt, P.C. (1987). Heterogeneous DNA damage and repair in the mammalian genome. *Cancer Research* **47**, 6426–6436.

Borowy-Borowski, H., Lipman, R., Chowdary, D. & Tomasz, M. (1990a). Duplex oligonucleotides crosslinked by mitomycin C at a single site: synthesis, properties and crosslink reversibility. *Biochemistry* **29**, 2992–2999.

Borowy-Borowski, H., Lipman, R., Chowdary, D. & Tomasz, M. (1990b). Recognition between mitomycin C and specific DNA sequences for crosslink formation. *Biochemistry* **29**, 2999–3006.

Bose, D.S., Thompson, A.S., Ching, J., Hartley, J.A., Berardini, M.D., Jenkins, T.C., Neidle, S., Hurley, L.H. & Thurston, D.E. (1992). Rational design of a highly efficient non-reversible DNA interstrand crosslinking agent based on the pyrrolobenzodiazepine ring system. *Journal of the American Chemical Society*, **114**, 4939–4941.

Broggini, M., Erba, E., Ponti, M., Ballinari, D., Geroni, C., Spreafico, F. & D'Incalci, M. (1991). Selective DNA interaction of the novel distamycin derivative FCE 24517. *Cancer Research* **51**, 199–204.

Broggini, M., Ponti, M., Ottolenghi, S., D'Incalci, M., Mongelli, M. & Mantovani, R. (1989). Distamycins inhibit the binding of OTF-1 and NFE-1 transcription factors to their conserved DNA elements. *Nucleic Acids Research* **17**, 1051–1059.

Capranico, G., Zunino, F., Kohn, K.W. & Pommier, Y. (1990). Sequence selective topoisomerase II inhibition by anthracycline derivatives in SV40 DNA: relationship with DNA binding affinity and cytotoxicity. *Biochemistry* **29**, 562–569.

Chaires, J.B., Herrera, J.E. & Waring, M.J. (1990). Preferential binding of daunomycin to 5′T/ACG and 5′T/AGC sequences revealed by footprinting titration experiments. *Biochemistry* **29**, 6145–6153.

Chen, K., Gresh, N. & Pullman, B. (1985). A theoretical investigation on the sequence selective binding of daunomycin to double-stranded polynucleotides. *Molecular Pharmacology* **30**, 279–286.

Chen, K., Gresh, N. & Pullman, B. (1986). A theoretical investigation on the sequence selective binding of Adriamycin to double-stranded polynucleotides. *Nucleic Acids Research* **14**, 2251–2267.

Coll, M., Aymami, J., van der Marel, J.A., van Boom, J.H., Rich, A. & Wang, A.H.-J. (1989). Molecular structure of the netropsin-d(CGCGATATCGCG) complex: DNA conformation in an alternating AT segment. *Biochemistry* **28**, 310–320.

Coll, M., Frederick, C.A., Wang, A.H.-J. & Rich, A. (1987). A bifurcated hydrogen-bonded conformation in the d(AT) base pairs of the DNA dodecamer d(CGCAAATTTGCG) and its complex with distamycin. *Proceedings of the National Academy of Sciences USA* **84**, 8385–8389.

Dabrowiak, J.C. & Goodisman, J. (1989). Quantitative footprinting analysis of drug–DNA interactions. In Kallenback, NR (ed.) *Chemistry and Physics of DNA-Ligand Interactions*, pp. 143–174. Adenine Press, New York.

Dervan, P.B. (1986). Design of sequence-specific DNA-binding molecules. *Science* **323**, 464–471.

Dolnick, B.J. (1991). Antisense agents in cancer research and therapeutics. *Cancer Investigation* **9**, 185–194.

Drew, H.R. (1984). Structural specificities of five commonly used DNA nucleases. *Journal of Molecular Biology* **176**, 535–557.

Frederick, C.A., Williams, L.D., Ughetto, G., van der Marel, G.A., van Boom, J.H., Rich, A. & Wang, A.H.-J. (1990). Structural comparison of anticancer drug–DNA complexes: adriamycin and daunomycin. *Biochemistry* **29**, 2538–2549.

Futscher, B.W. & Erickson, L.C. (1990). Changes in c-*myc* and c-*fos* expression in a human tumor cell line following exposure to bifunctional alkylating agents. *Cancer Research* **50**, 62–66.

Govan, H.L., Valles-Ayoub, Y. & Braun, J. (1990). Fine-mapping of DNA damage and repair in specific genomic segments. *Nucleic Acids Research* **18**, 3823–3830.

Gralla, J.D., Sasse-Dwight, S. & Poljak, L.G. (1987). Formation of blocking lesions at identical DNA sequences by the nitrosourea and platinum class of anticancer drugs. *Cancer Research* **47**, 5092–5096.

Hartley, J.A., Berardini, M., Ponti, M., Gibson, N.W., Thompson, A.S., Thurston, D.E. Hoey, B.M. & Butler, J. (1991a). DNA crosslinking and sequence selectivity of aziridinylbenzoquinones. A unique reaction at 5'-GC-3' sequences with 3,6-diaziridinyl-1,4-benzoquinone upon reduction. *Biochemistry* **30**, 11719–11724.

Hartley, J.A., Berardini, M. & Souhami, R.L. (1991b). An agarose gel method for the determination of DNA interstrand crosslinking applicable to the measurement of the rate of total and 'second-arm' crosslink reactions. *Analytical Biochemistry* **193**, 131–134.

Hartley, J.A., Bingham, J.P. & Souhami, R.L. (1991c). DNA sequence selectivity of guanine-N7 alkylation by nitrogen mustards is preserved in intact cells. *Nucleic Acids Research* **20**, 3175–3178.

Hartley, J.A., Forrow, S.M. & Souhami, R.L. (1990). Effect of ionic strength and cationic DNA affinity binders on the DNA sequence selective alkylation of guanine-N7 positions by nitrogen mustards. *Biochemistry* **29**, 2985–2991.

Hartley, J.A., Gibson, N.W., Kohn, K.W. & Mattes, W.B. (1986). DNA sequence selectivity of guanine-N7 alkylation by three antitumour chloroethylating agents. *Cancer Research* **46**, 1943–1947.

Hemminki, K. & Ludlum, D.B. (1984). Covalent modification of DNA by antineoplastic agents. *Journal of the National Cancer Institute* **73**, 1021–1028.

Hertzberg, R.P., Hecht, S.M., Reynolds, V.L., Molineux, I.J. & Hurley, L.H. (1986). DNA sequence specificity of the pyrrolo[1,4] benzodiazepine antitumour antibiotics. Methidium-EDTA-Iron(II) footprinting analysis of DNA binding sites for anthramycin and related drugs. *Biochemistry* **25**, 1249–1258.

Hopkins, P.B., Millard, J.T., Woo, J., Weidner, M.F., Kirchner, J.J., Sigurdsson, S. Th. & Raucher, S. (1991). Sequence preferences of DNA interstrand cross-linking agents: importance of minimal DNA structural reorganization in the cross-linking reactions of mechlorethamine, cisplatin and mitomycin C. *Tetrahedron* **47**, 2475–2489.

Hurley, L.H. & Thurston, D.E. (1984). Pyrrolo[1,4] benzodiazepine antitumour antibiotics: chemistry, interaction with DNA and biological implications. *Pharmaceutical Research* **2**, 52.

Hurley, L.H., Reck, T., Thurston, D.E., Langley, D.R., Holden, K.G., Hertzberg, R.P., Hoover, R.E., Gallagher, G., Faucelle, L.F., Mong, S.M. & Johnson, R.K.

(1988). Pyrrolo[1,4] benzodiazepine antitumor antibiotics: relationship of DNA alkylation and sequence specificity to the biological activity of natural and synthetic compounds. *Chemical Research and Toxicology* **1,** 258–268.

Hurley, L.H., Reynolds, V.L., Swenson, D.H. & Scahill, T. (1984). Reaction of the antitumor antibiotic CC-1065 with DNA: structure of a DNA adduct with DNA sequence specificity. *Science* **226,** 843–844.

Hurley, L.H., Warpehoski, M.A., Lee, C-S., McGovren, J.P., Scahill, T.A., Kelly, K.C., Wicnieski, N.A., Gebhard, I. & Bradford, V.S. (1990). Sequence specificity of DNA alkylation by the unnatural enantiomers of CC-1065 and its synthetic analogs. *Journal of the American Chemical Society* **112,** 4633–4649.

Jones, G.B., Davey, C.L., Jenkins, T.C., Kamal, A., Kneale, G.C., Neidle, S., Webster, G.D. & Thurston, D.E. (1990). The non-covalent interaction of pyrrolo[2,1-c] [1,4] benzodiazepine-5,11-diones with DNA. *Anticancer Drug Design* **5,** 249–264.

Karlin, S. (1986). Significant potential secondary structure in the Epstein–Barr virus genome. *Proceedings of the National Academy of Sciences USA* **83,** 6915–6919.

Kissinger, K., Krowicki, K., Dabrowiak, J.C. & Lown, J.W. (1987). Molecular recognition between oligopeptides and nucleic acids: monocationic lexitropsins that display enhanced GC sequence dependent DNA binding. *Biochemistry* **26,** 5590–5595.

Kohn, K.W., Hartley, J.A. & Mattes, W.B. (1987). Mechanisms of DNA sequence selective alkylation of guanine-N7 positions by nitrogen mustards. *Nucleic Acids Research* **15,** 10531–10549.

Koo H.-S., Wu, H.-M. & Crothers, D.M. (1986). DNA bending at adenine thymine tracts. *Nature* **320,** 501–506.

Kopka, M.L., Yoon, C., Godsell, D., Pjura, P. & Dickerson, R.E. (1985). The molecular origin of DNA drug specificity in netropsin and distamycin. *Proceeedings of the National Academy of Sciences USA* **82,** 1376–1380.

Krowicki, K., Balzarini, J., De Clercq, E., Newman, R.A. & Lown, J.W. (1988). Novel DNA groove binding alkylators. Design, synthesis and biological evaluation. *Journal of Medicinal Chemistry* **31,** 341–345.

Lane, M.J., Dabrowiak, J.C. & Vournakis, J.N. (1983). Sequence specificity of actinomycin D and netropsin binding to pBR322 DNA analysed by protection from DNase I. *Proceedings of the National Academy of Sciences USA* **80,** 3260–3264.

Lavery, R., Pullman, A. & Pullman, B. (1982). The electrostatic field of B-DNA. *Theoretica Chimica Acta* **62,** 93.

Le Doan, R., Perrouault, L., Praseuth, D., Habhoub, N., Decout J.-L., Thuong, N.T., Lhomme, J. & Helene, C. (1987). Sequence-specific recognition, photocrosslinking and cleavage of the DNA double helix by an oligo-[α]-thymidylate covalently linked to an azidoproflavine derivative. *Nucleic Acids Research* **15,** 7749–7760.

Lee, C.-S., Sun, D., Kizu, R. & Hurley, L.H. (1991). Determination of the structural features of (+)-CC-1065 that are responsible for bending and winding of DNA. *Chemical Research and Toxicology* **4,** 203–209.

Lee, M., Hartley, J.A., Pon, R.T., Krowicki, K. & Lown, J.W. (1988a). Sequence specific molecular recognition by a monocationic lexitropsin of the decadeoxyribonucleotide d-[CATGGCCATG]: structural and dynamic aspects deduced from high field 'H-NMR studies. *Nucleic Acids Research* **16,** 665–684.

Lee, M., Krowicki, K. Hartley, J.A., Pon, R.T. & Lown, J.W. (1988b). Molecular recognition between oligopeptides and nucleic acids: influence of van der Waal's contacts in determining the 3'-terminus of DNA sequences read by monocationic lexitropsins. *Journal of the American Chemical Society* **110,** 3641–3649.

Lee, M., Krowicki, K., Shea, R.G., Pon, R.T. & Lown, J.W. (1989). Molecular recognition between oligopeptides and nucleic acids: specificity of binding of a monocationic *bis*-furan lexitropsin to DNA deduced from footprinting and ^{1}H-NMR studies. *Journal of Molecular Recognition* **2**, 84–93.

Leupin, W. (1990). Experimental proofs of a drug DNA sequence specificity. In Pullman, B. & Jortner, J. (eds.) *Molecular Basis of Specificity in Nucleic Acid–Drug Interactions*, pp. 579–603. Kluwer Academic Publishers, Dordrecht.

Li, V.-S. & Kohn, H. (1991). Studies on the bonding specificity for mitomycin C-DNA monoalkylation processes. *Journal of the American Chemical Society* **113**, 275–283.

Low, C.M.L., Drew, H.R. & Waring, M.J. (1984). Sequence-specific binding of echinomycin to DNA: evidence for conformational changes affecting flanking sequences. *Nucleic Acids Research* **12**, 4865–4879.

Lown, J.W. (1988). Lexitropsins: rational design of DNA sequence reading agents as novel anticancer agents and potential cellular probes. *Anticancer Drug Design* **3**, 25–40.

Lown, J.W. (1990). Molecular mechanisms of DNA sequence recognition by groove binding ligands: biochemical and biological consequences. In Pullman, B. & Jortner, J. (eds.). *Basis of Specificity in Nucleic Acid–Drug Interactions*, pp. 103–122. Kluwer Academic Publishers, Dordrecht.

Lown, J.W., Krowicki, K., Balzarini, J., Newman, R.A. & De Clercq, E. (1989). Novel linked antiviral and antitumor agents related to netropsin and distamycin: synthesis and biological evaluation. *Journal of Medicinal Chemistry* **32**, 2368–2375.

Lown, J.W., Krowicki, K., Bhat, V.G., Skorobogaty, A., Ward, B. & Dabrowiak, J.C. (1986). Molecular recognition between oligopeptides and nucleic acids: novel imidazole-containing oligopeptides related to netropsin that exhibit altered DNA sequence specificity. *Biochemistry* **25**, 7408–7416.

McLean, M.J. & Waring, M.J. (1988). Chemical probes reveal no evidence of Hoogsteen base-pairing in complexes formed between echinomycin and DNA in solution. *Journal of Molecular Recognition* **1**, 138–151.

McLean, M.J., Seela, F. & Waring, M.J. (1989). Echinomycin-induced hypersensitivity to osmium tetroxide of DNA fragments incapable of forming Hoogsteen base pairs. *Proceedings of the National Academy of Sciences USA* **86**, 9687–9691.

Madhani, H.D., Bohr, V.A. & Hanawalt, P.C. (1986). Differential DNA repair in transcriptionally active and inactive proto-oncogenes: c-*abl* and c-*mos*. *Cell* **45**, 417–423.

Maher, L.J., Wold, B. & Dervan, P.B. (1989) Inhibition of DNA binding proteins by oligonucleotide-directed triple helix formation. *Science* **245**, 725–730.

Mattes, W.B. (1990). Lesion selectivity in blockage of lambda exonuclease by DNA damage. *Nucleic Acids Research* **18**, 3723–3730.

Mattes, W.B., Hartley, J.A. & Kohn, K.W. (1986a). DNA sequence selectivity of guanine N7 alkylation by nitrogen mustards. *Nucleic Acids Research* **14**, 2971–2987.

Mattes, W.B., Hartley, J.A. & Kohn, K.W. (1986b). Mechanism of DNA strand breakage by piperidine at sites of N7-alkyl-guanines. *Biochimica Biophysica Acta* **868**, 71–76.

Mattes, W.B., Hartley, J.A., Kohn, K.W. & Matheson, D.W. (1988). GC-rich regions in genomes as targets for DNA alkylation. *Carcinogenesis* **9**, 2065–2072.

Millard, J.T., Raucher, S. & Hopkins, P.B. (1990). Mechlorethamine cross-links deoxyguanosine residues at 5'-GNC sequences in duplex DNA fragments. *Journal of American Chemical Society* **112**, 2459–2460.

Mitchell, M.A., Johnson, P.D., Williams, M.G. & Aristoff, P.A. (1989). Interstrand DNA crosslinking with dimers of spirocyclopropylalkylating moeity of CC-1065. *Journal of American Chemical Society* **111**, 6428–6429.

Moore, M.H., Hunter, W.N., Langlois d'Estaintot, B. & Kennard, O. (1989). DNA–drug interactions. The crystal structure of d(CGATCG) complexed with daunomycin. *Journal of Molecular Biology* **206,** 693–705.

Moser, H.E. & Dervan, P.B. (1987). Sequence-specific cleavage of double helical DNA by triple helix formation. *Science* **238,** 645–650.

Myers, C.E., Mimnaugh, E.G., Grace, C.Y. & Sinha, B.K. (1988). Biochemical mechanisms of tumour cell kill by anthracyclines. In Lown, J.W. (ed.) *Anthracycline and Anthracinedione-based Anticancer Agents*, pp. 528–570. Elsevier, Amsterdam.

Neidle, S., Pearl, L.H. & Skelly, J.V. (1987). DNA structure and perturbation by drug binding. *Biochemical Journal* **243,** 1–13.

Pelton, J.G. & Wemmer, D.E. (1989). Structural characterization of a 2:1 distamycinA: d(CGCAAATTGGC) complex by two-dimensional NMR. *Proceedings of National Academy of Sciences USA* **86,** 5723–5727.

Pelton, J.G. & Wemmer, D.E. (1990). Binding modes of distamycin A with d(CGCAAATTTGCG)$_2$ determined by two-dimensional NMR. *Journal of the American Chemical Society* **112,** 1393–1399.

Phillips, D.R., Cullinane, C., Trist, H. & White, R.J. (1990). *In vitro* transcription analysis of the sequence specificity of reversible and irreversible complexes of adriamycin with DNA. In Pullman, B. & Jortner, J. (eds.) *Molecular Basis of Specificity in Nucleic Acid–Drug Interactions*, pp. 137–155. Kluwer Academic Publishers, Dordrecht.

Pieper, R.O. & Erickson, L.C. (1990). DNA adenine adducts induced by nitrogen mustards and their role in transcription termination *in vitro*. *Carcinogenesis* **11,** 1739–1746.

Pieper, R.O., Futscher, B.W. & Erickson, L.C. (1989). Transcription terminating lesions induced by bifunctional alkylating agents *in vitro*. *Carcinogenesis* **10,** 1307–1314.

Ponti, M., Forrow, S.M., Souhami, R.L., D'Incalci, M. & Hartley, J.A. (1991a). Measurement of the sequence specificity of covalent DNA modification by antineoplastic agents using *Taq* DNA polymerase. *Nucleic Acids Research* **19,** 2929–2933.

Ponti, M., Souhami, R.L., Fox, B.W. & Hartley, J.A. (1991b). DNA interstrand crosslinking and sequence selectivity of dimethanesulphonates. *British Journal of Cancer* **63,** 743–747.

Portugal, J. (1989). Footprinting analysis of sequence-specific DNA–drug interactions. *Chemico-Biological Interactions* **71,** 311–324.

Pullman, A. & Pullman, B. (1981). Molecular electrostatic potential of the nucleic acids. *Quarterly Review of Biophysics* **14,** 289–380.

Pullman, B. (1989). Molecular mechanisms of specificity in DNA–antitumour drug interactions. *Advances in Drug Research*, **18,** 1–113.

Quigley, G.J., Ughetto, G., van der Marel, G.A., van Boom, J.H., Wang, A.H. & Rich, A. (1986). Non-Watson–Crick GC and AT base pairs in a DNA–antibiotic complex. *Science* **232,** 1255–1258.

Quigley, G.L., Wang, A., Ughetto, G., van der Marel, G., van Boom, J.H. & Rich, A. (1980). Molecular structure of an anticancer drug–DNA complex: daunomycin plus d(CpGpTpApCpG). *Proceedings of the National Academy of Sciences USA* **77,** 7204–7208.

Rao, K.E., Shea, R.G., Yadagiri, B. & Lown, J.W. (1990). Molecular recognition between oligopeptide and nucleic acids: DNA sequence specificity and binding properties of thiazole-lexitropsins incorporating the concepts of base site acceptance and avoidance. *Anti-Cancer Drug Design* **5,** 3–20.

Rehfuss, R., Goodisman, J. & Dabrowiak, J.C. (1990). Quantitative footprinting analysis of actinomycin D-DNA interaction, In Pullman, B. & Jortner, J. (eds.) *Molecular Basis of Specificity in Nucleic Acid–Drug Interactions*, pp. 157–166. Kluwer Academic Publishers, Dordrecht.

Reynolds, V.L., Molineux, L.J., Kaplan, D., Swenson, D.H. & Hurley, L.H. (1985). Reaction of the antitumour antibiotic CC-1065 with DNA, location at the site of thermally induced strand breakage and analysis of DNA sequence specificity. *Biochemistry* **24**, 6228–6237.

Rich, A., Nordheim, A. & Wang, A.H.-J. (1984). The chemistry and biology of left-handed Z-DNA. *Annual Review of Biochemistry* **53**, 791–846.

Royer-Pokora, B., Gordon, L.K. & Haseltine, W.A. (1981). Use of exonuclease III to determine the site of stable lesions in defined sequences of DNA: the cyclobutane pyrimidine dimer and *cis* and *trans* dichlorodiammine platinum II examples. *Nucleic Acids Research* **9**, 4595–4609.

Schult, P.G. & Dervan, P.B. (1984). Distamycin and penta-*N*-methylpyrrolo-carboxamide binding sites on native DNA, a comparison of methidiumpropyl-EDTA-Fe(II) footprinting and DNA affinity cleaving. *Journal of Biomolecular Structure and Dynamics* **1**, 1133–1147.

Scott, E.V., Jones, R.L., Banville, D.L., Zon, G., Marzilli, L.G. & Wilson, W.D. (1988). ^{1}H and ^{31}P NMR investigations of actinomycin D binding selectivity with oligodeoxyribonucleotides containing multiple adjacent d(GC) sites. *Journal of the American Chemical Society* **27**, 915–923.

Teng, S.P., Woodson, S.A. & Crothers, D.M. (1989). DNA sequence specificity of mitomycin cross-linking. *Biochemistry* **28**, 3901–3907.

Thurston, D.E. & Hurley, L.H. (1983). A rational basis for the development of antitumor agents in the pyrrolo[1,4] benzodiazepine group. *Drugs of the Future* **8**, 957–971.

Thurston, D.E., Jones, G.B. & Davies, M.E. (1990). Synthesis and reactivity of a novel oxazolo[2,3-c] [1,4] benzodiazepine ring system with DNA recognition potential: a new class of anthramycins. *Journal of the Chemical Society Chemical Communications* **12**, 874–876.

Tomasz, M., Lipman, R. Chowdary, C., Pawlak, J., Verdine, G.L. & Nakanishi, K. (1987). Isolation and structure of a covalent cross-link adduct between mitomycin C and DNA. *Science* **235**, 1204–1208.

van Dyke, M.W. & Dervan, P.B. (1984). Echinomycin binding sites on DNA. *Science* **225**, 1122–1127.

van Dyke, M.W., Hertzberg, R.P. & Dervan, P.B. (1982). Map of distamycin, netropsin and actinomycin binding sites on heterogeneous DNA: DNA cleavage-inhibition patterns with methidium propyl-EDTA-Fe(II). *Proceedings of the National Academy of Sciences USA* **79**, 5470–5474.

Vos, J.-M. & Hanawalt, P.C. (1987). Processing of psoralen adducts in an active human gene: repair and replication of DNA containing monoadducts and interstrand cross-links. *Cell* **50**, 789–799.

Wang, A.H.-J., Kujii, S., van Boom, J.H. & Rich, A. (1982). Molecular structure of the octamer d(G-G-C-C-G-G-C-C): modified A-DNA. *Proceedings of the National Academy of Sciences USA* **79**, 3968–3972.

Wang, A.H.-J., Liaw, Y.-C., Robinson, H. & Gao, Y.-G. (1990). Mutual conformational adaptation of both ligand and receptor in antitumor drug-DNA complexes. In Pullman, B. & Jortner, J. (eds.) *Molecular Basis of Specificity in Nucleic Acid–Drug Interactions*, pp. 1–21. Kluwer Academic Publishers, Dordrecht.

Wang, A.H.-J., Quigley, G.J., Kolpak, F.J., Crawford, J.L., van Boom, J.H., van der Marel, G.A. & Rich, A. (1979). Molecular structure of a left-handed double helical

DNA fragment at atomic resolution. *Nature* **282**, 680–686.

Wang, A.H.-J., Ughetto, G., Quigley, G.J. & Rich, A. (1987). Interactions between an anthracycline antibiotic with DNA: molecular structure of daunomycin complexed to d(CpGpTpApCpG) at 1.2A resolution. *Biochemistry* **26**, 1152–1163.

Waring, M.J. (1990). The molecular basis of specific recognition between echinomycin and DNA. In Pullman, B. & Jortner, J. (eds.) *Molecular Basis of Specificity in Nucleic Acid–Drug Interactions*, pp. 225–245. Kluwer Academic Publishers, Doredrecht.

Warpehoski, M.A. & Hurley, L.H. (1988). Sequence selectivity of DNA covalent modifications. *Chemical Research and Toxicology* **1**, 315–333.

Warpehoski, M.A., McGovren, P., Mitchell, M.A. & Hurley, L.H. (1990). Contrasting mechanisms for the sequence recognition of DNA by (+) and (−)-CC-1065. In Pullman, B. & Jortner, J. (eds.) *Molecular Basis for Specificity in Nucleic Acid–Drug Interactions*, pp. 531–550. Kluwer Academic Publishers.

Wassermann, K., Kohn, K.W. & Bohr, V.A. (1990). Heterogeneity of nitrogen mustard-induced DNA damage and repair at the level of the gene in Chinese hamster ovary cells. *Journal of Biological Chemistry* **265**, 13906–13913.

Weidner, M.F., Sigurdsson, S.Th. & Hopkins, P.B. (1990). Sequence preferences of DNA interstrand crosslinking agents: dG-to-dG crosslinking at 5′-CG by structurally simplified analogues of mitomycin C. *Biochemistry* **29**, 9225–9233.

Wells, R.D. & Harvey, S.C. (eds) (1987). *Unusual DNA Structures*. Springer-Verlag, New York.

Wing, R., Drew, H., Takano, T., Broka, C., Tanaka, S., Itakura, K. & Dickerson, R.G. (1980). Crystal structure analysis of a complete turn of B-DNA. *Nature* **287**, 755–758.

Zerial, M., Salinas, J., Filipski, J. & Berardini, G. (1986). Gene distribution and nucleotide sequence organization in the human genome. *European Journal of Biochemistry* **160**, 479–485.

Ziegler, J.L. (1981). Burkitt's lymphoma. *New England Journal of Medicine* **305**, 735–745.

Zimmer, C. & Wahnert, U. (1986). Non-intercalating DNA-binding ligands: specificity of the interaction and their use as tools in biophysical, biochemical and biological investigations of the genetic material. *Progress in Biophysics and Molecular Biology* **47**, 31–112.

Chapter 11
Mechanism of sequence-specific oxidative DNA damage by neocarzinostatin and other enediyne-containing antitumour antibiotics

Irving H. Goldberg

Introduction

With the demonstration 30 years ago that antinomycin D interferes with transcription by binding to DNA (Goldberg & Rabinowitz, 1962) in a specific manner (Goldberg *et al.*, 1962) and the realization that a wide variety of antitumour antibiotics alter the structure and function of DNA by complex formation (Ward *et al.*, 1965), it has been generally accepted that the chemotherapeutic properties of such agents depend on their interaction with DNA. The validity of this assumption has not been convincingly demonstrated in all instances, although much circumstantial support has been offered. The case for DNA as the chemotherapeutic target has been better made where the agent not only forms a physical complex with the DNA but also modifies it chemically (Goldberg & Friedman, 1971; Goldberg, 1987; Fisher & Aristoff, 1988; Hurley, 1989).

Most antitumour agents that carry out chemistry on their target DNA do so primarily by interacting with the nucleic acid bases. This results often in the formation of drug-base adducts involving various functional groups on the DNA base. Other agents, such as neocarzinostatin (NCS) (Goldberg, 1987) and bleomycin (Stubbe & Kozarich, 1987), damage DNA virtually exclusively by attacking the deoxyribose moiety in the DNA, resulting in the formation of direct strand breaks or alkali-labile, abasic sites. Whereas bleomycin (and ionizing radiation) exerts its deoxyribose-damaging activity via some species (not yet convincingly identified) of drug-bound reactive oxygen, NCS-induced damage is due to a diradical species of the drug itself, oxygen playing a secondary role in expression of the damage. Both agents exhibit DNA sequence requirements in their interaction with DNA. Although the sequence specificity for bleomycin appears to be rather stringent (G_p pyrimidine, with the pyrimidine as the attack site); that for NCS is more complex. In fact, for the latter the precise sequence plays an important role in the determination of the chemistry of the deoxyribose damage. Further, it controls whether the lesions involve one or both strands of the DNA. These very complexities in the nature of the interaction between NCS and DNA and in the pattern of DNA damage generated, make it a useful probe in the elucidation of DNA microstructure.

This chapter will focus on aspects of the chemistry of NCS and its activation mechanism that provide it with unprecedented properties as a DNA-damaging agent and biochemical tool. More recently discovered enediyne-containing agents, such as the calicheamicins (Lee *et al.*, 1987a,b), esperamicins (Golik *et al.*, 1987a,b) and dynemicin (Konishi *et al.*, 1989), that involve analogous mechanisms and hold promise as potent antitumour agents will be mentioned for comparative purposes. Further, since rather comprehensive reviews of NCS action have recently appeared (Goldberg *et al.*, 1981, 1990; Goldberg, 1987), this article will centre on remaining questions and more speculative aspects of its action that will hopefully lead to ideas for the development of other agents with novel properties.

Drug structure and mechanism of activation: diradical formation

The study of the mechanism of action of NCS has been marked by unexpected and rather surprising findings. NCS was first discovered by Ishida *et al.* (1965) over 25 years ago and identified as a protein-containing antitumour antibiotic. The protein has been sequenced (Hirayama *et al.*, 1986 and references therein) and recent ^{1}H nuclear magnetic resonance (NMR) and crystallographic studies (Saito *et al.*, 1989b; Adjadj *et al.*, 1990; Remerowski *et al.*, 1990) have revealed its secondary structure. Although NCS was almost immediately found to interfere with DNA synthesis and lead to DNA degradation (Ono *et al.*, 1966), it was not until several years later that it was appreciated that DNA strand scission was a primary effect in cells (Beerman & Goldberg, 1974; Hatayama & Goldberg, 1979) and that this reaction could be reproduced in the test tube provided that an activating cofactor, such as thiol, was included in the reaction (Beerman & Goldberg, 1974). It was not obvious, however, how a 'protein' antibiotic of mol. wt *c.* 11 000 entered cells and was targetted to the cell nucleus to exert its DNA-damaging activity. In fact, there were studies showing that NCS was cytotoxic under conditions (attached to insoluble supports) where it was unable to penetrate cells (Nakamura & Ono, 1974; Lazarus *et al.*, 1977). Further, the *in vitro* DNA scission reaction was markedly stimulated by agents, such as organic solvents or other protein-denaturing chemicals (Kappen & Goldberg, 1979), that would have been expected to inactivate the protein. These findings raised the possibility that the active material was not the well-characterized protein but rather, an as yet undetected small molecule carried by the protein, that was released upon its unfolding (Napier et al., 1980). This proved to be the situation, since methanol treatment of the holoantibiotic resulted in the extraction of a non-protein chromophoric substance that possessed all the biologic activity of the parent material (Napier et al., 1979; Kappen et al., 1980a; Ohtsuki et al., 1980; Suzuki et al., 1980). The isolated chromophore (NCS-Chrom) was extremely labile in aqueous solution at neutral or higher pHs but was protected from degradation by very tight binding to its apoprotein (K_D c. 10^{-10} M) or to a DNA substrate (K_D c.10^{-6} M) (Povirk & Goldberg, 1980).

How then does NCS-Chrom get inside a cell; is it released from the apoprotein before or after cell membrane pentration? Further, since the binding to apoprotein is much tighter than to DNA, how can it attack DNA, since while complexed to the apoprotein it is inactive as a DNA cleaving agent (Kappen et al., 1980a)? Conclusive answers to these questions are not yet forthcoming. Evidence has been reported to show that the protein is taken up by the cell (Oda & Maeda, 1987), but is not yet clear that NCS-Chrom remain associated. Free NCS-Chrom can penetrate cells (Kappen & Goldberg, 1980) and cells multiply-resistant to a number of antitumour agents are also resistant to NCS-Chrom (L.S. Kappen and I.H. Goldberg, unpublished data, cited in Kappen et al., 1987), suggesting that they share common mechanisms for efflux of the chromophore. If it is the holoantibiotic that is presented to nuclear DNA, how is NCS-Chrom released from the apoprotein? Since thio-activated NCS-Chrom binds less tightly to apoprotein (K_D c. 10^{-6} M) (Povirk & Goldberg, 1980), perhaps this is the species that is released to interact with the DNA.

As will be emphasized later, since thiol activates NCS-Chrom by nucleophilic addition (Hensens et al., 1983) the structure of the activated drug varies with the particular thiol, and thus may account for the thiol structure-dependency of the DNA damage process. Thiol also appears to be essential for drug activation in vivo, since glutathione depletion greatly reduces NCS cytotoxicity, mutagenicity and DNA strand breakage in mammalian cells (DeGraff & Mitchell, 1985; DeGraff et al., 1985; Kappen et al., 1987). Of interest in terms of chemotherapeutic considerations is the observation that 'normal' cell lines appeared to be more resistant to glutathione depletion than 'cancer' cells and thus were more resistant to the toxic effects of NCS, raising the possibility of enhancing the therapeutic index of NCS by selective thiol depletion (Russo et al., 1986).

The apoprotein carrier possesses a hydrophobic cleft where NCS-Chrom is believed to reside (Saito et al., 1989b; Adjadj et al., 1990; Remerowski et al., 1990) and is protected from degeneration. Other related antitumour protein antibiotics that cleave DNA (Kappen et al.,

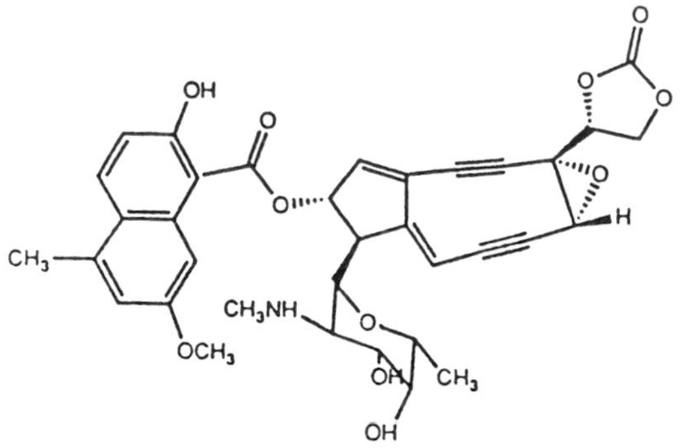

Neocarzinostatin

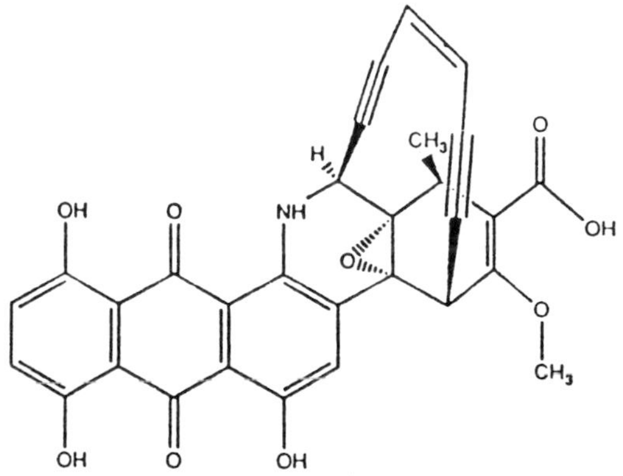

Dynemicin

Fig. 11.1. Structures of enediyne antibiotics.

1979; 1980b), macromycin (auromomycin) and actinoxanthine, possess homologous primary and secondary protein structures (Pletnev *et al.*, 1982; Samy *et al.*, 1983; Van Roey & Beerman, 1989) to NCS, but the non-protein chromophoric substances appear to be different, although they remain incompletely studied (Kumada *et al.*, 1983). The interaction between chromophore and apoprotein appears to be specific, since the NCS apoprotein is far superior in protecting NCS-Chrom from degradation that the apoproteins of the related agents (Kappen & Goldberg, 1980).

At the time, the structure of NCS-Chrom was unique for a natural (and even synthetic) product in that it possessed a bicyclic ring system containing two acetylenic bonds in the nine-membered ring (Fig. 11.1) (Henscns *et al.*, 1983, 1989; Edo *et al.*, 1985). Form A of NCS-Chrom, the major species, consists of three subunits: a 5-methyl-7-methoxy napthoate, a 2,6-dideoxy-2-methyl-amino-galactose moiety and an interconnecting highly unsaturated C_{12}-subunit bearing a cyclic carbonate and an epoxide.

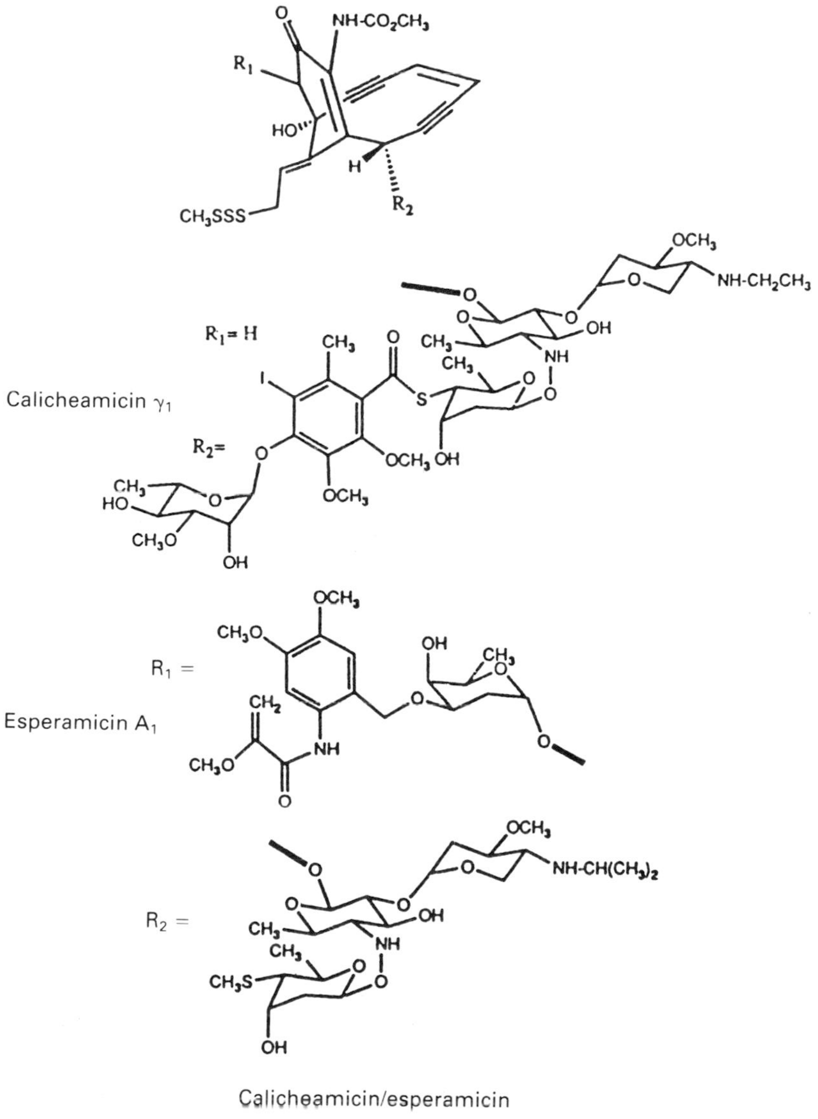

Calicheamicin γ_1

Esperamicin A_1

Calicheamicin/esperamicin

Fig. 11.1. *Continued.*

The C_{12}-subunit consists of a novel, highly strained bicyclic (7,3,0) dode-cadiyne system. The absolute stereochemistry of the molecule has been recently determined (Myers *et al.*, 1988). Two analogues of the NCS epoxide, the chlorohydrin and the diol monomethyl ether have been prepared; the latter is inactive, although it can bind to DNA, while the former is about half as active in various systems as the parent epoxide (Lee & Goldberg, 1988). Two other forms of NCS Chrom A resulting from alteration in the cyclic carbonate (1,3-dioxolan-2-one) moiety have been identified: form C, the methyl ester, results from storage of NCS-Chrom in methanol, whereas form B, the open diol decarboxylation product, is present in the material used clinically at a level of 10% of form A (Napier *et al.*, 1981a,b). Form C is active both *in vitro* and *in vivo*, whereas form B is active only *in vitro*. The cyclic carbonate moiety appears not to be essential for DNA damage, but may be required for entry of the drug into mammalian cells. Both B and C are somewhat more stable than A. Other enediyne-containing antibiotics (calicheamicins, esperamicins and dynemicins) (Fig. 11.1), which are not associated with a protein carrier, have since been described, and analogy with the chemistry of their transformation to inactive species by a Bergman-type rearrangement has provided insight into the mechanism of NCS-Chrom activation. These agents are among the most potent antitumour agents known; calicheamicin has been found to about 1000-fold more active than adriamycin in tests against murine tumours (Zein *et al.*, 1988). The structure of dynemicin is fascinating, since it is a hybrid molecule combining the structures of two types of antitumour agents: enediyne and anthraquinone (Konishi *et al.*, 1989).

As will be described later, there was compelling evidence that DNA deoxyribose damage by NCS-Chrom involved a radical species of the activated drug; in fact; it had been proposed that thiol activation converted NCS-Chrom into a diradical form before its enediyne structure was known (Kappen & Goldberg, 1985). Based on ^{1}H NMR and mass spectroscopy (MS) of the thiol- and borohydride-reacted chromophore (Hensens *et al.*, 1983) and in analogy with the Bergman-type aromatization of the calicheamicin/esperamicin class of antibiotics to form benzenoid diradicals (Golik *et al.*, 1987a; Lee *et al.*, 1987b), Myers (1987) proposed a mechanism for NCS-Chrom activation shown in Fig. 11.2 involving a cumulene intermediate, in the generation of an indacene diradical. The latter species is presumably involved in hydrogen atom abstraction from deoxyribose. In the proposed mechanism, thiol attacks C-12 of NCS-Chrom by nucleophilic addition. This results in opening of the epoxide and rearrangement to form the cumulene precursor (Myers & Proteau, 1989) of the diradical with radical centres at C-2 and C-6. The bicyclic dienediyne core and a leaving group at C-5 (epoxide of chloro group) are required for diyl formation (Lee & Goldberg, 1988). This reactive intermediate can then either abstract hydrogen from DNA to form a final stable product or abstract hydrogen from elsewhere, borohydride or thiol, in the absence of DNA to form the same product. The thiol attacks C-12 of NCS in trans configuration to the naphthoate (Hensens & Goldberg, 1989). Evidence in support of this formulation comes from experiments showing that in the absence of DNA deuterium is incorporated from borodeuteride in deuteriated solvent into C-12, C-6 and C-2 of NCS-Chrom, whereas in its presence deuterium is incorporated only into C-12 and hydrogen into C-6 and C-2 (Chin *et al.*, 1988). These results indicate that DNA is the source of hydrogen donation to the two radical centres

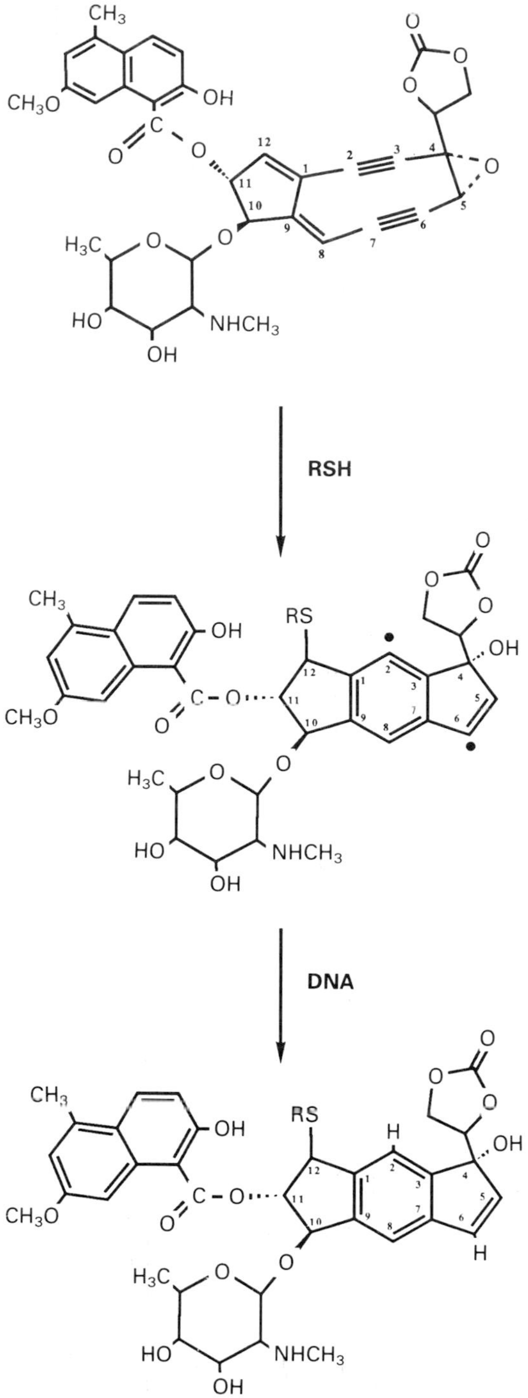

Fig. 11.2. Mechanism of neocarzinostatin (NCS) activation and action. RSH, activating thiol species.

of the activated chromophore at C-6 and C-2 and provide additional support for a diradical mechanism. They also suggest that labelling of a specific attack site in the DNA minor groove will lead to labelling of *either* C-6 *or* C-2 of the chromophore. The outcome of such an experiment involving deuterium labelling of C-5′ of a specific T residue in an oligo-nucleotide and its implication for the structure of the activated drug-DNA complex will be described later.

To date the only compounds found to serve as activators of NCS-Chrom in DNA cleavage are thiols and sodium borohydride (Kappen & Goldberg, 1978). For reasons, not yet obvious, other strong nucleophiles, such as cyanide, fail to activate the drug to a species capable of hydrogen atom abstraction from DNA deoxyribose (L.S. Kappen and I.H. Goldberg, unpublished date). As will be noted later, it would be advantageous in further elucidation of the mechanism to find an *activator* of NCS-Chrom that does not also act as a *reductant* in the expression of the DNA sugar damage. An effort to separate these two activities is underway.

The esperamicin/calicheamicin group of drugs undergoes reductive cleavage of the allylic trisulphide (1, Fig. 11.3) by thiol to give a thiolate anion which undergoes a Michael addition to the α,β-unsaturated ketone to generate the dihydrothiophene (2) in which the acetylenes are closer together. This facilitates the Bergman aromatization to form the diradical (1,4-diyl intermediate) species (3) (Zein *et al.*, 1988; Long *et al.*, 1989). The mechanism of activation of dynemicin to its diradical species is less clear, but it has been proposed that opening of the epoxide ring, following reduction of the quinone, leads to quinone methide formation and subsequent Bergman aromatization (Snyder & Tipsword, 1990; Sugiura *et al.*, 1990).

Mechanisms of DNA damage

It has been known for some time that NCS-Chrom binds DNA by a process involving intercalation of its naphthoate moiety between the DNA base pairs and electrostatic interaction of its positively charged amino-sugar and the negatively charged sugar phosphate backbone (Napier & Goldberg, 1983; Dasgupta *et al.*, 1985). The DNA helix is unwound by 21° and the DNA is lengthened by 3.3 Å, equivalent to one base pair, by each molecule of bound chromophore (Povirk *et al.*, 1981). Further, it was shown that the chrompohore lies in the minor groove of the DNA (Dasgupta & Goldberg, 1985) where its activated form has ready access to hydrogen atoms of the sugars of both DNA strands.

Early work on *in vitro* DNA scission showed that NCS-Chrom produces primarily single strand breaks (and abasic sites) and that there was *base* but little clear-cut *sequence* specificity (Takeshita *et al.*, 1981; Lee & Goldberg, 1989; Lee *et al.*, 1989). NCS-Chrom generated breaks mainly

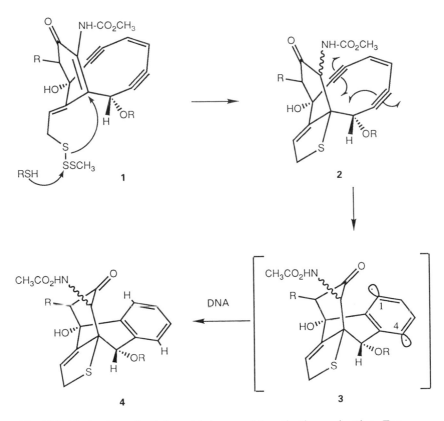

Fig. 11.3. Mechanism of calicheamicin/esperamicin activation and action. For further details see text.

at T residues (T > A ≫ C > G); about 75% of the lesions were at T residues (Poon *et al.*, 1977). The chemistry of the scissions at the T residue was shown to consist of a break, producing DNA fragments with 3′-phosphate and 5′-thymidine 5′-aldehyde ends (Kappen *et al.*, 1982; Kappen & Goldberg, 1983). This lesion was shown to result from the selective abstraction of a hydrogen atom by the activated drug from C-5′ of thymidylate in DNA (Charnas & Goldberg, 1984; Kappen & Goldberg, 1985) (Fig. 11.4, pathway b). Using $^{18}O_2$, it was found that dioxygen adds to the carbon-centred radical at C-5′ to form a peroxyradical species (pathway c) (Chin *et al.*, 1984) and, following reduction by thiol, results in the formation of the nucleoside 5′-aldehyde and a strand break (pathway e). This mechanism accounts for over 80% of the breaks produced by NCS-Chrom due to 5′ chemistry.

Fewer than 20% of the breaks appear to result from 5′ chemistry in which the peroxyradical species possibly converts to an oxyradical (pathway f) that undergoes β fragmentation with cleavage between C-4′

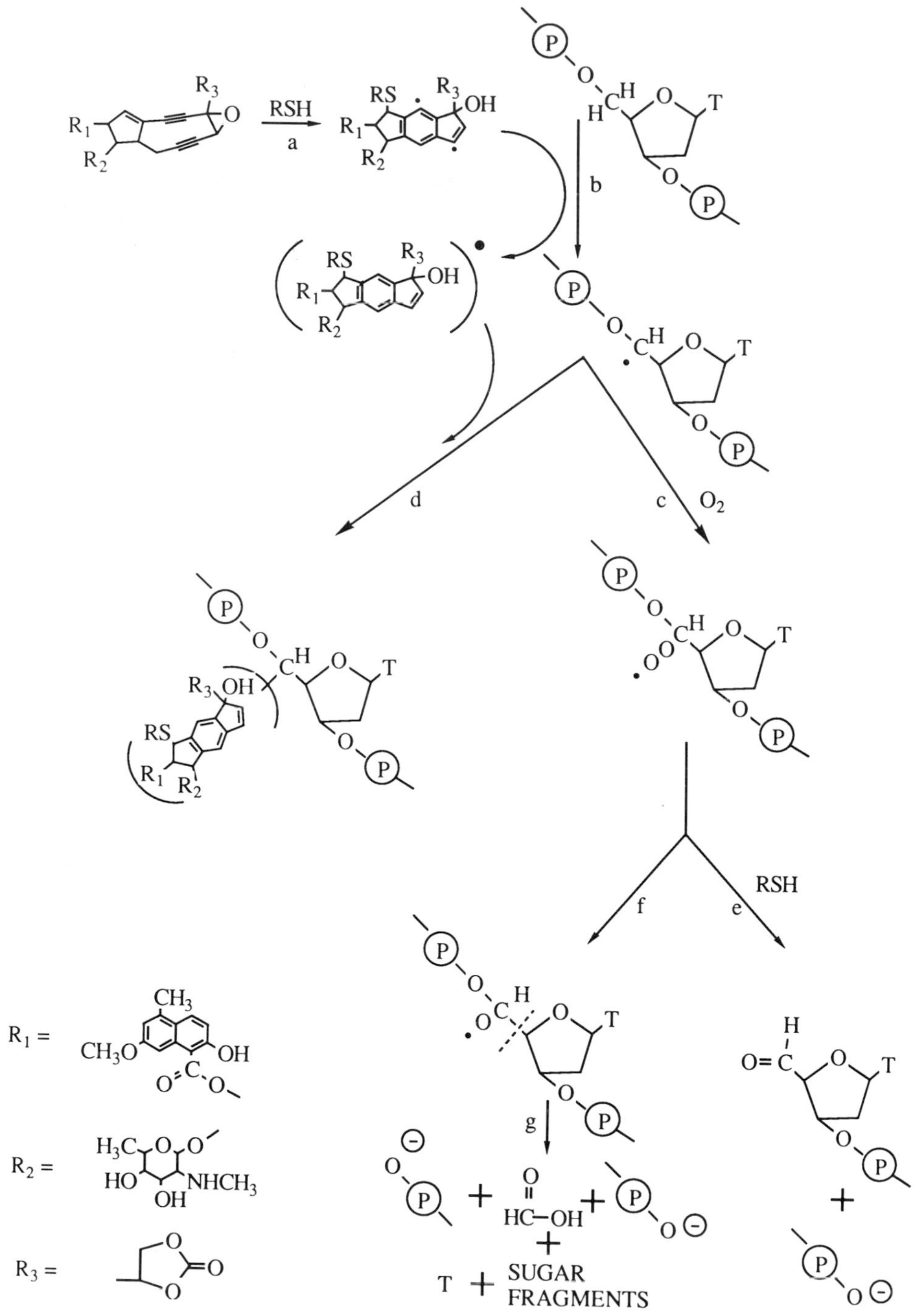

Fig. 11.4. Mechanism of neocarzinostatin (NCS)-induced damage at C-5′ of deoxy-ribose of thymidylate in DNA.

and C-5′ (pathway g). This results in the generation of a 3′-formyl-phosphate-ended fragment, a high-energy formyl donor, that either spontaneously hydrolyses to form formate and a 3′-phosphate-ended fragment (pathway g) or donates the formyl moiety to an available nucleophile, such as the amino group of nearby proteins (Chin *et al.*, 1987). Labelling of histone H1 by C-5′ of NCS-treated mammalian cell nuclei has, in fact, been found (P.C. Dedon and I.H. Goldberg, unpublished date). The sugar product resulting from the remaining four carbons of the deoxyribose has recently been identified and quantified (Kawabata *et al.*, 1989).

Similar chemistry occurs as the major lesion when the radiation sensitizer misonidazole is used as an oxygen substitute (Fig. 11.5). When misonidazole substitutes for dioxygen in the NCS–DNA reaction, the attack site specificity is the same as in dioxygen, but in the presence of misonidazole, base release and gap formation (with 3′- and 5′-phosphoryl termini) predominate (Kappen & Goldberg, 1984). The amount of DNA damage produced varies with the one-electron redox potential of the nitroaromatic compound, with the more electron-affinic compounds being more effective. Despite the difference in the distribution of the final DNA damage products, abstraction of 5′-hydrogen by thiol-activated drug to form a carbon-centred radical on C-5′ of deoxyribose appears to be a common initial step in both the dioxygen- and misonidazole-dependent reactions. In fact, there appears to be a competition between the misonidazole-dependent and the oxygen-dependent pathways, as revealed by cleavage patterns on DNA-sequencing gels. Under anaerobic conditions in the presence of misonidazole a reactive form of formate from C-5′ of deoxyribose of thymidylate is generated, and the formate can be transferred to available nucleophiles. These results, plus the evidence that misonidazole reduction is DNA-dependent, suggest a mechanism (Fig. 11.5) in which the carbon-centred radical formed at C-5′(*1*) by hydrogen atom abstraction by thiol-activated NCS reacts anaerobically with misonidazole to form a nitroxide radical adduct intermediate (2) (reaction 1), which unexpectedly cleaves between the oxygen and nitrogen (reaction 2) to produce an oxyradical at C-5′ (*3*). β-scission (reaction 3) results in cleavage between C-5′ and C-4′, with the generation of 3′-formyl phosphate ended DNA (*4*), a high-energy form of formate. The latter spontaneously hydrolyses, releasing formate (*6*) and creating a 3′-phosphate-end (*7*), or transfers the formyl moiety to available nucleophiles (Chin *et al.*, 1987). Strong evidence for a nitroxide radical adduct intermediate formed between the nitro group of misonidazole and the carbon-centred radical at C-5′ comes from experiments in which both oxygens of the nitro group contain ^{18}O and the carbonyl oxygen of the formate product becomes labelled with the ^{18}O (Kappen *et al.*, 1989).

In the absence of oxygen there is little, if any, DNA strand breakage; instead, it appears that the carbon-centred radical at C-5′ can interact with

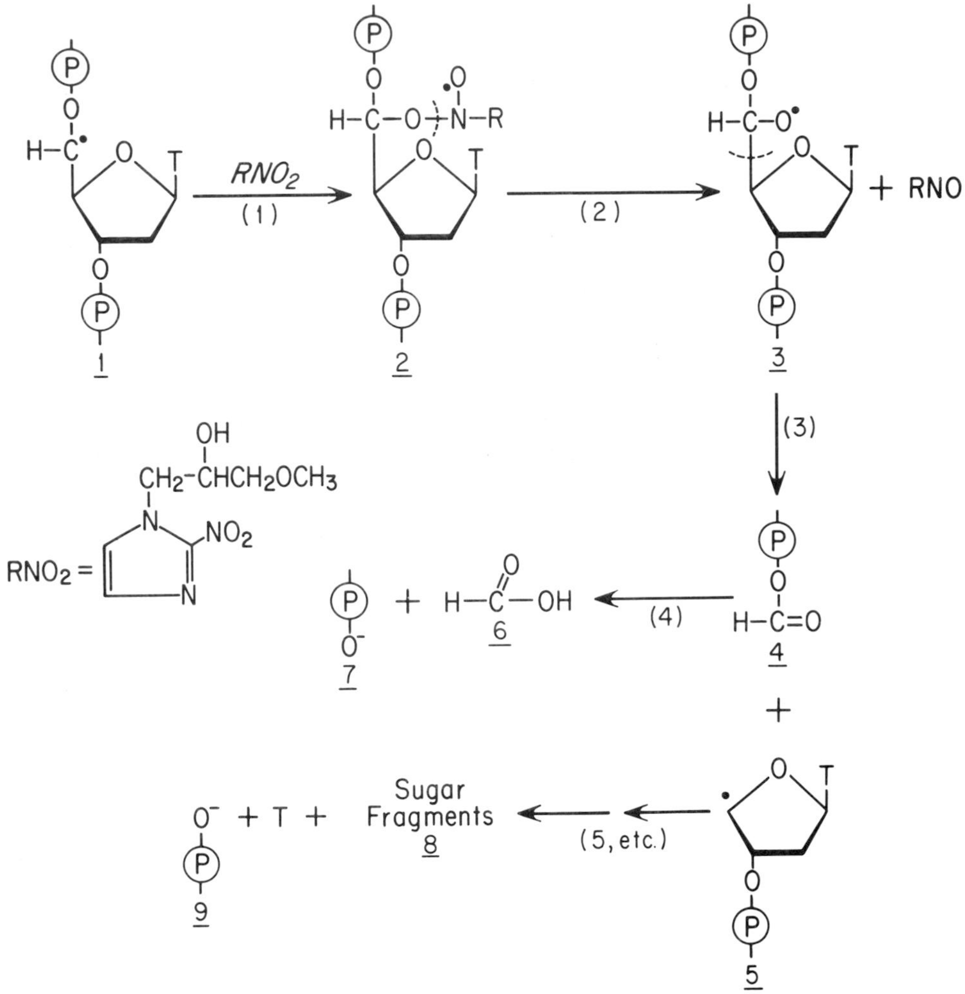

Fig. 11.5. Mechanism of involvement of misonidazole (RNO_2) in neocarzinostatin (NCS)-induced damage at C-5′.

the bound chromophore to form a covalent drug–DNA adduct (Fig. 11.4, pathway d) (Povirk & Goldberg, 1984). The biological implications of this novel lesion (e.g. on DNA replication and transcription) involving a drug-*deoxyribose* adduct remain to be explored. Such adducts had not been described before. Clearly, in order to generate an adduct on the deoxyribose moiety, one of its carbons must first be 'activated'. By mapping the adducts as exonuclease termination sites in defined-sequence DNA, it has been shown that stable adducts occurred with the same base specificity as for strand break formation (Povirk & Goldberg, 1985a). The similarity in sequence specificity of adducts and strand breaks suggests that a common form of nascent DNA damage may be a precursor to both lesions. A chromophore-induced carbon-centred radical on deoxyribose, subject to competitive fixation by addition reactions with either oxygen or chromophore, is the most likely candidate for such a precursor.

Sequence-specific bistranded lesions

Until recently there was uncertainty as to the mechanism involved in the formation of double-strand (DS) breaks, which are likely the cytotoxic lesions in mammalian cells (Hatayama & Goldberg, 1979). It had been found that in mammalian cells the ratio of single-strand (SS) to DS breaks was on the order of 5 : 1 (Hatayama & Goldberg, 1979), but when DNA strand cleavage was characterized *in vitro* the ratio was 30–50 : 1 (Poon *et al.*, 1977; Dedon & Goldberg, 1990). The latter values gave rise to the conjecture that DS breaks result from the random placement of SS breaks at closely opposed sites and that DS breakage as a discrete event occurred rarely, if at all. The paradox existing between the *in vivo* and *in vitro* data was resolved once it was appreciated that the difference in ratios of SS to DS breaks might be related to the fact that glutathione is the thiol *in vivo* and 2-mercaptoethanol was used *in vitro* (Dedon & Goldberg, 1990). In fact, when glutathione was used *in vitro*, the SS to DS ratio was found to be 6 : 1, closer to that found *in vivo*. Further, the number of DS breaks increased seven-fold. Analysis of a number of NCS-treated restriction fragments for DS cleavage sites revealed that DS breaks were sequence-specific and that most of the lesions occurred at the T residue of a GT step, especially at AGT·ACT sequences, resulting in a DS break with a two base pair stagger to the cleavage site.

Elucidation of the chemistry at the DS break (Dedon & Goldberg, 1990) showed that at the T residue of ACT 5'-chemistry resulted in the formation of 5'-nucleoside 5'-aldehyde- and 3'-phosphate-ended fragments (Fig. 11.6), whereas at the T residue of AGT, two nucleotides to the 3'-side of the break on the other strand, there is mainly 4'-chemistry (Fig. 11.6) resulting in fragments with 3'-phophoglycolate and 5'-phosphate ends. Detailed study of the 4'-chemistry occurring at the T residue of a GT step was facilitated by using DNA or oligodeoxynucleotides selectively labelled with deuterium at either C-4' or C-5' of the T residue (Frank *et al.*, 1991; Kappen *et al.*, 1991). Direct evidence for C-4' hydrogen atom abstraction was provided by the finding of a significant isotope selection effect ($k_D/k_H = 4$) at this site. Further, labelling C-4' with deuterium resulted in a partial shift in attack site to C-5', showing that the radical centre on the drug can choose between the closely positioned sites at C-4' and C-5' based on kinetic isotope selection. Strand breakage involving 3'-phosphoglycolate formation classically occurs with

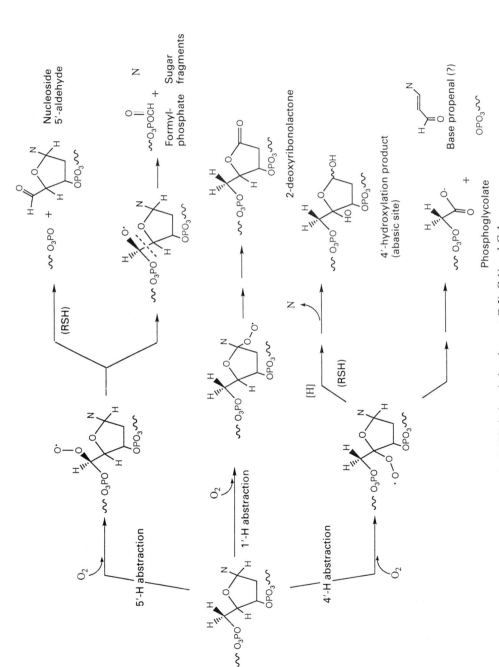

Fig. 11.6. Mechanism of neocarzinostatin (NCS)-induced chemistry at C-5′, C-1′ and C-4.

bleomycin (Stubbe & Kozarich, 1987); the concomitant generation of base-propenal from the remaining 4-carbon fragment, as found with bleomycin, however, has not yet been identified for NCS-Chrom, leaving open the possibility that the mechanism of product formation following hydrogen atom abstraction are basically different for the two agents. In addition to 3'-phosphoglycolate, both agents generate an abasic site due to a 4'-hydroxylation product, but the mechanism of its formation differs for the two agents. With bleomycin, oxygen is not required for its formation after the C-4' hydrogen atom abstraction reaction (Stubbe & Kozarich, 1987). By contrast, oxygen (or misonidazole) *is* required for abasic site formation with NCS-Chrom. It appears that a deoxyribose peroxyradical intermediate formed by NCS-Chrom partitions to generate both products with NCS-Chrom (Kappen *et al.*, 1991). Interestingly, it has been found that the partitioning between the two products depends on the thiol used as activator/reductant.

Bistranded lesions involving an abasic site, due to 4'-chemistry, at the *T* residue of AG*T* and a direct strand break at the *T* residue of the complementary strand AC*T* are also produced (Z.-w Jiang and I.H. Goldberg, unpublished data). Acidic thiols produce more glycolate product (Frank *et al.*, 1991; Kappen *et al.*, 1991); 4-hydroxythiolphenol, used first by Saito *et al.* (1989a) to show formation of the 4'-hydroxylation product, produces little, if any, glycolate and results in very few DS breaks, raising the possibility that its adducted form of activated NCS-Chrom does not bind with the correct geometry to generate bistranded lesions (Frank *et al.*, 1991; Kappen *et al.*, 1991). Since the size, shape and charge of the activated drug will differ depending upon the particular thiol, these differences might be expected to result in change in binding to the DNA minor groove, as well as in the orientation of the diradical species for attack on the DNA deoxyribose.

The bistranded lesions at AG*T* · AC*T*, involving breaks (or abasic site and break) at *T* residues two nucleotides apart to the 3' side on opposite DNA strands to generate a DS break, are analogous to an earlier described bistranded lesion involving 1' chemistry (Fig. 11.6) at the *C* residue of AG*C* · GC*T* and 5' chemistry at the *T* residue on the complementary strand (Povirk & Goldberg, 1985b; Kappen *et al.*, 1988, 1990; Kappen & Goldberg, 1989). The latter lesion has been shown to be responsible for GC to AT transitions in lambda phage and *Escherichia coli* (Povirk & Goldberg, 1986). 1' chemistry at the *C* residue results in the formation of an abasic site consisting of a 2-deoxyribonolactone moiety (Kappen & Goldberg, 1989), and 5' chemistry produces a strand break due to nucleoside 5'-aldehyde formation (Kappen *et al.*, 1988; Povirk *et al.*, 1988). Every abasic site at the *C* residue is accompanied by a direct break at the *T* residue on the complementary strand, suggesting that it occurs as part of

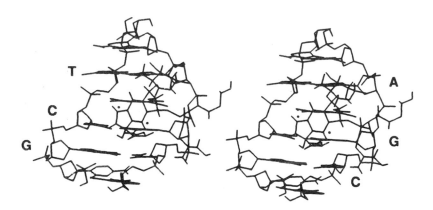

Fig. 11.7. Stereodrawings of optimized structure of reacted form of neocarzinostatin (NCS) complexed with AGC · GCT containing oligodeoxynucleotide. C-2 and C-6 of NCS are labelled with a dot. Glutathione is attached to C-12 of NCS. (Modified from Galat & Goldberg, 1990.)

a bistranded lesion due to the concerted action of the two radical centres at C-2 and C-6 of a single NCS-Chrom molecule (Porvirk *et al.*, 1988).

Molecular model building based on energy minimization and molecular dynamics simulations has led to a model of the activated NCS-Chrom-AGC·GC*T* complex in which the radical centre at C-6 abstracts a hydrogen atom from C-5′ of the *T* residue and C12 abstracts a hydrogen atom from C-1′ of the *C* residue (Fig. 11.7) (Galat & Goldberg, 1990). In the model the naphthoate moiety of NCS-Chrom is intercalated between the A : T and G : C base pairs and the indacene diradical lies in the DNA minor groove, projecting towards the 3′ end of the (+) strand. The intercalated naphthoate adds the equivalent of a base pair to the interaction site so that separation of the lesions on each strand by two rather than three (as with the non-intercalating calicheamicin) base pairs represents the shortest distance across the DNA minor groove (essentially at 90° with the two DNA strands). The model also shows that the glutathione adduct at C-12 of the chromophore forces the radical centre at C-2 deeper into the minor groove so as to be able to attack C-1′ of the deoxyribose of the *C* residue, perhaps accounting for the increased formation of the abasic lesion with this thiol. To corroborate the model and to further clarify the underlying mechanism the C-5′ position of the deoxyribose of the *T* residue was labelled with deuterium and the deuterium incorporation into the spent NCS-Chrom was analyzed by ¹H NMR (Meschwitz & Goldberg, 1991). These studies showed that the deuterium was incorporated only into C-6 of the chromophore, as predicted by the model. A similar experiment done with calicheamicin has shown that only C-4 (Fig. 11.3) of the spent drug was labelled with deuterium from C-5′ of its cytidylate target

(De Voss *et al.*, 1990). This result supports the proposed model for the calicheamicin–DNA complex (Hawley *et al.*, 1989).

The DS nature of the NCS-Chron-induced lesion at $AGC \cdot GCT$ probably accounts for its mutagenicity. The abasic lesion has been found to be a relatively poor site for the initiation or repair by apurinic/apyrimidinic endonucleases as compared with the ordinary acid-produced apurinic site (Povirk & Goldberg, 1985b), possibly because of the deoxyribonolactone structure, but more likely due to the break at the T residue on the complementary strand, since these enzymes have a strict requirement for duplex DNA. Further, if a break were placed by a repair endonuclease at this site, it would, in effect, be generating a DS break, a possibly lethal lesion. It is likely, therefore, that the direct break at the T residue would be repaired first, resulting in a A residue usually being mistakenly placed opposite the non–encoding abasic site (Boiteux & Laval, 1982; Sagher & Strauss, 1983; Schaaper *et al.*, 1983) and in the reconstitution of the duplex structure. Replacement of the abasic site can then proceed and results in insertion of a T residue opposite the A residue, completing the G : C to A : T transition This is a novel type of mutagenesis that results from the repair process and occurs in the absence of DNA replication.

The two types of bistranded lesions induced by NCS-Chrom involve different DNA sequence requirements and result from different chemical mechanisms depending on whether a C or a T residue is 3′ to a G residue. The importance of DNA microstructure is further emphasized by the finding that substitution of an I residue for this G residue virtually eliminates both 1′ and 4′ chemistry at the pyrimidine (C and T, respectively) immediately 3′ (Kappen *et al.*, 1988, 1991). Further, replacement of the G on the opposite strand with an I residue ($AGC \cdot ICT$) markedly enhances abasic site formation (Kappen *et al.*, 1988). Thus, the simple removal of a 2-amino group of a G residue in the minor groove has profound effects on the drug–DNA interaction. Clearly DNA microstructure, as represented by nucleotide sequence and the presence of functional groups in the minor groove, plays a critical role in determining the chemical mechanisms involved in oxidative deoxyribose damage. While such influences are usually identified with specific DNA sequences, it must be emphasized that it is the *geometry* of the formed complex that is the critical factor. Thus, it has been found that cleavage of DNA by NCS (and other cleaving-intercalating agents) is especially prominent immediately 3′ to a single-base bulge on the opposite strand, *independent of the sequence involved* (Williams & Goldberg, 1988).

All mechanisms of NCS-induced damage of DNA involve hydrogen atom abstraction reactions, whether from C-5′, C-1′ or C-4′, followed by dioxygen addition to the carbon-centred radical generated on the deoxyribose. The nitroaromatic radiation sensitizer misonidazole can in each case substitute for dioxygen to form a nitroxide radical adduct species that can undergo oxyradical formation as shown in Fig. 11.5 for C-5'. It should be noted that using NCS as a specific agent to form deoxyribose radical species has, for the first time, enabled mechanistic studies on the action of the nitroaromatic radiation sensitizers that probably have relevance for how these compounds sensitize radioresistant hypoxic tumour cells to ionizing radiation. Because of the complexity of lesions induced in DNA by ionizing radiation, involving both base and sugar, the effort to determine their mechanisms in this system has led to relatively little success (Wardman, 1987).

Unlike NCS-Chrom, calicheamicin/esperamicin activation by thiol does not result in the thiol becoming part of the activated drug and thus the particular thiol might not be expected to have an important influence on the extent of bistranded lesion formation (Zein *et al.*, 1988; Long *et al.*, 1989). Further, since calicheamicin lacks an intercalating moiety, it is expected that its bistranded lesions are separated by three, rather than two, base pairs (Zein *et al.*, 1988,1989b). The preferred sequence cleaved by calicheamicin is TCCT with the C residue undergoing 5' chemistry and nucleoside 5'-aldehyde formation. A break occurs on the complementary strand three nucleotides to the 3' side; the specific nature of the attacked residue on this strand appears not to be crucial and may involve 4' chemistry. Other homopyrimidine · homopurine sequences also appear to be good attack sites. No clear-cut sequence requirement has been reported for esperamicin, although breaks occur more often at pyrimidine bases in oligopyrimidine regions (Shiraki & Sugiura, 1989). Dynemicin appears to cleave preferentially on the 3' side of purine bases (Sugiura *et al.*, 1990).

Efforts at rational drug design

Elucidation of the unprecedented mechanisms by which the enediyne-containing antitimour antibiotics act has stimulated an enormous interest in the design and synthesis of simplified molecules working by similar mechanisms. Recent efforts based on the NCS-Chrom mechanism has led to the preparation of simple acyclic eneyneallenes that generate diradical species (Myers *et al.*, 1989; Nagata *et al.*, 1989, 1990; Nakatani *et al.*, 1990). Synthesis of the parent bicyclic core of NCS-Chrom has also been accomplished (Wender *et al.*, 1988), as well as analogues possessing the ability to form diradicals (Wender *et al.*, 1990). Similar efforts are underway to develop agents based on the calicheamicin/esperamicin mechanism (Danishefsky *et al.*, 1988; Nicolaou *et al.*, 1988a,b, 1990; Haseltine *et al.*, 1989). So far the synthetic work has focused on diradical formation, not on the DNA-complexation aspect of the problem. This has resulted in the generation of some potentially interesting molecules that appear to undergo a Bergman-type rearrangement to form diradicals, but the concentrations required for DNA cleavage are extremely high. Until the chemical synthesis can be worked out sufficiently to permit the attachment of DNA-binding moieties, it will not be possible to determine their usefulness as either antitumour agents or as tools in DNA structure determination.

Biological effects

Many of the biological effects of the enediyne antibiotics resemble those of ionizing radiation (Goldberg, 1987). Low doses of NCS selectively inhibit DNA replicon initiation in mammalian cells, but have little effect on chain elongation; at higher levels of drug, elongation is also affected (Povirk & Goldberg, 1982). There is a quantitative correlation between NCS-induced inhibition of replicon initiation and the generation of sufficient strand breakage to relax domains of supercoiling in mammalian DNA (target size of about 10^9 Da). These data imply that a single event, presumably a strand break; is adequate to disrupt DNA structure sufficiently to interrupt replicon initiation. Preferential cleavage of DNA by NCS has been found to occur in actively transcribed genes (Beckermann et al., 1987).

Human ataxia telangiectasia cells are more sensitive to killing by NCS than normal human fibroblasts and DNA synthesis in the mutant cells is also inhibited to a lesser extent (Povirk & Goldberg, 1982; Shiloh & Becker, 1982). In these respects, as well as in its mutagenic action, NCS resembles ionizing radiation. Further, as has been reported for other DNA-damaging agents, NCS has been found to induce neuronal morphology in mouse neuroblastoma cells in culture (Schor, 1989).

The usefulness of the enediyne antibiotics and their synthetic congeners in cancer chemotherapy remains to be demonstrated. Efforts to improve the pharmacological properties of NCS by its chemical conjugation to a copolymer of styrene and maleic acid (smancs) has led to reports of enhanced antitumour activity in animals and man (see Oda & Maeda, 1987 for details and references). The presence of a carrier protein in the case of NCS complicates its usefulness for immunological and other reasons. Substitution of the apoprotein of NCS by a non-protein carrier molecule having a protective hydrophobic pocket, such as exists in substances like the cyclodextrins, might offer advantages for drug delivery. The calicheamicin/esperamicin and dynemicin group of agents lack a carrier protein, are more stable than NCS-Chrom, and are amongst the most potent antititumour agents known. Advantage has been taken of this high level of toxicity by conjugating calicheamicin/esperamicin with tumour-specific antibodies with preliminary encouraging results in animal tumour systems (Wallace et al., 1990). The study of enediyne-containing drugs as antitumour agents is only at the beginning. While it is not yet clear what role they will finally play in cancer chemotherapy, they do represent a novel class of agents working by interesting and unusual mechanisms. They have already proven to be useful tools in the study of the structure and function of DNA, in revealing a novel mechanism of mutagenesis and in studies on the mechanism of action or radiation sensitizers.

References

Adjadj, E., Mispelter, J., Quiniou, E., Dimicoli, J.-L., Favaudon, V. & Lhoste, J.-M. (1990). Proton NMR studies of apo-neocarzinostatin from *Streptomyces carzinostaticus*. Sequence-specific assignment and secondary structure. *European Journal of Biochemistry* **190**, 263–271.

Beckermann, R.P., Agostino, M.J., McHugh, M.M., Sigmund, R.D. & Beerman, T.A. (1987). Assessment of preferential cleavage of an actively transcribed retroviral hybrid gene in murine cells by deoxyribonuclease I, bleomycin, neocarzinostatin, or ionizing radiation. *Biochemistry* **26**, 5409–5415.

Beerman, T.A. & Goldberg, I.H. (1974). DNA strand scission by the anti-tumor protein, neocarzinostatin. *Biochemical and Biophysical Research Communications* **59**, 1254–1261.

Boiteux, S. & Laval, J. (1982). Coding properties of poly(deoxycytidylic acid) templates containing uracil or apyrimidinic sites: *in vitro* modulation of mutagenesis by DNA repair enzymes. *Biochemistry* **21**, 6746–6751.

Charnas, R.L. & Goldberg, I.H. (1984). Neocarzinostatin abstracts a hydrogen during formation of nucleotide 5′-aldehyde on DNA. *Biochemical and Biophysical Research Communications* **122**, 642–648.

Chin, D.-H., Carr, S.A. & Goldberg, I.H. (1984). Incorporation of $^{18}O_2$ into thymidine 5′-aldehyde in neocarzinostatin chromophore-damaged DNA. *Journal of Biological Chemistry* **259**, 9975–9978.

Chin, D.-H., Kappen, L.S. & Goldberg, I.H. (1987). 3′-formyl phosphate-ended DNA: high energy intermediate in antibiotic-induced DNA sugar damage. *Proceedings of the National Academy of Sciences USA* **84**, 7070–7074.

Chin, D.-H., Zeng, C.-H., Costello, C.E. & Goldberg, I.H. (1988). Sites in the diyne-ene bicyclic core of neocarzinostatin chromophore responsible for hydrogen abstraction from DNA. *Biochemistry* **27**, 8106–8114.

Danishefsky, S.J., Mantlo, N.B., Yamashita, D.S. & Schulte, G. (1988). A concise route to the calicheamicin/esperamicin series: the crystal structure of a core subunit. *Journal of the American Chemical Society* **110**, 6890–6891.

Dasgupta, D. & Goldberg, I.H. (1985). Mode of reversible binding of neocarzinostatin chromophore to DNA: evidence for binding via the minor groove. *Biochemistry* **24**, 6913–6920.

Dasgupta, D., Auld, D.S. & Goldberg, I.H. (1985). Cryospectrokinetic evidence for the mode of reversible binding of neocarzinostatin chromophore to poly(deoxyadenylic-deoxythymidylic acid). *Biochemistry* **24**, 7049–7054.

Dedon, P.C. & Goldberg, I.H. (1990). Sequence-specific double-strand breakage of DNA by neocarzinostatin involves different chemical mechanisms within a staggered cleavage site. *Journal of Biological Chemistry* **265**, 14713–14716.

DeGraff, W.G. & Mitchell, J.B. (1985). Glutathione dependence of neocarzinostatin cytotoxicity and mutagenicity in Chinese hamster V-79 cells. *Cancer Research* **45**, 4760–4762.

DeGraff, W.G., Russo, A. & Mitchell, J.B. (1985). Glutathione depletion greatly reduces neocarzinostatin cytotoxicity in Chinese hamster V79 cells. *Journal of Biological Chemistry* **260**, 8312 8315.

De Voss, J.J., Townsend, C.A., Ding, W.-D., Morton, G.O., Ellestad, G.A., Zein, N., Tabor, A.B. & Schreiber, S.L. (1990). Site-specific atom transfer from DNA to a bound ligand defines the geometry of a DNA-calicheamicin γ_1^1 complex. *Journal of the American Chemical Society* **112**, 9669–9670.

Edo, K., Mizugaki, M., Koide, Y., Seto, H., Furihata, K., Otake, N. & Ishida, N. (1985). The structure of neocarzinostatin chromophore possessing a novel bicyclo [7,3,0] dodecadiyne system. *Tetrahedron Letters* **26**, 331–334.

Fisher, J.F. & Aristoff, P.A. (1988). The chemistry of DNA modification by antitumor antibiotics. *Progress in Drug Research* **32**, 411–498.

Frank, B.L., Worth, L. Jr, Christner, D.F., Kozarich, J.W., Stubbe, J., Kappen, L.S. & Goldberg, I.H. (1991). Isotope effects on the sequence-specific cleavage of DNA by neocarzinostatin: kinetic partitioning between 4' and 5'-hydrogen abstraction at unique thymidine sites. *Journal of the American Chemical Society*, **113**, 2271–2275.

Galat, A. & Goldberg, I.H. (1990). Molecular models of neocarzinostatin damage of DNA: analysis of sequence dependence in 5'GAGCG : 5'CGCTC. *Nucleic Acids Research* **18**, 2093–2099.

Goldberg, I.H. (1987). Free radical mechanisms in neocarzinostatin-induced DNA damage. *Free Radical Biology and Medicine* **3**, 41–54.

Goldberg, I.H. & Friedman, P.A. (1971). Antibiotics and nucleic acids. *Annual Review of Biochemistry* **40**, 775–810.

Goldberg, I.H. & Rabinowitz, M. (1962). Actinomycin D inhibition of deoxyribonucleic acid-dependent synthesis of ribonucleic acid. *Science* **136**, 315–316.

Goldberg, I.H., Hatayama, T., Kappen, L.S., Napier, M.A. & Povirk, L.F. (1981). Protein antibiotics as DNA-damaging agents. In Sartorelli, A.C., Bertino, J.R. & Lazo, J.S. (eds) *Molecular Actions and Targets for Cancer Chemotherapeutic Agents*, pp. 163–191. Academic Press, New York.

Goldberg, I.H., Kappen, L.S., Chin, D.-H. & Lee, S.H. (1990). Bistranded oxidative DNA sugar damage by targeted antibiotic diradicals. In Makriyannis, A. (ed.) *New Methods in Drug Research. Site Specific Recognition by DNA Active Ligands*, Vol. 3, pp. 27–42. J.R. Prous Science, Barcelona, Spain.

Goldberg, I.H., Rabinowitz, M. & Reich, E. (1962). Basis of actinomycin action. I. DNA binding and inhibition of RNA-polymerase synthetic reactions by actinomycin. *Proceedings of the National Academy of Sciences USA* **48**, 2094–2101.

Golik, J., Clardy, J., Dubay, G., Groenewold, G., Kawaguchi, H., Konishi, M., Krishnan, B., Ohkuma, H., Saitoh, K.-I. & Doyle, T.W. (1987a). Esperamicins, a novel class of potent antitumor antibiotics. II. Structure of esperamicin X. *Journal of the American Chemical Society* **109**, 3461–3462.

Golik, J., Dubay, G., Groenewold, G., Kawaguchi, H., Konishi, M., Krishnan, B., Ohkuma, H., Saitoh, K. & Doyle, T.W. (1987b). Esperamicins, a novel class of potent antitumor antibiotics. III. Structures of esperamicins A_1, A_2, A_{1b}. *Journal of the American Chemical Society* **109**, 3462–3464.

Haseltine, J.N., Danishefsky, S.J. & Schulte, G. (1989). Experimental modeling of the priming mechanism of the calicheamicin/esperamicin antibiotics: actuation by the addition of intramolecular neuclephiles to the bridgehead double bond. *Journal of the American Chemical Society* **111**, 7638–7640.

Hatayama, T. & Goldberg, I.H. (1979). DNA damage and repair in relation to cell killing in neocarzinostatin-treated HeLa cells. *Biochimica et Biophysica Acta* **563**, 59–71.

Hawley, R.C., Kiessling, L.L. & Scheiber, S.L. (1989). Model of the interactions of calicheamicin γ_1 with a DNA fragment from pBR322. *Proceedings of the National Academy of Sciences USA* **86,** 1105–1109.

Hensens, O.D. & Goldberg, I.H. (1989). Mechanism of activation of the antitumor antibiotic neocarzinostatin by mercaptan and sodium borohydride. *Journal of Antibiotics* **42,** 761–768.

Hensens, O.D., Dewey, R.S., Liesch, T.M., Napier, M.A., Reamer, R.A., Smith, J.L., Albers-Schonberg, G. & Goldberg, I.H. (1983). Neocarzinostatin chromophore: presence of a highly strained ether ring and its reaction with mercaptan and sodium borohydride. *Biochemical and Biophysical Research Communications* **113,** 538–547.

Hensens, O.D., Giner, J.-L. & Goldberg, I.H. (1989). Biosynthesis of NCS Chrom A, the chromophore of the antitumor antibiotic neocarzinostatin. *Journal of the American Chemical Society* **111,** 3295–3299.

Hirayama, K., Ando, T., Takahashi, R. & Murais, A. (1986). A revised primary structure of neocarzinostatin using the combination of endopeptidase, carboxypeptidase Y, and fast atom bombardment mass spectrometry. *Bulletin of the Chemical Society of Japan* **59,** 1371–1378.

Hurley, L.H. (1989). DNA and associated targets for drug design. *Journal of Medicinal Chemistry* **32,** 2027–2033.

Ishida, N., Miyazaki, K., Kumagai, K. & Rikimaru, M. (1965). Neocarzinostatin, an antitumor antibiotic of high molecular weight. *Journal of Antibiotics* **18,** 68–76.

Kappen, L.S. & Goldberg, I.H. (1978). Activation and inactivation of neocarzinostatin-induced cleavage of DNA. *Nucleic Acids Research* **5,** 2959–2967.

Kappen, L.S. & Goldberg, I.H. (1979). Mechanism of the effect of organic solvents and other protein-denaturants on neocarzinostatin activity. *Biochemistry* **18,** 5647–5653.

Kappen, L.S. & Goldberg, I.H. (1980). Stabilization of neocarzinostatin nonprotein chromophore activity by interaction with apoprotein and with HeLa cells. *Biochemistry* **19,** 4786–4790.

Kappen, L.S. & Goldberg, I.H. (1983). Deoxyribonucleic acid damage by neocarzinostatin chromophore: strand breaks generated by selective oxidation of C-5′ of deoxyribose. *Biochemistry* **22,** 4872–4878.

Kappen, L.S. & Goldberg, I.H. (1984). Nitroaromatic radiation sensitizers substitute for oxygen in NCS-induced DNA damage. *Proceedings of the National Academy of Sciences USA* **81,** 3312–3316.

Kappen, L.S. & Goldberg, I.H. (1985). Activation of neocarzinostatin chromophore and formation of nascent DNA damage do not require molecular oxygen. *Nucleic Acids Research* **13,** 1637–1648.

Kappen, L.S. & Goldberg, I.H. (1989). Identification of 2-deoxyribonolactone at the site of neocarzinostatin-induced cytosine release in the sequence d(AGC). *Biochemistry* **28,** 1027–1032.

Kappen, L.S., Chen, C.-Q. & Goldberg, I.H. (1988). Atypical abasic sites generated by neocarzinostatin at sequence-specific cytidylate residues in oligodeoxynucleotides. *Biochemistry* **27,** 4331–4340.

Kappen, L.S., Ellenberger, T.E. & Goldberg, I.H. (1987). Mechanism and base specificity of DNA breakage in intact cells by neocarzinostatin. *Biochemistry* **26,** 384–390.

Kappen, L.S., Goldberg, I.H., Frank, B.L., Worth, L.J., Christner, D.F., Kozarich, J.W. & Stubbe, J. (1991). Neocarzinostatin-induced hydrogen atom abstraction from C-4′ and C-5′ of the T residue at a d(GT) step in oligonucleotides: shuttling between deoxyribose attack sites based on isotope selection effects. *Biochemistry* **30,** 2034–2042.

Kappen, L.S., Goldberg, I.H. & Liesch, J.M. (1982). Identification of thymidine 5′-aldehyde at DNA strand breaks induced by neocarzinostatin chromophore. *Proceedings of the National Academy of Sciences USA* **79,** 744–748.

Kappen, L.S., Goldberg, I.H. & Samy, T.S. (1979). Contrasts in the actions of protein antibiotics on DNA structure and function. *Biochemistry* **18**, 5123–5127.

Kappen, L.S., Goldberg, I.H., Wu, S.H., Stubbe, J., Worth, L. Jr, & Kozarich, J.W. (1990). Isotope effects on the sequence-specific cleavage of dC in d(AGC) sequences by neocarzinostatin: elucidation of chemistry of minor lesions. *Journal of the American Chemical Society* **112**, 2797–2798.

Kappen, L.S., Lee, T.R., Yang, C.-C. & Goldberg, I.H. (1989). Oxygen transfer from the nitro group of a nitroaromatic radiosensitizer to a DNA sugar damage product. *Biochemistry* **28**, 4540–4542.

Kappen, L.S., Napier, M.A. & Goldberg, I.H. (1980a). Roles of chromophore and apoprotein in neocarzinostatin action. *Proceedings of the National Academy of Sciences USA* **77**, 1970–1974.

Kappen, L.S., Napier, M.A., Goldberg, I.H. & Samy, T.S.A. (1980b). Requirement for reducing agents in deoxyribonucleic acid strand scission by the purified chromophore of auromycin. *Biochemistry* **19**, 4780–4785.

Kawabata, H., Takeshita, H., Fujiwara, T., Sugiyama, H., Matsuura, T. & Saito, I. (1989). Chemistry of neocarzinostatin-mediated degradation of d(GCATGC). Mechanism of spontaneous thymine release. *Tetrahedron Letters* **30**, 4263–4266.

Konishi, M., Ohkuma, H., Matsumoto, K., Tsuno, T., Kamei, H., Miyaki, T., Oki, T. & Kawaguchi, H. (1989). Dynemicin A, a novel antibiotic with the anthraquinone and 1,5-diyne-3-ene subunit. *Journal of Antibiotics* **42**, 1449–1452.

Kumada, Y., Miwa, T., Naoi, N., Watanabe, K., Naganawa, H., Takita, T., Umezawa, H., Nakamura, H. & Iitaka, Y. (1983). A degradation product of the chromophore of auromomycin. *Journal of Antibiotics* **36**, 200–202.

Lazarus, H., Raso, V. & Samy, T.S.A. (1977). *In vitro* inhibition of human leukemic cells (CCRF-CEM) by agarose-immobilized neocarzinostatin. *Cancer Research* **35**, 3731–3736.

Lee, S.H. & Goldberg, I.H. (1988). Role of epoxide in NCS chromophore stability and action. *Molecular Pharmacology* **33**, 396–401.

Lee, S.H. and Goldberg, I.H. (1989). Sequence-specific, strand-selective, and directional binding of neocarzinostatin chromophore to oligodeoxyribonucleotides. *Biochemistry* **28**, 1019–1026.

Lee, M.D., Dunne, T.S., Chang, C.C., Ellestad, G.A., Siegel, M.M., Morton, G.O., McGahren, W.J. & Borders, D.B. (1987a). Calicheamicins, a novel family of antitumor antibiotics. II. Chemistry and structure of calicheamicin γ-1. *Journal of the American Chemical Society* **109**, 3466–3468.

Lee, M.D., Dunne, T.S., Marshall, M.S., Chang, C.C., Morton, G.O. & Borders, D.B. (1987b). Calicheamicins, a novel family of antitumor antibiotics. I. Chemistry and partial structure of calicheamicin γ-1. *Journal of the American Chemical Society* **109**, 3464–3466.

Lee, S.H., Thivierge, J.O. & Goldberg, I.H. (1989). DNA microstructural requirements for neocarzinostatin by mercaptan and sodium borohydride. *Nucleic Acids Research* **17**, 5809–5825.

Long, B.H., Golik, J., Forenza, S., Ward, B., Rehfuss, R., Dabrowiak, J.C., Catino, J.J., Musial, S.T., Brookshire, K.W. & Doyle, T.W. (1989). Esperamicins, a class of potent antitumor antibiotics: mechanism of action. *Proceedings of the National Academy of Sciences USA* **86**, 2–6.

Meschwitz, S.M. & Goldberg, I.H. (1991). Selective abstraction of ^{2}H from C5' of thymidylate in oligodeoxynucleotide by radical center at C6 of diradical species of neocarzinostatin: chemical evidence for structure of activated drug–DNA complex. *Proceedings of the National Academy of Sciences USA* **88**, 3047–3051.

Myers, A.G. (1987). Proposed structure of the neocarzinostatin chromophore-methyl thioglycolate adduct: a mechanism for the nucleophilic activation of neocarzinostatin. *Tetrahedron Letters* **28**, 4493–4496.

Myers, A.G. & Proteau, P.J. (1989). Evidence for spontaneous, low-temperature biradical formation from a highly reactive neocarzinostatin chromophore-thiol conjugate. *Journal of the American Chemical Society* **111**, 1146–1147.

Myers, A.G., Kuo, E.Y. & Finney, N.S. (1989). Thermal generation of α,3-dehydrotoluene from (Z)-1,2,4-heptatrien-6-yne. *Journal of the American Chemical Society* **111**, 8057–8059.

Myers, A.G., Proteau, P.J. & Handel, T.M. (1988). Stereochemical assignment of neocarzinostatin chromophore. Structures of neocarzinostatin chromophore-methyl thioglycolate adducts. *Journal of the American Chemical Society* **110**, 7212–7214.

Nagata, R., Yamanaka, H., Murahashi, E. & Saito, I. (1990). DNA cleavage by acyclic eneyne-allene systems related to neocarzinostatin and esperamicin-calicheamicin. *Tetrahedron Letters* **31**, 2907–2910.

Nagata, R., Yamanaka, H., Okazaki, E. & Saito, I. (1989). Biradical formation from acyclic conjugated eneyne-allene system related to neocarzinostatin and esperamicin-calicheamicin. *Tetrahedron Letters* **30**, 4995–4998.

Nakamura, H. & Ono, K. (1974). Inhibition of cell growth by sepharose-bound neocarzinostatin. In *Proceedings of the Japanese Cancer Association, 33rd Annual Meeting* p. 13.

Nakatani, K., Arai, K., Hirayama, N., Matsuda, F. & Terashima, S. (1990). Synthesis and cytoxicity of the acyclic (E)- and (Z)-dienediyne systems related to neocarzino statin chromophore. *Tetrahedron Letters* **31**, 2323–2326.

Napier, M.A. & Goldberg, I.H. (1983). Neocarzinostatin chromophore: Assignment of spectral properties and structural requirements for binding to DNA. *Molecular Pharmacology* **23**, 500–510.

Napier, M.A., Goldberg, I.H., Hensens, O.D., Dewey, R.S., Liesch, J.M. & Albers-Schonberg, G. (1981a). Neocarzinostatin chromophore: presence of a cyclic carbonate subunit and its modification in the structure of other biologically active forms. *Biochemical and Biophysical Research Communications* **100**, 1703–1712.

Napier, M.A., Holmquist, B., Strydom, D.J. & Goldberg, I.H. (1979). Neocarzinostatin: spectral characterization and separation of a non-protein chromophore. *Biochemical and Biophysical Research Communications* **89**, 635–642.

Napier, M.A., Holmquist, B., Strydom, D.J. & Goldberg, I.H. (1981b). Neocarzinostatin chromophore: purification of the major active form and characterization of its spectral and biological properties. *Biochemistry* **20**, 5602–5608.

Napier, M.A., Kappen, L.S. & Goldberg, I.H. (1980). Effect of non-protein chromophore removal on neocarzinostatin action. *Biochemistry* **19**, 1767–1773.

Nicolaou, K.C., Maligres, P., Shin, J., de Leon, E. & Rideout, D. (1990). DNA cleavage and antitimor activity of designed molecules with conjugated phosphine oxide-allene-ene-yne functionalities. *Journal of the American Chemical Society* **112**, 7825–7826.

Nicolaou, K.C., Ogawa, Y., Zuccarello, G. & Kataoka, H. (1988a). DNA cleavage by a synthetic mimic of the calicheamicin-esperamicin class of antibiotics. *Journal of the American Chemical Society* **110**, 7247–7248.

Nicolaou, K.C., Zuccarello, G., Ogawa, Y., Schweiger, E.J. & Kumazawa, T. (1988b). Cyclic conjugated enediynes related to calicheamicins and esperamicins: calculations, synthesis, and properties. *Journal of the American Chemical Society* **110**, 4866–4868.

Oda, T. & Maeda, H. (1987). Binding to and internalization by cultured cells of neocarzinostatin and enhancement of its actions by conjugation with lipophilic styrene-maleic acid copolymer. *Cancer Research* **47**, 3206–3211.

Ohtsuki, K. & Ishida, N. (1980). The biological effects of a nonprotein component removed from neocarzinostatin (NCS). *Journal of Antibiotics* **33**, 744–750.

Ono, Y., Watanabe, Y. & Ishida, N. (1966). Mode of action of neocarzinostatin: inhibition of DNA synthesis and degradation of DNA in *Sarcina lutea*. *Biochimica et Biophysica Acta* 119, 46–58.

Pletnev, V.Z., Kuzin, A.P., Trakhanov, S.D. & Kostetsky, P.V. (1982). Three-dimensional structure of antinoxanthin. *Biopolymers* 21, 287–300.

Poon, R., Beerman, T.A. & Goldberg, I.H. (1977). Characterization of DNA strand breakage *in vitro* by the antitumor protein neocarzinostatin. *Biochemistry* 16, 486–493.

Povirk, L.F., Dattagupta, N., Warf, B.C. & Goldberg, I.H. (1981). Neocarzinostatin chromophore binds to deoxyribonucleic acid by intercalation. *Biochemistry* 20, 4007–4014.

Povirk, L.F. & Goldberg, I.H. (1980). Binding of the nonprotein chromophore of neocarzinostatin to deoxyribonucleic acid. *Biochemistry* 19, 4773–4780.

Povirk, L.F. & Goldberg, I.H. (1982). Inhibition of mammalian DNA synthesis by neocarzinostatin: selective effect on replicon initiation in CHO cells and resistant synthesis in ataxia telangiectasia fibroblasts. *Biochemistry* 21, 5857–5862.

Povirk, L.F. & Goldberg, I.H. (1984). Competition between anaerobic covalent linkage of neocarzinostatin chromophore to deoxyribose in DNA and oxygen-dependent strand breakage and base release. *Biochemistry* 23, 6295–6299.

Povirk, L.F. & Goldberg, I.H. (1985a). Detection of neocarzinostatin chromophore-deoxyribose adducts as exonuclease-resistant sites in defined-sequence DNA. *Biochemistry* 24, 4035–4040.

Povirk, L.F. & Goldberg, I.H. (1985b). Endonuclease-resistant apyrimidinic sites formed by neocarzinostatin at cytosine residues in DNA: evidence for a possible role in mutagenesis. *Proceedings of the National Academy of Sciences USA* 82, 3182–3186.

Povirk, L.F. & Goldberg, I.H. (1986). Base substitution mutations induced in the cI gene of lambda phage by neocarzinostatin chromophore: Correlation with depyrimidination hotspots at the sequence AGC. *Nucleic Acids Research* 14, 1417–1426.

Povirk, L.F., Houlgrave, C.W. & Han, Y.-H. (1988). Neocarzinostatin-induced DNA base release accompanied by staggered oxidative cleavage of the complementary strand. *Journal of Biological Chemistry* 263, 19263–19266.

Remerowski, M.L., Glaser, S.J., Sieker, L.C., Samy, T.S.A. & Drobny, G.P. (1990). Sequential ¹H NMR assignments and secondary structure of apo-neocarzinostatin in solution. *Biochemistry* 29, 8401–8409.

Russo, A., De Graff, W., Friedman, N. & Mitchell, J.B. (1986). Selective modulation of glutathione levels in human normal versus tumor cells and subsequent differential response to chemotherapy drugs. *Cancer Research* 46, 2845–2848.

Sagher, D. & Strauss, B. (1983). Insertion of nucleotides opposite apurinic/apyrimidinic sites in deoxyribonucleic acid during *in vitro* synthesis: uniqueness of adenine nucleotides. *Biochemistry* 22, 4518–4526.

Saito, I., Kawabata, H., Fujiwara, T., Sugiyama, H. & Matsuura, T. (1989a). A novel ribose C-4′ hydroxylation pathway in neocarzinostatin-mediated degradation of oligonucleotides. *Journal of the American Chemical Society* 111, 8302–8303.

Saito, K., Y., Edo, K., Akiyami, M.Y., Koide, Y., Ishida, N. & Mizugaki, M. (1989b). Characterization of secondary structure of neocarzinostatin apoprotein. *Chemistry and Pharmacology Bulletin* 37, 3078–3082.

Samy, T.S.A., Hahm, K.-S., Modest, E.J., Lampman, G.W., Keutmann, H.T., Umezawa, H., Herlihy, W.C., Gibson, B.W., Carr, S.A. & Biemann, K. (1983). Primary structures of macromycin, an antitumor antibiotic protein. *Journal of Biological Chemistry* 258, 183–191.

Schaaper, R.M., Kunkel, T.A. & Loeb, L.A. (1983). Infidelity of DNA synthesis associated with bypass of apurinic sites. *Proceedings of the National Academy of Sciences USA* **80,** 487–491.

Schor, N.F. (1989). Neocarzinostatin induces neuronal morphology of mouse neuroblastoma in culture. *Journal of Pharmacology and Experimental Therapeutics* **249,** 906–910.

Shiloh, Y. & Becker, Y. (1982). Reduced inhibition of replicon initiation and chain elongation by neocarzinostatin in skin fibroblasts from patients with ataxia telangiectasia. *Biochimica et Biophysica Acta* **721,** 485–488.

Shiraki, T. & Sugiura, Y. (1989). DNA binding and cleavage by enediyne antitumor antibiotics, esperamicin and dynemicin. *Nucleic Acid Research* **21,** 53–54.

Snyder, J.P. & Tipsword, G.E. (1990). Proposal for blending classical and biradical mechanisms in antitumor antibiotics: dynemicin A. *Journal of the American Chemical Society* **112,** 4040–4042.

Stubbe, J. & Kozarich, J.W. (1987). Mechanisms of bleomycin-induced DNA degradation. *Chemical Reviews* **87,** 1107–1136.

Sugiura, Y., Shiraki, T., Konishi, M. & Oki, T. (1990). DNA intercalation and cleavage of an antitumor antibiotic dynemicin that contains anthracycline and enediyne cores. *Proceedings of the National Academy of Sciences USA* **87,** 3831–3835.

Suzuki, H., Mura, K., Kumada, T., Takeuchi, T. & Tanaka, N. (1980). Biological activities of non-protein chromophores of antitumor antibiotics: auromomycin and neocarzinostatin. *Biochemical and Biophysical Research Communications* **94,** 255–261.

Takeshita, M., Kappen, L.S., Grollman, A.P., Eisenberg, M. & Goldberg, I.H. (1981). Strand scission of deoxyribonucleic acid by neocarzinostatin, auromomycin, and bleomycin: studies on base release and nucleotide sequence specificity. *Biochemistry* **20,** 7599–7506.

Van Roey, P. & Beerman, T.A. (1989). Crystal structure analysis of auromomycin apoprotein (macromomycin) shows importance of protein side chains to chromophore binding selectivity. *Proceedings of the National Academy of Sciences USA* **86,** 6587–6591.

Wallace, R.E., Hinman, L.H., Hamann, P., Upeslacis, J. & Durr, F.E. (1990). Calicheamicin immunoconjugates: activity against human tumors in athymic mice. *Proceedings of the American Association for Cancer Research* **31,** 285.

Ward, D., Reich, E. & Goldberg, I.H. (1965). Base specificity in the interaction of polynucleotides with antibiotic drugs. *Science* **149,** 1259–1263.

Wardman, P. (1987). The mechanism of radiosensitization by electron-affinic compounds. *Radiation Physics and Chemistry* **30,** 423–432.

Wender, P.A., Harmata, M., Jeffrey, D., Mukai, C. & Suffert, J. (1988). Studies on DNA-active agents: the synthesis of the parent carbocyclic subunit of neocarzinostatin chromophore A. *Tetrahedron Letters* **29,** 909–912.

Wender, P.A., McKinney, J.A. & Mukai, C. (1990). General methodology for the synthesis of neocarzinostatin chromophore analogues: intramolecular chromium-mediated closures for strained-ring synthesis. *Journal of the American Chemical Society* **112,** 5369–5370.

Williams, L.D. & Goldberg, I.H. (1988). Selective strand scission by intercalating drugs at DNA bulges. *Biochemistry* **27,** 3004–3011.

Zein, N., McGahren, W.J., Morton, G.O., Ashcroft, J. & Ellestad, G.A. (1989a). Exclusive abstraction of nonexchangeable hydrogens from DNA by calicheamicin $\gamma 1^1$. *Journal of the American Chemical Society* **111,** 6888–6890.

Zein, N., Poncin, M., Nilakantan, R. & Ellestad, G.A. (1989b). Calicheamicin $\gamma 1^1$ and DNA: molecular recognition process responsible for site-specificity. *Science* **244,** 697–699.

Zein, N., Sinha, A.M., McGahren, W.J. & Ellestad, G.A. (1988). Calicheamicin $\gamma 1^1$: an antitumor antibiotic that cleaves double-stranded DNA site specificity. *Science* **240,** 1198–1201.

Chapter 12
Tumour endothelium as a target for solid tumour therapy

John S. Lazo, Claire M. Tenny and Robert H. Connamacher

Introduction

Solid tumours remain largely an unconquered target of chemotherapy. We now recognize the essential role of the vasculature in the biology of solid tumours and in the pathogenesis of neoplasia. Consequently, there has been growing interest in exploring methods of targetting tumour vasculature for antineoplastic therapy. Endothelial cell damage by chemotherapeutic agents may represent a novel approach for the desired destruction of solid tumours. The growth of solid tumours is angiogenesis-dependent; inhibition of tumour vascularization impairs tumour growth and decreases metastatic potential (Folkman, 1990). Thus, agents that exhibit antiangiogenic actions may also be useful and novel antineoplastic drugs. Vascular damage has been noted following irradiation, photodynamic therapy, cytokine administration and with certain clinically used cytotoxic chemotherapeutic agents. In addition, modulation of tumour blood flow with vasoactive agents may enhance antitumour activity of existing therapeutic agents. Selectivity may be possible because of the apparent differences in endothelial populations (McCarthy et al., 1991). The goal of this review is to discuss agents that affect angiogenesis and to examine the vascular actions of existing and potential antineoplastic therapies. We will also highlight information regarding known and/or potential mechanisms, which mediate selective damage to the tumour vasculature.

Antiangiogenic factors

The mechanisms of angiogenesis have been well reviewed (Arnold & Kumar, 1985; Folkman, 1990; Schartz *et al.*, 1990) and will only be briefly summarized here. Neovascularization of tissue normally occurs during embryogenesis as well as during wound healing. Additionally there are several pathological conditions that require angiogenesis. These include solid tumour development, diabetic retinopathy, corneal neovascularization, rheumatoid arthritis and psoriasis. In each case, the basic mechanisms appear to be the same, although different angiogenic factors may act on different vessels (Yang & Moses, 1990). The initiation of angiogenesis is under humoral control; many natural factors have been identified that promote angiogenesis. Most of these are proteins or polypeptides, including cytokines and growth factors, such as tumour necrosis factor α (TNF-α) (Liebovich *et al.*, 1987), endothelial-derived growth factor (EDGF) (Ishikawa *et al.*, 1989), acidic and basic fibroblast growth factors (aFGF and bFGF) (Maciag *et al.*, 1979; Mignatti *et al.*, 1989), transforming growth factor β (TGF-β) (Yang & Moses, 1990), and interferons (Sidsky & Borden, 1987). Another protein, angiogenin has been found to stimulate angiogenesis but not cell replication; it has a very similar homology to a ribonuclease and has some RNase activity (Fett *et al.*, 1985). Because it is present in normal tissues in relatively high concentrations, angiogenin is believed to be a pro-enzyme that needs to be activated by a yet unknown factor.

A number of factors that affect endothelial cell replication have been isolated from tumours, platelets, mast cells and other tissues. The substance most commonly associated with tumours is the tumour angiogenesis factor (TAF) (Greenblatt & Shubik, 1968). It now appears that there are a variety of tumour angiogenic factors, many of which may belong to the family of heparin-binding growth factors and include aFGF, bFGF, *hst* and *int* 2 (Gospodarowicz *et al.*, 1976; Maciag *et al.*, 1979; Schwartz *et al.*, 1990). Although these factors work by promoting and maintaining the replication of endothelial cells, the exact mechanism by which this occurs remains uncertain.

Several factors, both endogenous and synthetic, can prevent normal neovascularization (e.g. Folkman, 1990). In animal tumour models, these agents have been generally shown to inhibit the growth of solid but not ascites tumours. The effect is dramatic, with significant shrinkage of the tumour and virtually complete loss of peritumour vascularization. While many of these compounds are not curative, tumour growth was markedly suppressed by some promising new synthetic analogues of fumagillin (Ingber *et al.*, 1990).

Antiangiogenic agents can be divided mechanistically into two major areas: (i) antimigratory; and (ii) antiproliferative substances. Many of the specific antiangiogenic agents under investigation as antineoplastic agents have a greater effect on cell migration than on proliferation. This may be because so many of them appear to affect the cell matrix or collagen production rather than affecting the endothelial cells themselves. Both endogenous substances as well as synthetic substances appear to have the pharmacophore for antiangiogenesis and we have discussed these below.

Endogenous factors

Several naturally occurring substances have been identified that inhibit angiogenesis. Bagavondoss and Wilks (1990) found a thrombospondin-like protein, which inhibits the proliferation of endothelial cell cultures from a wide variety of tissues. These effects were reversed by monoclonal antibodies against thrombospondin. Recombinant platelet factor 4 inhibits angiogenesis both in chorioallantoic membrane preparations (Maione et al., 1990) and in mouse tumours (Sharpe et al., 1990). Endothelial cell migration was inhibited by platelet factor 4, although the concentration required was similar to that affecting cell proliferation (Sharpe et al., 1990). Antiangiogenic activity was confined to the carboxylic end of the 70 amino acid molecule and this offers a potential for developing synthetic analogues. Other antiangiogenic compounds have been isolated from human chondrosarcoma cells (Takigawa et al., 1990b) and from shark cartilage (Oikawa et al., 1990b), but these have not been fully characterized. Lastly, it has been suggested that interferons may be capable of suppressing neovascularization; interferons have been shown to strongly inhibit the vessel formation in mice inoculated with tumour cells in skin or cornea (Sidsky & Borden, 1987). A better understanding of the endogenous factors and mechanisms that regulate angiogenesis may allow for the utilization of endogenous antiangiogenic factors for antineoplastic therapies.

Promoters of cell differentiation

Substances that promote endothelial cell differentiation also appear to inhibit angiogenesis. Retinoids, for example, have been shown both to promote differentiation and inhibit angiogenesis and tumour growth in the chorioallantoic membrane (Ingber & Folkman, 1988). More recently, Oikawa et al. (1990c) found that active analogues of vitamin D_3 1,25-dihydroxyvitamin D and 22-oxo-1,25-dihydroxyvitamin D (an active synthetic analogue) inhibit angiogenesis in chick chorioallantoic membranes in a concentration-dependent manner while vitamin D_3 itself was inactive. Lastly, the antibiotic herbimycin was found to inhibit angiogenesis in both the chorioallantoic membrane and rabbit cornea preparations and in cell culture (Yamashita et al., 1989). Whereas proliferation of several types of cells could be inhibited, capillary endothelial cells were at least one order of magnitude more sensitive than others. Endothelium of solid tumours comprises predominantly small vessels; selective sensitivity of these endothelial cells may be therapeutically useful.

Heparin, steroids and fumagillin

The effect of heparin on angiogenesis was deduced from observations that mast cells accumulate at the site of tumour vascularization. When secretions from mast cells were tested, however, only heparin promoted angiogenesis (Azizkhan *et al.*, 1980); this effect was inhibited by protamine (Folkman, 1990). Cortisol and cyclo-oxygenase inhibitors have also been shown to inhibit angiogenesis in animal models (Lee *et al.*, 1987); however, the effects of these agents on tumour angiogenesis when administered alone has been disappointing. Synergistic inhibition of angiogenesis has been reported with chorioallantoic membranes with the combination of cortisol and heparin (Folkman *et al.*, 1983); this may be mediated by a decrease in collagen synthesis (Maragoudakis *et al.*, 1989). The combination of cortisol and heparin has been shown to be effective in animal tumour models and has been tried clinically (Maione & Sharpe, 1990). Folkman *et al.* (1989) searching for heparin analogues reported that β-cyclodextrin could replace heparin in potentiating the antiangiogenesis activity of cortisol. While it had no activity alone, β-cyclodextrin was strongly inhibitory when combined with cortisol in the rabbit cornea and the chick chorioallantoic membrane. The inhibition was correlated with decreased endothelial cell migration (Stokes *et al.*, 1990). It seems likely that during the next few years the search for heparin analogues will yield new compounds that maintain antiangiogenic activity but lack unacceptable toxicities. Fumagillin, an antibiotic effective against intestinal amoebae, was accidently found to inhibit angiogenesis (Ingber *et al.*, 1990). Because fumagillin has high toxicity, semisynthetic products of fumagillin were tested. AGM-1470, a chloroacetylcarbamoyl derivative, were found to be 50 times more potent and significantly less toxic than the parent compound using chorioallantoic membrane, mouse dorsal air sac, rat sponge implantation and endothelial cell culture assays (Ingber *et al.*, 1990; Kasuka *et al.*, 1991). Inhibition was due to depressed endothelial cell migration and microtube formation rather than inhibition of cell growth. Ingber *et al.* (1990) reported that fumagillin and its analogue also inhibit tumour growth in mice, confirming the original report of DiPaolo *et al.* in 1958.

Inhibitors of cell matrix

The actions of cortisol and heparin on the synthesis of collagen (Maragoudakis *et al.*, 1989) may plan a role in their antiangiogiogenic activity. It had been shown that tube formation by endothelial cells during angiogenesis is stabilized by luminal collagen IV synthesis (Folkman, 1985). Other compounds that affect basement membrane also inhibit angiogenesis. A quinolizinium salt 8,9-dihydroxy-7-methyl-benzo(b)quinolizinium-bromide (GPA1734) inhibits both basement membrane biosynthesis (Maragoudakis *et al.*, 1988) and angiogenesis (Missirlin *et al.*, 1990), although toxic concentrations were required for the antiangiogenesis. Another compound, tricyclodecan-9-yl-xanthate (D609), also inhibits both basement membrane biosyntheses and angiogenesis but at more tolerable concentrations. Although the results using the chick chorioallantoic membrane are difficult to interpret due to simultaneous addition of cortisol, D609 was active alone against Walker 256 carcinoma in rats with a clear antiangiogenic response. While GPA1734 and D609 prevented the synthesis of collagen, another antiangiogenesis compound appears to act by inhibiting collagen breakdown. Endogenous compounds, e.g. TIMP and TIMP-2 (tissue inhibitors of metalloproteinases), inhibit the breakdown of collagen and simultaneously block spermine-induced angiogenesis in the chick yolk sac (Takigawa *et al.*, 1990a). Minocycline, a clinically used antibiotic, strongly inhibits new vessel formation (Tamargo *et al.*, 1991). This action is specific to endothelial cells with no affect on three different tumour cell lines and may be mediated by inhibition of collagenase activity (Golub *et al.*, 1984).

Copper and D-penicillamine

Copper induces angiogenesis in various tissues; this is possibly due to its promotion of fibronectin synthesis (Hannan & McAuslan, 1982). Brem *et al.* (1990) studied the effect of dietary deprivation of copper or D-penicillamine chelation of copper on the rate of growth of cerebrally-implanted VX2 carcinoma cells in rabbit brain. Copper deprivation greatly slowed the rate of tumour growth and penicillamine appeared to potentiate the effect. Vascular density of tumour-associated vessels was severely depressed. Unfortunately, although growth was slowed, the length of survival of the rabbits was unchanged, and severe brain oedema was noted in these animals.

Antineoplastic agents

Very little literature is available concerning the effect of clinically important antineoplastic agents on angiogenesis. Methotrexate has been shown to inhibit cultures of umbilical vein endothelial cells with concentrations far below those showing cytotoxic activity (Hirata *et al.*, 1989). Medroxyprogesterone also inhibits angiogenesis, possibly related to its inhibition of plasminogen activator (Ashino-Fuse *et al.*, 1989). Bleomycin is inhibitory to angiogenesis in chick chorioallantoic membranes in concentrations as low as 1 ng/egg and is even more potent when administered as its copper complex (Oikawa *et al.*, 1990b). Cyclosporine A also inhibits proliferation of cultured human endothelial cells, but this is probably secondary to an effect on production of bFGF (Sharpe *et al.*, 1989). Currently there is no evidence as yet that any of these angiogenic effects play a role in the antineoplastic activity of these drugs but this should be examined in the future.

Vascular endothelium as a direct target of toxicity

Irradiation

The effects of X-irradiation on vascular endothelium have been well characterized. In normal, slowly proliferating tissues, microvascular damage is an early manifestation of radiation injury, and is a mediator of the fibrosis and atrophy seen later. Initial changes in capillary endothelial cells include irregularity of the plasma membranes, increase or decrease in the number of organelles, swelling of cells, followed by the development of platelet and fibrin thrombi (Witte *et al.*, 1989). Studies with cultured endothelial cells have revealed that one of the earliest changes occurring after irradiation is slowing of endothelial cell progression through the cell cycle (Rubin *et al*, 1990). Given the high proliferation rate of endothelial cells in tumours compared to normal tissue, it has been hypothesized that irradiation might have a more pronounced effect on vasculature function in tumours than in normal tissues. Irradition also induces polymorphonuclear leucocyte and platelet adhesion and increases vascular permeability. Cultured endothelial cells surviving irradiation have increased lactate dehydrogenase and ZnCu superoxide dismutase activity, suggesting changes towards anaerobic metabolism and increased anti-oxidant activity in surviving cells. Endothelial cells release FGF after irradiation (Witte *et al.*, 1989), which may have a role in endothelial cell repair of radiation-induced damage, as well as in the pathogenesis of post radiation fibrosis.

Cytokines

Cytokines have a broad range of biological activities, including effects on the haematopoietic, immunological and vascular systems. TNF-α has been identified as the causative agent in the induction of haemorrhagic necrosis of tumours produced by endotoxin (Bevilacqua *et al.*, 1986). Although TNF-α exhibits direct cytotoxicity to tumour cells in culture, the overall antitumour mechanism *in vivo* is not fully understood. The haemorrhagic necrosis of tumours in mice that follows TNF-α and interleukin-1 (IL-1) administration has stimulated extensive research on the effects of cytokines on endothelial cells and tumour vasculature. It is likely that the procoagulant, immunological and direct inhibitory effects of these cytokines are all involved in mediation of antitumour activity.

TNF-α induces pronounced morphological changes and growth inhibition in vascular endothelial cells in culture (Sato *et al.*, 1986). Perturbations in the actin-based cytoskeleton are accompanied by cell retraction. Within 1–3 h after exposure to TNF-α, there is an increase in endothelial permeability to macromolecules and lower mol. wt solutes. In addition, TNF-α has a direct cytotoxic effect on bovine capillary endothelial cells, which was not seen in large vessel endothelia (Sato *et al.*, 1986). Tumour neovascularization generally arises from capillaries and postcapillary venules (Schlingemann, 1990) and they may be relatively sensitive to the effects of TNF-α.

The vascular endothelium is a key regulator of coagulation; in the quiescent state it maintains a non–thrombogenic surface. Both TNF-α and IL-1 modulate endothelial cell haemostatic activity, inducing procoagulant activity (Bevilacqua *et al.*, 1986; Nawroth *et al.*, 1986). Synthesis and expression of tissue factor, a cofactor initiating coagulation via the intrinsic cascade, are induced by TNF-α in bovine aortic and human umbilical vein endothelial cells, and by IL-1 in rabbit aortic endothelium. In addition, TNF-α and IL-1 suppress endothelial cell-dependent protein C activation (Stern *et al.*, 1985; Nawroth *et al.*, 1986). Thus exposure to TNF-α and/or IL-1 results in a shift in the endothelial cell to a state where procoagulant mechanisms predominate. These changes undoubtedly contribute to the thrombus formation seen in tumours following administration of these agents.

The endothelium is the major regulator of cellular traffic from the blood stream to sites of inflammation or immunological challenge. Leucocytes bind to endothelial cells via specific cell adhesion molecules, which are expressed both constitutively and in response to inflammatory stimuli, including cytokines such as TNF-α, IL-1 and granulocyte-macrophage colony-stimulating factor (GM-CSF) (Gamble *et al.*, 1989). Leucocyte binding induced by cytokines appears to be mediated by one or more receptors expressed in response to cytokine stimulation. Vascular cell adhesion molecule-1, a member of the integrin family of adhesion molecules that bind lymphocytes, is induced on the surface of endothelial cells by IL-1 and TNF-α within hours of stimulation and remains at high levels for 72 h (Osborn *et al.*, 1989). IL-1 and TNF-α also promote binding and transendothelial migration of neutrophils *in vitro* (Moser *et al.*, 1989).

The effects of TNF-α on tumour vasculature in mice have been examined directly using a sight glass implanted in the animals. Effects on tumour vasculature included haemorrhaging at 1–2 h, congestion at 4–6 h and blood circulation blockade at 24 h (Watanabe *et al.*, 1988). Histological examination revealed thrombus formation at 4 h; suppression of thrombus formation by heparin had no effect on the antitumour activity of TNF-α. Histological examination of vessels from skin, pulmonary aorta and abdominal vena cava from treated mice showed no abnormalities in the vascular endothelial cells.

In vitro studies have revealed susceptibility of endothelial cells in the growing/motile state to the procoagulant effects of TNF-α (Gerlach *et al.*, 1989). This appears to be related to the presence of high affinity receptors for TNF-α, which were present on cells in preconfluent, but not postconfluent, cultures. Expressions of the high-affinity binding-sites appears to be related to the cytoskeletal configuration of cells proliferating and motile cells, as exposure to microtubule poisons, which result in changes in cell shape and cytoskeletal configuration, also leads to induction of high-affinity TNF-α receptors.

The exposure of high-affinity receptors on activated endothelium may be one mechanism that explains the localized effects seen in the vascular tree following cytokine administration. Ultrastructural studies of tumour endothelium reveal several morphological changes that are characteristic of activated endothelium, including hypertrophic cytoplasm showing signs of active protein synthesis, infolding of the luminal surface, fenestrations, saccular luminal membrane processes and microvilli, and an irregular, thickened basement membrane (Schlingemann, 1990). These findings may account for the localization of vascular damage to tumours following *in vivo* administration of TNF-α.

Cytotoxic chemotherapeutic agents: bleomycin and cyclophosphamide

Many antineoplastic agents act by destroying rapidly proliferating cells, without regard for the malignant phenotype. The doubling time of normal tissue endothelium is 20–2000 times longer than that of tumour endothelium (Hobson & Denekamp, 1984); it has been hypothesized that some of the activity of current antineoplastic agents against solid tumours may be secondary to damage to rapidly proliferating capillary endothelium (Lazo, 1986). There is also evidence that some of the toxicity of chemotherapeutic agents is due to damage to the endothelium of normal tissues. For example, morphological changes in pulmonary vascular endothelium seem after bleomycin injection include the formation of blebs, followed by oedema and subsequent detachment of endothelium (Lazo, 1986). Cyclophosphamide can induce similar damage in the pulmonary endothelium. This endothelial injury precedes the pulmonary fibrosis that may occur after administration of bleomycin and cyclophosphamide. The molecular mechanism responsible for these endothelial-specific changes is unexplained, although it has been suggested that the susceptibility of the endothelium to bleomycin may correlate with low levels of bleomycin hydrolase. Whether the antitumour activity of these agents is due in part to damage to the tumour vasculature has not been examined.

Flavone acetic acid (FAA)

Considerable interest has been generated by a mechanistically unique agent, FAA, which may have selective toxicity for the endothelium of solid tumours. FAA is a synthetic flavonoid with a number of interesting characteristics. It is active against a number of refractory murine carcinomas and human colorectal carcinoma xenografts (Finlay et al., 1988). It has greater activity against solid tumours than either leukaemias or early tumours, and low potency as a cytotoxic agent in vitro. It has been proposed that the antitumour effects of FAA are indirect and may be mediated by effects on the tumour vasculature (Finlay et al., 1988).

FAA induces haemorrhaging necrosis in adenocarcinomas within 2 h of administration. This is accompanied by a reduction in tumour plasma volume and complete vascular shutdown (Bibby et al., 1989). Additional studies evaluating tumour blood flow in subcutaneous colon 38 tumours in mice using a fluorescent dye revealed a 50% reduction in tumour blood flow within 3 h of FAA administration, and complete inhibition at 24 h (Zwi et al., 1989). In vitro studies of the effect of FAA on cultured human umbilical vein endothelial cells have shown that FAA produces a dose-dependent increase in tissue factor (Murray et al., 1990); this may contribute to the vascular effects seen with FAA. Other effects of FAA, which may contribute to its antitumour activity, include its biological response modifier functions. FAA augments natural killer (NK) cell activity in normal and tumour-bearing mice, and in human cancer patients (Hornung et al., 1988). Augmentation of splenic NK cell activity appears to be secondary to FFA-induced increases of serum interferon (IFN) levels; administration of anti-IFN antibodies to FAA-treated mice inhibited drug-induced increases in NK activity. FAA induces TNF-α as well as IFN-γ and interferon-α mRNA expression in splenic leucocytes (Mace et al., 1990). IFN and TNF-α levels were detectable in the serum immediately following appearance of mRNA in FAA-treated mice. Cytokine release was strictly dose-dependent, with significant induction occurring at FAA doses of greater than or equal to 150 mg/kg. There was no induction of TNF-β, IL-1 or IL-2 expression. Interestingly, FAA at doses of greater than 150 mg/kg interacts synergistically with IL-2 in the treatment of murine renal tumours; lower doses exhibit little therapeutic effect, suggesting that the biological effects of FAA are responsible for the enhanced activity seen.

To evaluate the significance of tumour vascularization and host immune factors in cytotoxic activity of FAA, mice bearing intramuscular

EMT-6/Ak tumours and mice implanted with intraperitoneal EMT-6/Ak multicellular spheroids were treated with FAA (Zwi *et al.*, 1989). A small decrease in the number of clonogenic cells obtained from the spheroids occurred after FAA treatment; this effect was minimal compared to the 1000-fold fall in clonogenicity seen with treatment of the intramuscular tumours. The avascular EMT-6/Ak spheroids were extensively infiltrated with host immune cells. These studies suggest that inhibition of tumour blood flow, and/or other direct effects on tumour endothelium, such as local cytokine production, are necessary for the antitumour activity of FAA. Clinical trials of FAA to date have been disappointing. In a Phase I study of 38 patients with refractory malignancies, no responses were seen (Havlin *et al.*, 1991). Hypertension was the dose-limiting toxicity, occurring at $10 \, g/m^2$. It has been demonstrated in mice that both protraction of dose over 5–7 h and pretreatment with bicarbonate (which has been routinely used in clinical trials to prevent crystallization of drug in the renal tubules) reduced antitumour efficacy (Denekamp *et al.*, 1990). These findings may explain the lack of response in clinical trials. The preclinical findings of synergistic effects of FAA with IL-2 and TNF-α also need to be explored (Murray *et al.*, 1990).

Vasoactive agents

Reduction of tumour blood flow may enhance the effects of some chemotherapeutic agents. Vasoactive drugs administered at the time of maximal chemotherapeutic levels in the tumour may prolong tumour exposure to the cytotoxic agent. Decreasing blood flow may also increase tumour hypoxia and enhance the cytotoxicity of bioreductive agents. Hydralazine significantly enhanced the cytotoxicity of melphalan towards the KHT tumour in mice (Stratford *et al.*, 1988). The greatest effect occurred when hydralazine was given 15 min after melphalan administration, which corresponds to the time at which peak plasma levels are obtained. There was a small increase in systemic toxicity; however, the enhancement was considerably less than the enhancement ratio observed for tumour response. The enhancement did not appear to be due to hypoxia; administration of BW12C, a drug which increases tumour hypoxia by increasing the O_2 affinity of haemoglobin, did not penetrate the effects of melphalan. Misonidazole has also been used as a chemosensitizer in combination with melphalan. The mechanism for this potentiation is not well understood, but recent data suggest that alterations in tumour blood flow may be responsible (Murray *et al.*, 1987; Murray & Randhawa, 1988). Following misonidazole administration to mice, blood flow in tumours decreased by 60% within 2 h. Only slight changes were seen in muscle blood flow and none in the kidneys.

The chemosensitization seen with vasoactive drugs may result from significant changes in the pharmacokinetics of cytotoxic agents. Although most vasoactive drugs have systemic effects, the inability of tumour vasculature to respond to changes in perfusion may result in more pronounced abnormalities in tumour perfusion, which can then be exploited to maximise antineoplastic effects and decrease systemic toxicity of cytotoxic agents.

Conclusion

The tumour vasculature represents a novel and largely ignored target for the development of future antineoplastic therapies. Several potential targets have been identified and a number of prototype agents are being evaluated. Current strategies include inhibiting tumour neovascularization with antiangiogenic agents and altering tumour perfusion with cytokines, vasodilators and new drugs, such as FAA. In addition, the endothelial cell is recognized as a key mediator of cellular traffic and as such plays a major role in immunological approaches to antitumour therapy. The great increases in our understanding of the biology of the endothelium, especially that of tumours, promise exciting avenues for future research.

References

Arnold, F. & Kumar, S. (1985). Restraint of metastasis and antiangiogenesis. *Reviews of Endocrine-Related Cancer* **22,** 19–23.

Ashino-Fuse, H., Takano, J., Oikawa, T., Shimamura, M. & Iwaguchi, T. (1989). Medroxyprogesterone acetate, an anti-cancer and anti-angiogenic steroid, inhibits the plasminogen activator in bovine endothelial cells. *International Journal of Cancer* **44,** 859–864.

Azizkhan, R.G., Azizkhan, J.C., Zetter, B.R. & Folkman, J. (1980). Mast cell heparin stimulates migration of capillary endothelial cells *in vitro*. *Journal of Experimental Medicine* **152,** 931–944.

Bagavondoss, P. & Wilks, J.W. (1990). Specific inhibition of endothelial cell proliferation by thrombospondin. *Biochemical Biophysical Research Communications* **170,** 867–872.

Bevilacqua, M.P., Pober, J.S., Majeau, G.R., Fiers, W. & Cotran, R.S. (1986). Recombinant tumor necrosis factor induces procoagulant activity in cultured human vascular endothelium: characterization and comparison with the actions of interleukin 1. *Proceedings of the National Academy of Sciences USA* **83,** 4533–4537.

Bibby, M.C., Double, J.A., Loadman, P.M. & Duke, C.V. (1989). Reduction of tumor blood flow by flavone acetic acid: a possible component of therapy. *Journal of the National Cancer Institute* **81,** 216–220.

Brem, S.S., Zagzag, D., Tsanaclis, A.M.C., Gately, S., Elkouby, M.P. & Brien, S.E. (1990). Inhibition of angiogenesis and tumor growth in the brain: suppression of endothelial cell turnover by penicillamine and the depletion of copper, an angiogenic cofactor. *American Journal of Pathology* **137,** 1121–1142.

Denekamp, J., Hill, S.A. & Williams, K.B. (1990). Scheduling details in the clinical application of FAA and other vasoactive agents. In Moore, J.V. & West, D.C. (eds)

Proceedings of the 16th LH Gray Conference: Vasculature as a Target for Anti-Cancer Therapy, Manchester, England.

DiPaolo, J.A., Tarbell, D.S. & Moore, G.E. (1958). Studies on the carcinolytic activity of fumagillin and some of its derivatives. *Antibiotic Annual 1958* 541–546.

Fett, J.W., Strydom, D.J., Lobb, F.R., Alderman, E.M., Bethune, J.L., Riordan, J.F. & Vallee, B.L. (1985). Isolation and characterization of angiogenin, an angiogenic protein from human carcinoma cells. *Biochemistry* **24**, 5480–5487.

Finlay, G.J., Smith, G.P., Fray, L.M. & Baguley, B.C. (1988). Effect of flavone acetic acid on Lewis lung carcinoma: evidence for an indirect effect. *Journal of the National Cancer Institute* **80**, 241–245.

Folkman, J. (1985). Regulation of angiogenesis: a new function of heparin. *Biochemical Pharmacology* **34**, 905–909.

Folkman, J. (1990). What is the evidence that tumors are angiogenesis dependent? *Journal of the National Cancer Institute* **82**, 4–6.

Folkman, J., Langer, R., Linhardt, R.J., Haudenschild, C. & Taylor, S. (1983). Angiogenesis inhibition and tumor regression caused by heparin or a heparin fragment in the presence of cortisone. *Science* **221**, 719–725.

Folkman, J., Weisz, P.B., Joullie, M.M., Li, W.W. & Ewing, W.R. (1989). Control of angiogenesis with synthetic heparin substitutes. *Science* **243**, 1490–1493.

Gamble, J.R., Elliot, M.J., Jaipargas, E., Lopez, A.F. & Vadas, M.A. (1989). Regulation of human monocyte adherence by granulocyte-macrophage colony-stimulating factor. *Proceedings of the National Academy of Sciences USA* **86**, 7169–7173.

Gerlach, H., Lieberman, H., Bach, R., Godman, G., Brett, J. & Stern, D. (1989). Enhanced responsiveness of endothelium in the growing/motile state to tumor necrosis factor/cachectin. *Journal of Experimental Medicine* **170**, 913–931.

Golub, L.M., Ramamurthy, N.S., McNamara, T.F., Gomes, B., Wolff, M., Casino, A., Kapoor, A., Zambon, J., Ciancio, S., Schneir, M. & Perry, H. (1984). Tetracyclines inhibit tissue collagenase activity. *Journal of Periodontal Research* **19**, 651–655.

Gospodarowicz, D., Moran, J., Braun, D. & Birdwell, C. (1976). Clonal growth of bovine vascular endothelial cells: fibroblast growth factor as a survival agent. *Proceedings of the National Academy of Sciences* **73**, 4120–4124.

Greenblatt, M. & Shubik, P. (1968). Tumour angiogenesis: transfilter diffusion studies in the hamster by the transparent chamber technique. *Journal of the National Cancer Institute* **41**, 111–124.

Hannan, G.N. & McAuslan, B.R. (1982). Modulation of synthesis of specific proteins in endothelial cells by copper, cadmium, and disulfiram: an early response to an angiogenic inducer of cell migration. *Journal of Cellular Physiology* **111**, 207–212.

Havlin, K.A., Kuhn, J.G., Craig, J.B., Boldt, D.H., Weiss, G.R., Koeller, J., Harman, G., Schwartz, R., Clark, G.N. & Von Hoff, D.D. (1991). Phase I clinical and pharmacokinetic trial of flavone acetic acid. *Journal of the National Cancer Institute* **83**, 124–128.

Hirata, S., Matsubara, T., Saura, R., Tateishi, H. & Hirohata, K. (1989). Inhibition of *in vitro* vascular endothelial cell proliferation and *in vivo* neovascularization by low-dose methotrexate. *Arthritis and Rheumatism* **32**, 1065–1073.

Hobson, B. & Denekamp, J. (1984). Endothelial proliferation in tumors and normal tissues: continuous labelling studies. *British Journal of Cancer* **49**, 405–413.

Hornung, R.L., Young, H.A., Urba, W.J. & Wiltrout, R.H. (1988). Immunomodulation of natural killer cell activity by flavone acetic acid: occurrence via induction of interferon alpha/beta. *Journal of the National Cancer Institute* **80**, 1226–1231.

Ingber, D. & Folkman, J. (1988). Inhibition of angiogenesis through modulation of collagen metabolism. *Laboratory Investigation* **59**, 44–51.

Ingber, D., Fujita, T., Kishimoto, S., Sudo, K., Kanamaru, T., Brem, H. & Folkman,

J. (1990). Synthetic analogs of fumagillin that inhibit angiogenesis and suppress tumour growth. *Nature* **348**, 555–557.

Ishikawa, F., Miyazono, K., Hellman, U., Drexler, H., Wernstedt, C., Hagiwara, K., Usuki, K., Takaku, F., Risau, W. & Heldin, C.H. (1989). Identification of angiogenic activity and the cloning and expression of platelet-derived endothelial cell growth factor. *Nature (London)* **338**, 557–562.

Kasuka, M., Sudo, K., Fujita, T., Marui, S., Itoh, F., Ingber, D. & Folkman, J. (1991). Potent anti-angiogenic action of AGM-1470: comparison to the fumagillin parent. *Biochemical and Biophysical Research Communications* **174**, 1070–1076.

Lazo, J.S. (1986). Endothelial injury caused by antineoplastic agents. *Biochemical Pharmacology* **35**, 1919–1923.

Lee, K.E., Erturk, R., Mayer, R. & Cockett, A.T.K. (1987). Efficacy of antitumor chemotherapy in C3H mice enhanced by the antiangiogenesis steroid, cortisone acetate. *Cancer Research* **47**, 5021–5024.

Liebovich, S.J., Polverini, P.J., Shepard, H.M., Wiseman, D.M., Shively, V. & Nuseir, N. (1987). Macrophage-induced angiogenesis is mediated by tumour necrosis factor-α. *Nature (London)* **329**, 630–632.

McCarthy, S.A., Kuzu, I., Gatter, K.C. & Bicknele, R. (1991). Heterogeneity of the endothelial cell and its role in organ preference of tumour metastasis. *Trends in Pharmacological Science* **12**, 462–467.

Mace, K.F., Hornung, R.L., Wiltrout, R.H. & Young, H.A. (1990). Correlation between *in vivo* induction of cytokine gene expression by flavone acetic acid and strict dose dependency and therapeutic efficacy against murine renal cancer. *Cancer Research* **50**, 1741–1747.

Maciag, T., Cerundolo, J., Ilsley, S., Kelly, P.R. & Forand, R. (1979). An endothelial cell growth factor from bovine hypothalamus. Identification and partial characterization. *Proceedings of the National Academy of Sciences USA* **76**, 5674–5678.

Maione, T.E., Gray, G.S., Pietro, J., Hunt, A.J., Donner, A.L., Bauer, S.I., Carson, H.F. & Sharpe, R.J. (1990). Inhibition of angiogenesis by recombinant human platelet factor-4 and related peptides. *Science* **247**, 77–79.

Maione, T.E. & Sharpe, R.J. (1990). Development of angiogenesis inhibitors for clinical applications. *Trends in Pharmacological Sciences* **11**, 457–461.

Maragoudakis, M.E., Sarmonika, M. & Panoutsacopoulou, M. (1989). Antiangiogenic action of heparin plus cortisone is associated with decreased collagenous protein synthesis in the chick chorioallantoic membrane system. *Journal of Pharmacology and Experimental Therapeutics* **251**, 679–682.

Maragoudakis, M.E., Sarmonika, M. & Panoutsacopoulou, M. (1988). Inhibition of basement membrane synthesis prevents angiogenesis. *Journal of Pharmacology and Experimental Therapeutics* **244**, 729–733.

Matsubara, T., Saura, R., Hirohata, K. & Ziff, M. (1989). Inhibition of human endothelial cell proliferation *in vitro* and neovascularization *in vivo* by D-penicillamine. *Journal of Clinical Investigation* **83**, 158–167.

Mignatti, P., Tsuboi, R., Robbins, E. & Rifkin, D.B. (1989). *In vitro* angiogenesis on the human amniotic membrane: requirement for basic fibroblast growth factor-induced proteinases. *Journal of Cell Biology* **108**, 671–682.

Missirlin, E., Karakiulakis, G. & Maragoudakis, M.E. (1990). Antitumor effect of GPA1734 in rat Walker 256 carcinoma. *Investigational New Drugs* **8**, 145–147.

Moser, R., Schleiffenbaum, B., Groscurth, P. & Fehr, J. (1989). Interleukin-1 and tumor necrosis factor stimulate human vascular endothelial cells to promote transendothelial neutrophil passage. *Journal of Clinical Investigation* **83**, 444–455.

Murray, J.C. & Randhawa, V.S. (1988). Misonidazole reduced blood flow in two experimental murine tumors. *British Journal of Cancer* **58**, 128–132.

Murray, J.C., Randhawa, V.S. & Denekamp, J. (1987). The effects of melphalan and misonidazole on the vasculature of a murine sarcoma. *British Journal of Cancer* **55**, 233–238.

Murray, J.C., Smith, K.A. & Stern, D. (1990). Flavone acetic acid and TNF-alpha act synergistically to promote endothelial procoagulant activity *in vitro* and inhibit tumor growth *in vivo*. In *Proceedings of the 16th LH Gray Conference: Vasculature as a Target for Anti-Cancer Therapy*, Manchester, England.

Nawroth, P.P., Handley, D.A., Esmon, C.T. & Stern, D.M. (1986). Interleukin-1 induces endothelial cell procoagulant while suppressing cell-surface anticoagulant activity. *Proceedings of the National Academy of Sciences USA* **83**, 3460–3464.

Oikawa, T., Ashino-Fuse, H., Shimamura, M., Koide, U. & Iwaguchi, T. (1990a). A novel angiogenic inhibitor derived from Japanese shark cartilage. (1) Extraction and estimation of inhibitory activities toward tumor and embryonic angiogenesis. *Cancer Letters* **51**, 181–186.

Oikawa, T., Hirotani, K., Ogasawara, H., Katayama, T., Ashino-Fuse, H., Shimamura, M., Iwaguchi, T. & Nakamura, O. (1990b). Inhibition of angiogenesis by bleomycin and its copper complex. *Chemical Pharmacology Bulletin* **38**, 1790–1792.

Oikawa, T., Hirotani, K., Ogasuwara, H., Katayama, T., Nakamura, O., Iwaguchi, T. & Hiragun, A. (1990c). Inhibition of angiogenesis by vitamin D3 analogs. *European Journal of Pharmacology* **178**, 247–250.

Osborn, L., Hession, C., Tizard, R., Vassallo, C., Luhowskyj, S., Chi-Rossi, G. & Lobb, R. (1989). Direct expression cloning of vascular cell adhesion molecule-1, a cytokine induced entothelial protein that binds to lymphocytes. *Cell* **59**, 1203–1211.

Rubin, D.B., Drab, E.A. & Ward, W.F. (1990). Physiological and biochemical markers of the endothelial cell response to irradiation. In *Proceedings of the 16th LH Gray Conference: Vasculature as a Target for Anti-Cancer Therapy*, Manchester, England.

Sato, N., Goto, T., Haranaka, K., Satomi, N., Nariuchi, H., Mano-Hirano, Y. & Sawasaki, Y. (1986). Actions of tumor necrosis factor on cultured vascular endothelial cells: morphologic modulation, growth inhibition and cytotoxicity. *Journal of the National Cancer Institute* **76**, 1113–1121.

Schlingemann, R.O. (1990). *Vascular Markers in Tumor Biology*, pp. 11–51. Thesis Nijmegen, The Netherlands.

Schwartz, S.M., Heimark, R.L. & Majesky, M.W. (1990). Developmental mechanisms underlying pathology of arteries. *Physiological Reviews* **70**, 1177–1209.

Sharpe, R.J., Arndt, K.A., Bauer, S.I. & Maione, T.E. (1989). Cyclosporine inhibits basic fibroblast growth factor-driven proliferation of human endothelial cells and keratinocytes. *Archives of Dermatology* **125**, 1359–1362.

Sharpe, R.J., Byers, H.R., Scott, C.F., Bauer, S.I. & Maione, T.E. (1990). Growth inhibition of murine melanoma and human colon carcinoma by recombinant human platelet factor 4. *Journal of the National Cancer Institute* **82**, 848–853.

Sidsky, Y.A. & Borden, E.C. (1987). Inhibition of angiogenesis by interferons: effect on tumor- and lymphocyte-induced vascular responses. *Cancer Research* **47**, 5155–5161.

Stern, D.M., Bank, I., Nawroth, P.P., Cassimeris, J., Kisiel, W., Fenton, J.W., Dinarello, C., Chess, L. & Jaffe, E.A. (1985). Self regulation of procoagulant events on the endothelial cell surface. *Journal of Experimental Medicine* **162**, 1223–1235.

Stokes, C.L., Weisz, P.B., Williams, S.K. & Lauffenburger, D.A. (1990). Inhibition of microvascular endothelial cell migration by B-cyclodextrin tetradecasulfate and hydrocortisone. *Microvascular Research* **40**, 279–284.

Stratford, I.J., Adams, G.E., Godden, J., Nolan, J., Howells, N. & Timpson, N. (1988). Potentiation of the anti-tumour effect of melphalan by the vasoactive agent, hydralazine. *British Journal of Cancer* **58**, 122–127.

Takigawa, M., Nishida, Y., Suzuki, F., Kishi, J., Yamashita, K. & Hayakawa, T.

(1990a). Induction of angiogenesis in chick yolk-sac membrane by polyamines and its inhibition by tissue inhibitors of metalloproteinases (TIMP and TIMP-2). *Biochemical Biophysical Research Communications* **171**, 1264–1271.

Takigawa, M., Pan, H-O, Enomoto, M., Kinoshita, A., Nishida, Y., Suzuki, F. & Tajima, K. (1990b). A clonal human chondrosarcoma cell line produces an antiangiogenic antitumor factor. *Anticancer Research* **10**, 311–315.

Tamargo, R.J., Bok, R.A. & Brem, H. (1991). Angiogenesis inhibition by minocycline. *Cancer Research* **51**, 672–675.

Watanabe, N., Niitsu, Y., Hiroshi, K., Neda, H. & Yamuchi, N. (1988). Toxic effect of tumor necrosis factor on tumor vasculature in mice. *Cancer Research* **48**, 2179–2183.

Witte, L., Fuks, Z., Haimovitz-Friedman, A., Vlodavsky, I., Goodman, D. & Eldor, A. (1989). Effects of irradiation on the release of growth factors from cultured bovine, porcine, and human endothelial cells. *Cancer Research* **49**, 5066–5072.

Yamashita, T., Sakai, M., Kawai, Y., Aono, M. & Takahashi, K. (1989). A new activity of herbimycin A: inhibition of angiogenesis. *Journal of Antibiotics* **42**, 1015–1017.

Yang, E.Y. & Moses, H.L. (1990). Transforming growth factor β-1-induced changes in cell migration, proliferation, and angiogenesis in the chicken chorioallantoic membrane. *Journal of Cell Biology* **111**, 731–741.

Zwi, L.J., Baguley, B.C., Gavin, J.B. & Wilson, W.R. (1989). Blood flow failure as a major determinant in the antitumor action of flavone acetic acid. *Journal of the National Cancer Institute* **81**, 1005–1013.

Chapter 13
Pharmacological approaches to the management of metastatic prostatic cancer

Gary D. Steinberg and John T. Isaacs

Introduction

During this year there will be 30 thousand deaths due to prostatic cancer in the USA (Boring *et al.*, 1992). This mortality rate makes prostatic cancer the second commonest fatal tumour in males in the USA. Besides a high annual mortality rate, prostatic cancer is the most commonly diagnosed malignancy in males of all ages in the USA. Approximately 122 000 new cases of prostatic cancer will be diagnosed this year in the USA (Boring *et al.*, 1992). These high annual incidence rates translate into the human reality that one of every 11 American white males will eventually develop clinical prostatic cancer during their lifetimes (Seidman *et al.*, 1985). Rates for American black males are even higher, such that the lifetime risk for cancer is one out of every 10 (Mettlin, 1983). In addition, the annual incidence rate of clinical prostatic cancer has increased steadily since the 1930s to the present time (Devesa & Silverman, 1978).

    Prostatic cancer varies widely in its clinical aggressiveness. In some patients, prostatic cancer metastasizes rapidly, killing the patient within 1 year of initial clinical presentation, while other patients may live for many years with localized disease without apparent metastases (Catalona & Scott, 1979). If prostatic cancer is truly localized, then radical prostatectomy can be used to cure the patient (Walsh & Jewett, 1980). Unfortunately, *c*. 60% of the 122 000 new cases of prostatic cancer detected this year in the USA will be non-organ confined at the time of initial diagnosis (Carter & Coffey, 1988). Thus the majority of prostatic cancer patients are not candidates for curative local surgery. Patients with non-organ confined disease eventually require systemic therapy, if they do not die of intercurrent disease. In this chapter, the presently used pharmacological approaches for such systemic therapy for metastatic prostatic cancer will be reviewed. An attempt will be made to focus upon the rationale, clinical effectiveness, and limitation of each approach. In addition, an overview to several new experimental approaches will be presented.

Rationale for androgen ablative therapy

The growth of any tissue, whether normal or cancerous, depends upon the quantitative relationship between the rate of cell proliferation and cell death. In normal adult tissues, these rates are usually balanced such that neither net continuous growth nor involution occurs. Studies in a large variety of different tissues have demonstrated that this balance is highly regulated by a series of tissue-specific growth factors. A fundamental characteristic of cancer cells is their change in responsiveness to these tissue-specific growth factors such that their rate of cell proliferation exceeds their rate of cell death and continuous growth occurs. This does not mean, however, that all cancer cells are completely unresponsive and therefore autonomous to such tissue-specific growth factors. On the contrary, many types of human cancers do respond to normal growth factors and often in a manner very similar to that of the normal tissue of tumour origin. For example, one of the critical tissue-specific growth factors involved in the regulation of cellular content of the normal prostate is androgen. In the normal prostate, androgen regulates the total cell number by chronically stimulating the rate of cell proliferation while simultaneously inhibiting the rate of cell death (Isaacs, 1984a). Like the normal prostate, prostatic cancers often retain a similar ability for androgenic regulation of their rate of cell proliferation and of cell death (Kyprianou *et al.*, 1990) and these cancers are thus often responsive to androgen ablation therapy (Scott *et al.*, 1980). Such androgen ablation therapy can be achieved by either surgical or pharmacological approaches. To understand the basis for these approaches, an overview of the regulation of systemic androgen levels is required.

Overview of regulation of systemic androgen levels

The organs involved in the regulation of androgen production are the hypothalamus, pituitary, testes and adrenal glands. The peptide hormones, luteinizing hormone-releasing hormone (LHRH) and cortico-tropin-releasing factor (CRF) are produced by the hypothalamus. These releasing hormones, via the hypothalamic–pituitary vascular network, reach the anterior pituitary where they stimulate respectively the release of luteinizing hormone (LH) and adrenocorticotropic hormone (ACTH) into the blood. LH and ACTH via the blood stimulates the testes and adrenal glands respectively. The Leydig cells of the testes under the influence of LH produce 95% of the circulating testosterone (T) while the adrenal under the influence of ACTH produces androstenedione and dehydro-epiandrosterone which can be converted within prostatic tissues to more active androgens (Coffey, 1986). More than 95% of the circulating T is bound to T–oestradiol-binding globulin and plasma albumin (Coffey, 1986). Feedback loops serve to modify the secretion of the anterior pitu-itary and the hypothalamus. Thus, serum T exerts a negative feedback in both the hypothalamus and pituitary, on the release of LHRH and LH respectively. Serum cortisol feeds back on the hypothalamus and pituitary and inhibits further production of CRF and ACTH. Adrenal androgens appear to be quite weak and do not appear to exert any negative feedback on the hypothalamic–pituitary axis (Swerdloff, 1986).

The goal of androgen ablation therapy in prostatic cancer is to deprive the androgen-dependent cancer cells of androgenic stimulation. This can be achieved by one or more combinations of four mechanisms:

1   surgical removal of the testes (i.e. bilateral orchiectomy) to eliminate testicular androgens and by hypophysectomy or adrenalectomy to elimi-nate adrenal androgens,

2   suppression of pituitary LH release, thereby inhibiting T production by the testes,

3   inhibition of androgenic synthesis in the testes and adrenals, and

4   inhibition of androgen action at the level of androgen-dependent prostatic cancer cells itself.

At present the 'gold standard' for androgen ablation therapy is bilat-eral orchiectomy (Huggins et al., 1941). Surgical removal of the testes results in a 95% reduction of circulating T. The advantages of this surgical approach include efficacy, assurance of patient compliance, cost effective-ness, minimal morbidity from the procedure and rapidity of symptomatic response. The disadvantages include the side effects of loss of libido, erectile impotence, hot flushes, occasional breast tenderness and possible psychological trauma of 'disfiguring' surgery. Based upon these disadvan-tages, substantial numbers of men with metastatic prostatic cancer choose alternative pharmacological approaches to produce androgen ablation. Presently, there are a large variety of pharmacological agents to achieve androgen ablation. These agents can be divided into two basic groups. The first group of agents produces androgen ablation indirectly by lowering the extracellular supply of androgen to the prostatic cancer cells by means

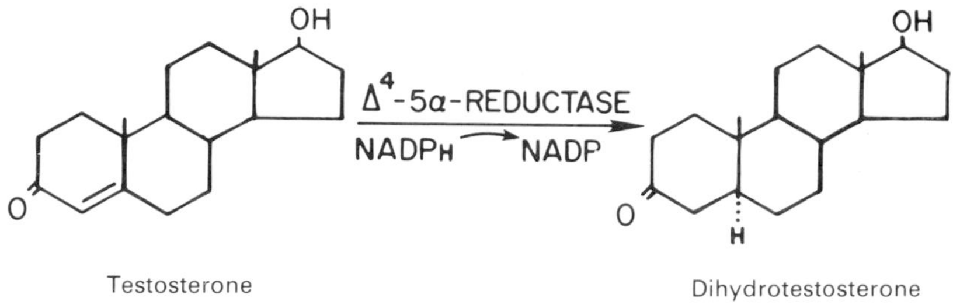

Fig. 13.1. Structure of testosterone and 5α-dihydrotestosterone.

of lowering the level of androgens in the blood. These agents include oestrogenic compounds, progestational agents and androgen synthesis inhibitors of various types. The second group of agents produce androgen ablation by inhibiting the intracellular response to androgen within androgen-dependent prostatic cancer cells. Quantitatively, the major circulating androgen in the blood is T. Within prostate cancer cells, however, T is converted to a series of metabolites, the major one being 5α-dihydro-testosterone (DHT) (Brendler *et al.*, 1984; Klein *et al.*, 1988). The enzyme responsible for the irreversible conversion of T to DHT is the membrane-bound nicotinamide–adenine dinucleotide phosphate (NADP)-dependent 5α-oxido-reductase (5α-reductase) (Bruchovsky & Wilson, 1968) (Fig. 13.1). Once formed by the 5α-reductase enzymes, DHT binds to the intracellular androgen receptor (Anderson & Liao, 1968). It is this DHT–androgen receptor binding which results in the trophic stimulation of proliferation and blockage of death of the hormone-dependent prostatic cancer cells (Kyprianou *et al.*, 1990). Thus, androgen ablation can be achieved at the prostatic cancer cell level either by inhibiting the production of DHT via 5α-reductase inhibitors or by preventing the binding of DHT to its receptor due to competitive inhibition by antiandrogen antagonists.

Pharmacological approaches to lower circulating androgen

Oestrogens

When the blood level of oestrogen rises to a pharmacologically sufficient concentration, inhibition of the release of LH from the pituitary results, thus decreasing T synthesis and release from the testes. Therefore, chronic maintenance of pharmacological blood levels of oestrogen can depress serum T to the same minimal level as that observed following surgical orchiectomy (Mackler *et al.*, 1972). When given orally, naturally occurring oestrogens (i.e. 17β-oestradiol and oestrone) (Fig. 13.2) are rapidly metabilized by the liver and are not able to sufficiently elevate the blood oestrogen levels to depress serum T. Diethylstilboestrol (DES) (3,4-*bis*

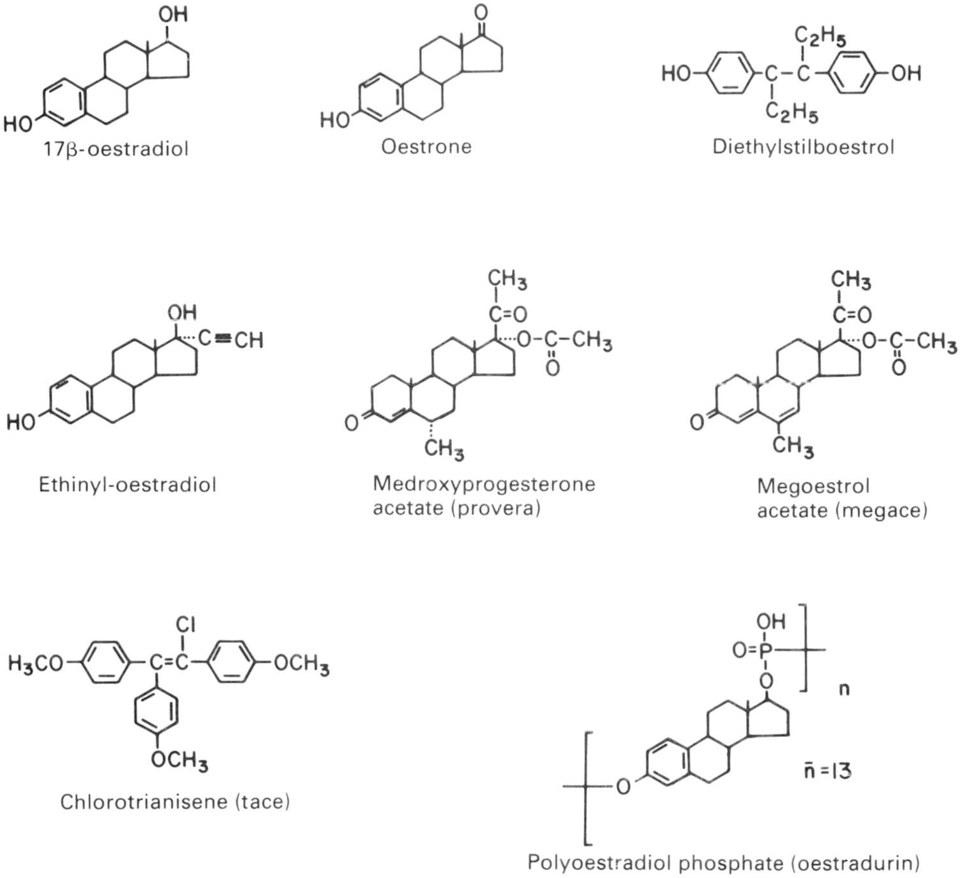

Fig. 13.2. Structures of a series of steroid and non-steroid oestrogens and progesterone analogues.

(*p*-hydroxyphenyl)-3-hexene) (Fig. 13.2) is a synthetic compound which has potent oestrogenic abilities and is capable of reaching sufficient blood levels following oral delivery to suppress LH release. DES, given orally at 3 mg/day chronically, is thus able to suppress serum T to castrate levels (Mackler *et al.*, 1972; Vermeulen *et al.*, 1982). For this reason, oral DES is the most commonly used form of oestrogen therapy for metastatic prostatic cancer. In addition to DES, there are other oral oestrogens available. For example, at the appropriate dose, the oral oestrogens premarin, provera (i.e. medroxyprogesterone acetate) and ethinyl oestradiol (Fig. 13.2) are as effective as DES. Chlorotrianisene (TACE) (tri-*p*-anisylchloroethylene) (Fig. 13.2) has produced (i.e. medroxyprogesterone acetate) (Fig. 13.2) clinical responses but does not completely suppress LH or T levels (Smith, 1987).

Unfortunately, the side effects of pharmacological amounts of oestrogens are numerous: nausea, vomiting, headaches, fluid retention, gynaecomastia, impotence, pedal oedema, thrombophlebitis, myocardial infarction and stroke (Blackard, 1975; Hedlund *et al.*, 1980; Glashan & Robinson, 1981). Byar and Corle (1988) reported on the long-term results of oestrogen therapy for prostate cancer based upon the studies of the Veterans Administration Cooperative Urological Research Group (VACURG). They concluded that:

1 oestrogen therapy provides significant palliation in most patients with advanced prostate cancer,

2 5 mg of DES/day is associated with significantly increased risk of cardiovascular death,

3 orchiectomy plus DES is no better than orchiectomy or DES alone,

4 1 mg/day of DES was equivalent in its effect on prostate cancer survival as 5 mg DES/day, however, 1 mg DES/day is not sufficient to depress serum T to castrate levels,

5 1 mg DES/day was associated with a decreased cardiovascular risk compared to 5 mg DES/day but still produced significant risk especially for elderly men with increased non-oestrogen risk factors, and

6 premarin or provera was no better than 1 mg DES/day.

Because of the significantly increased risk of cardiovascular complications associated with oral oestrogens, many physicians no longer prescribe them for their patients with prostatic cancer. The toxicity of oral oestrogens appears to be due to 'first pass' effects through the liver when absorption is via the portal route. These toxic effects can be eliminated if oestrogens are given parenterally; not orally. This has been clearly established by a large Finnish study of 477 men with prostatic cancer which demonstrated that increased cardiovascular risks can be eliminated with parenteral depot oestrogens (Aro, 1991). This study demonstrated that when 160 mg/month of polyoestradiol phosphate (PEP) (Fig. 13.2) is given as a slow release intramuscular depot, the treatment is effective for prostate cancer control and patients had significantly less cardiovascular deaths than men treated with orchiectomy or combination intramuscular and oral oestrogen therapy. In addition in this study, parenteral PEP had a protective effect on cardiovascular deaths. This may be due to the fact that, when given as a once-monthly intramuscular injection, parenteral PEP caused an increase in serum high-density lipoprotein (HDL) cholesterol and a decrease in total serum triglycerides and low-density lipoprotein (LDL) triglycerides (Agardh *et al.*, 1984; Rössner *et al.*, 1985; Aro *et al.*, 1991). Thus, the use of a parenteral depot of oesterogens given monthly as an intramuscular injection is an inexpensive and effective pharmacological approach to androgen ablation.

Megoestrol acetate (also called megace) (Fig. 13.2) is a progestational agent that acts primarily by suppressing pituitary release of LH while directly inhibiting steroidogenesis and weakly binding to androgen

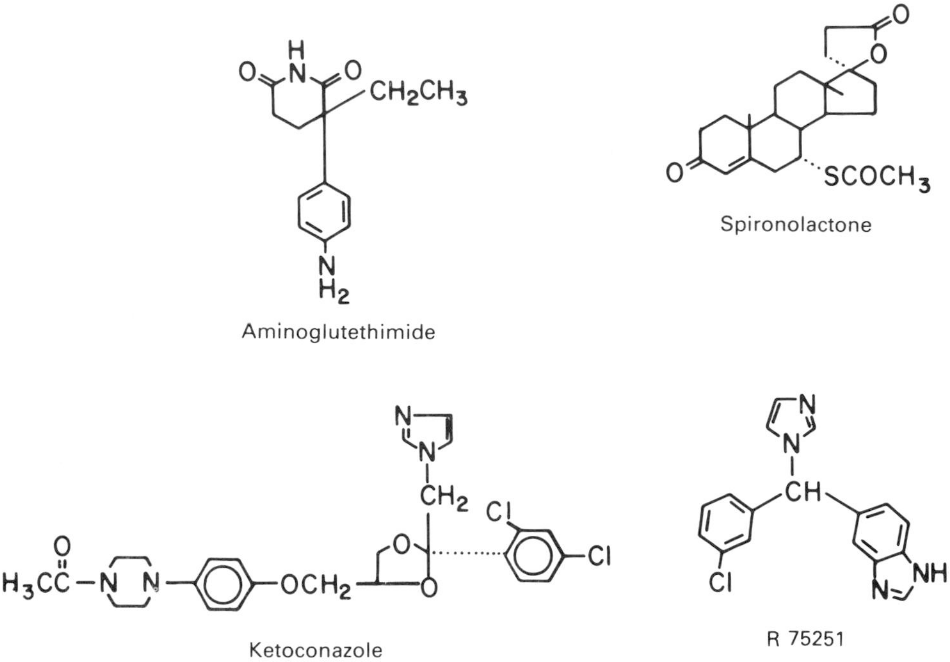

Aminoglutethimide

Spironolactone

Ketoconazole

R 75251

Fig. 13.3. Structure of a series of androgen synthesis inhibitors.

receptors in the prostate (Geller *et al.*, 1978). However, chronic clinical use of megoestrol acetate is limited because of the gradual return to normal serum T levels after 6 months of treatment. The mechanism of this escape is unknown. Magace does not cause fluid retention or increase cardiovascular side effects; however, it does cause impotence.

Androgen synthesis inhibiting agents

Aminoglutethimide (α-(p-aminophenyl)-α-ethylglutarimide) (Fig. 13.3) inhibits the 20,21-desmolase enzyme which converts cholesterol to pregnenolone in the testes and adrenal glands. Aminoglutethimide thus inhibits production of cortisol, aldosterone and androgen since pregnenolone is a critical early intermediate in the synthesis of these steroids (Worgul *et al.*, 1983; Ponder *et al.*, 1984; Murray & Pitt, 1985). Hydrocortisone must be administered with aminoglutethimide to prevent development of Addison's syndrome. The significant side effects of this agent include hypotension, nausea and vomiting, fatigue, anorexia, depression, oedema and skin rashes. Spironolactone (17-hydroxy-7α-mercapto-3-oxo-17α-pregn-4-ene-21-carboxylic acid γ-lactone, 7-acetate) (Fig. 13.3) inhibits testicular and adrenal cytochrome P450 enzyme activity with resultant blockade of 17α-hydroxylase and 17,20-desmolase enzymes thus suppressing serum levels of T (Walsh & Sitteri, 1975). Neither amino-glutethimide nor spironolactone is usually used as primary androgen ablation therapy. These agents are usually used as secondary approaches to block adrenal androgens once progression to testicular androgen ablation has occurred. Ketoconazole (*cis*-1-acetyl-4-[4-([2-(2,3-dichloro-phenyl)-2-(1H-imidazol-1-ylmethyl)-13-dioxolan-4-y]-methoxy)-phenyl]-piperazine) (Fig. 13.3) is commonly used as a broad-spectrum antifungal agent. It inhibits the conversion of lanenterol to ergosterol in fungi and to cholesterol in man via its ability to inhibit the testicular and adrenal cytochrome P450 enzymes. It produces a very rapid and sustained decrease in testicular and adrenal androgen production. At the usual dose of 200–300 mg every 8 h, ketoconazole reduces serum T to castrate levels in less than 24 h (Trachtenberg *et al.*, 1983; Trachtenberg, 1984; Mahler *et al.*, 1987; Pont, 1987; Johnson *et al.*, 1988). High-dose ketoconazole (i.e. 400 mg tid orally) although effective in lowering serum T, is not commonly used as first line androgen ablation therapy. This is because of the neces-sity of a strict every 8 h regimen to compensate for the short duration of its action coupled with poor compliance due to gastric intolerance.

Liarozole (the older name was R75251) (5-(3-chlorophenyl)-(1H-imi-dozol-1-ylmethyl)-1H-benzimidazole) (Fig. 13.3) is a new imidazole derivative which inhibits testicular and adrenal cytochrome P450 enzymes inhibiting the conversion of androgens to oestrogens, progestins to an-drostenedione and T, and of 11-deoxycorticosterone to corticosterone. As compared with high-dose ketoconozole, liarozole (i.e. 300 mg bid) is as efficacious in inhibiting serum T levels without significantly decreasing adrenal androgens (Bruynseels *et al.*, 1990). Experimental studies using serially transplantable rat prostatic cancers have demonstrated that oral feeding of liarozole exerts an antitumoural effect independent of its inhibi-tor of androgen biosynthesis (Van Ginckel *et al.*, 1990). Recent studies have demonstrated that liarozole inhibits the metabolism of all trans-reti-noic acid (RA) *in vivo* leading to enhanced endogeneous plasma con-centrations of RA (Van Wauwe *et al.*, 1990). This may be very significant since treatment of rats with the synthetic retinoid, *N*-14-hydroxyphenyl, retinamide has been demonstrated to prevent the development of chemical carcinogen-induced prostatic cancers in rats (Pollard *et al.*, 1991). In an open pilot study in 31 stage D prostatic cancer patients in active progres-sion after surgical castration, liarozole induced subjective responses in the majority of evaluateable patients and partial remission (50% reduction in primary tumour or lymph node volume) in two out of two patients with measurable disease. After 3 months of treatment, prostate-specific antigen levels decreased by at least 50% in more than half of the patients (Denis, 1991).

LHRH analogues

LHRH is a decapeptide (i.e. 5-oxo-L-prolyl[1]-L-histidyl[2]-L-tryptophyl[3]-L-seryl[4]-L-tyrosyl[5]-glysyl[6]-L-leucyl[7]-L-arginyl[8]-L-prolyl[9]-L-glysyl[10]) which stimulates the release of LH by the anterior pituitary. LH stimulates the testes to release T. Substitutions at the sixth, ninth or tenth positions of the decapeptide LHRH result in synthetic agonist analogues with prolonged half-life and potency. For example the LHRH agonist analogue leuprolide has a D-leucine at position 6 and a N-ethyl-L-prolinamide at position 9 while the agonist analogue buserelin has a D-(t-butyl) serine at position 6 and a N-ethyl-L-prolinamide at position 9. Initial administration of these agonist analogues results in stimulation of LH and follicle-stimulating hormone (FSH) production, and T levels rise 140–170% within several days (Tolis *et al.*, 1980; The Leuprolide Study Group, 1984; Crawford *et al.*, 1989). This rise in serum T can result in patients with metastatic prostatic cancer undergoing a 'flare' response (The Leuprolide Study Group, 1984; Waxman *et al.*, 1985). This 'flare' response can result in increased bony pain, urinary obstruction, lymphoedema or spinal cord compression. The 'flare' response can be blocked by administering an antiandrogen for 1 week before the start of LHRH agonist treatment (Svensson *et al.*, 1986).

With chronic LHRH agonist administration (i.e. after *c.* 4 weeks of treatment), castrate levels of T are produced. This paradoxical T suppression by LHRH agonist analogues results from: (i) alterations in the central feedback control of LH release; (ii) desensitization of the testes to LH due to a decrease in LH receptor content; and (iii) direct testicular steroid enzyme inhibition. LHRH agonists are not active orally but can be administered as nasal sprays, subcutaneous injections daily or deep intramuscular depot injections monthly. The advantages of the LHRH agonists are that the side effects are minimal, although they include hot flushes and erectile impotence (Eisenberger *et al.*, 1986), and that the androgen ablation is reversible if the agonist is discontinued. The major disadvantages of the agonists are that: (i) chronic administration of LHRH agonists is required to inhibit LH release and to reduce the serum androgens to castration levels; (ii) such chronic agonist treatment can induce an initial 'flare' response; and (iii) the treatment is very costly (i.e. over US$3000/year/patient). Due to its low cardiovascular toxicity, LHRH agonists, particularly as time release depot preparations, are rapidly becoming the most commonly used alternative to surgical ablation even with the cost disadvantage.

In contrast to LHRH agonists, LHRH antagonists do not induce a 'flare' response and do not require dosing at as frequent an interval. A new LHRH antagonist, free of oedematogenic and anaphylactoid reaction, has

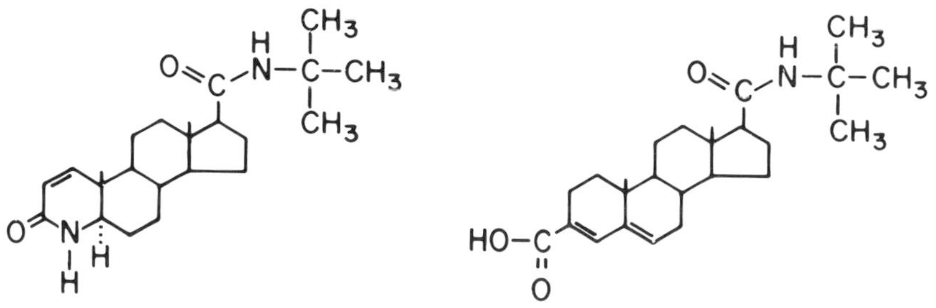

Finasteride   SK & F 105657

Fig. 13.4. Structures of 5α-reductase enzyme inhibitors.

been developed which contains the neutral hydrophilic D-ureidoalkyl-amino acid, D-citrulline, at position 6 and is termed SB-75 (i.e. N-Ac [3-(2-naphthyl)-D-alanyl[1] -4-chloro-D-phenylalanyl[2] -3-(3-pyridyl)-D-alanyl[3] -L-seryl[4]-L-trysosyl[5]-D-citrulline[6]-L-leucyl[7]-L-arginyl[8]-L-prolyl[9]-D-alanyl[10]] LHRH). SB-75 has been demonstrated experimentally to be effective in causing the suppression of serum T to castrate levels without causing an initial rise in serum T. It has likewise been shown to inhibit the growth of androgen-responsive rodent prostatic cancer *in vivo* (Korkut *et al.*, 1991).

Pharmacological approaches to blocking androgenic effects within prostatic cancer cells

5α-reductase inhibitors

DHT is believed to be the active intracellular androgen in stimulating growth and inhibiting cell death of androgen-dependent normal prostatic cells and presumably prostatic cancer cells (Coffey, 1986). Inhibiting DHT production without decreasing systemic T levels could be advantageous. T itself, without conversion to DHT, is capable of maintaining the anabolic effects of androgen upon muscle mass, male libido, as well as sperm maturation (George *et al.*, 1989). Theoretically, 5α-reductase inhibitors could inhibit the DHT-induced stimulation of androgen-dependent prostatic cancer growth without negating the effects of T on muscle mass, libido or erectile potence. Due to these quality of life issues, there is a great deal of clinical interest in developing effective and specific 5α-reductase inhibitors.

A series of steroid analogues have been synthesized which are capable of inhibiting the 5α-reductase catalysed production of DHT within cells. For example, finasteride (i.e. N-(2-methyl-2-propyl)-3-oxo-4-aza-5α-androst-1-ene-17β-carboxyamide) (Fig. 13.4) is a reversible competitive inhibitor of the interaction between T and the 5α-reductase enzyme. In experimental and human studies, the substrate inhibitor finasteride has been demonstrated to inhibit the 5α-reductase activity and to decrease the serum and tissue DHT content (Vermeulen *et al.*, 1982; Brooks *et al.*, 1986). *In vivo* treatment with finasteride eventually leads not only to a decrease in tissue DHT but also an increase in tissue T concentration (Brooks *et al.*, 1986). This increase in tissue T concentration could overcome some portion of the initial inhibition by this competitive substrate 5α-reductase inhibitor. Based upon this potential limitation and the sequential nature of the enzymatic 5α-reductase process (i.e. initial reduced NADP binding, followed by T binding, DHT conversion, then DHT leaving, and finally oxidized NADP$^+$ leaving to regenerate the 5α-reductase enzyme), 5α-reductase inhibitors have been synthesized which inhibit the enzyme in an uncompetitive manner versus T (Levy *et al.*, 1989). The uncompetitive inhibitors bind to the 5α-reductase enzyme– NADP$^+$ complex preventing its regeneration (i.e. dead end inhibition) and thus are not effected by the level of T. *In vitro* studies have demonstrated that such uncompetitive dead end 5α-reductase inhibitors like SKF105657 (i.e. 17β-*N*-(2-methyl-2-propyl)-carbamoyl-androst-3,5-dione-3-carboxylic acid) (Fig. 13.4) efficiently inhibit both the rat and human enzyme (Holt *et al.*, 1990). In rodent studies, treatment with SKF105657 has been demonstrated to decrease the prostatic DHT levels to that of a surgically castrated animal and to produce and maintain regression of the normal prostate (Lamb *et al.*, 1992a). Experimental studies using serially transplantable androgen-responsive rat and human prostatic cancers has likewise demonstrated that oral feeding of SKF105657 exerts a sustained antitumoural effect *in vivo* (Lamb *et al.*, 1992b). Presently, clinical trials are underway to test the efficiency of finasteride and SKF105657 as single agent therapy for metastatic prostatic cancer.

Antiandrogens

Antiandrogens can be of the 'pure' or 'non-pure' type. A 'pure' antiandrogen functions as an androgen antagonist by competitively inhibiting the binding of DHT or T with the androgen receptors within target cells without acting as an agonist and without decreasing serum T systemically. There are a series of 'pure' antiandrogens that have been developed. These include the steroidal antiandrogen cyproterone (1,2α-methylene-6-chloro-Δ^6-17α-hydroxyprogesterone), and non-steroidal antiandrogen, flutamide (4'-nitro-3'-trifluoromethyl isobutranilide) (Fig. 13.5). Since the 'pure' antiandrogens bind not only to androgen receptors in prostatic cancer cells but also to the androgen receptors in the hypothalamus and pituitary, these compounds block the negative feedback of androgens at the hypothalamic–pituitary level. Thus treatment with 'pure' antiandrogens eventually increases the level of LH released into circulation (Knuth *et al.*, 1984). This eventually leads to an increase in the serum T level, which

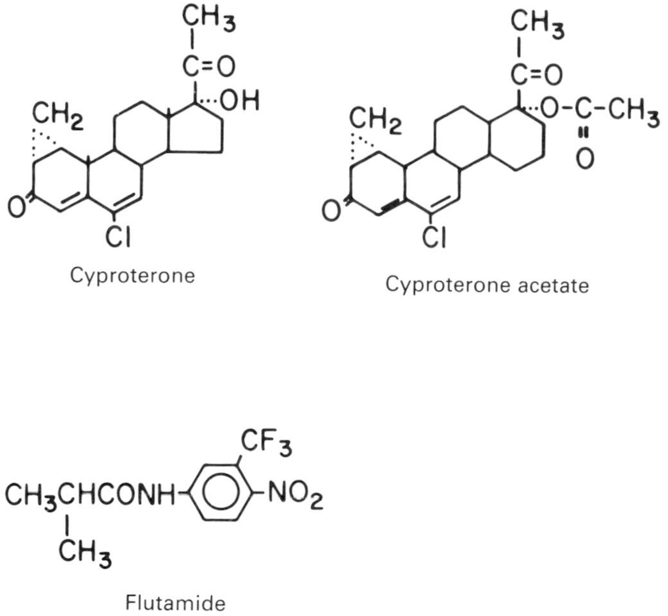

Cyproterone

Cyproterone acetate

Flutamide

Fig. 13.5. Structures of a series of 'pure' and 'non-pure' antiandrogens.

results in increased tissue levels of T and DHT which diminishes the ability of the 'pure' antiandrogen antagonist to compete for androgen receptor binding. Therefore 'pure' antiandrogens are rarely used as monotherapy. They are usually combined either with surgical castration or with LHRH analogues (Schroeder *et al.*, 1987; Crawford *et al.*, 1989; Beland *et al.*, 1990; Iversen *et al.*, 1990; Tyrrll *et al.*, 1991).

By addition of an acetate group to the 17α-hydroxy position, the 'pure' antiandrogen cyproterone becomes the 'non-pure' antiandrogen, cyproterone acetate (Fig. 13.5). Such an addition converts cyproterone acetate (CA) to a very potent progestational agent. As a potent progestational agent, CA inhibits the release of LH from the pituitary (Knuth *et al.*, 1984). CA still retains its androgen antagonist ability, like cyproterone, to directly compete with DHT for binding to the androgen receptor (Sufrin & Coffey, 1976). Thus CA functions both to decrease serum T systemically and to act as an androgen antagonist by competing for DHT binding to the androgen receptor within androgen-dependent prostatic cancer cells. Due to this dual ability, CA has been used as monotherapy for metastatic prostatic cancer with an efficiency equivalent to that for surgical castration (Jacobi *et al.*, 1980).

Limitations of androgen ablation therapy

As reviewed, there are now a large variety of alternative pharmacological approaches which can be used to produce androgen ablation. The multitude of options has the advantage of allowing the physician to choose the best pharmacological approach for androgen ablation therapy on an individual prostatic cancer patient basis. Unfortunately, however, the annual death rate from prostatic cancer has not decreased at all over the subsequent 50 years since androgen ablation has become standard therapy for metastatic disease (Boring et al., 1992). Over the last 50 years, the superficially benign nature of androgen ablation has disguised the fact that metastatic prostatic cancer is still a fatal disease for which no therapy is available which effectively increases survival (Lepor et al., 1982; Raghaven, 1988; Tyrell et al., 1991). Nearly all men with metastatic prostatic cancer treated by androgen ablation do respond, demonstrating that at least a portion of their cancer cells are androgen responsive (Scott et al., 1980). Unfortunately, however, essentially all of these patients eventually relapse to a state unresponsive to further antiandrogen therapy, no matter how aggressive or complete their androgen ablation treatment (Schulze et al., 1987a; Crawford et al., 1989; Tyrrell et al., 1991). The major reason for the inability of androgen ablation therapy to be curative is that the cancer within an individual metastatic patient is heterogeneously composed of clones of both androgen-dependent and androgen-independent prostatic cancer cells (Prout et al., 1976; Sinha et al., 1977; Smolev et al., 1977; Isaacs & Coffey, 1981).

Therapeutic implications of the tumour cell heterogeneity of prostatic cancer

Development of such tumour cell heterogeneity can occur by a variety of mechanisms (e.g. multifocal origin of the tumour, adaptation or genetic instability (Isaacs, 1982)). Regardless of the mechanism of development of such cellular heterogeneity, once androgen-independent cancer cells are present within individual prostatic cancer patients, the patient is no longer curable by androgen withdrawal therapy alone, no matter how complete, because this therapy kills only the androgen-dependent cells without eliminating pre-existing androgen-independent prostatic cancer cells (Schulze et al., 1987a). To affect all the heterogenous prostatic cancer cell populations within an individual patient, effective chemotherapy, specifically targetted against the androgen-independent cancer cells, must be simultaneously combined with androgen ablation to affect the androgen-dependent cells. The validity of each of these points has been demonstrated by a series of animal (Isaacs, 1984b; Ellis & Isaacs, 1985; Redding & Schally, 1985; Kung et al., 1988; Isaacs, 1989) and human studies (Schulze et al., 1987b). The animal studies demonstrated that only by giving such a combined chemohormonal treatment, is it possible to produce any reproducible level of cures in animals bearing prostatic cancer (Isaacs, 1989). To produce cures however, treatment must be started early in the course of the disease, the chemotherapy must have definitive efficacy against androgen-independent cancer cells, it must be given for a crucial period, and it must be begun simultaneously with, and not sequentially with, androgen ablation (Isaacs, 1989). Although the concept of early combinational chemohormonal therapy for prostatic cancer is valid, for such an approach to be therapeutically effective in humans, a chemotherapeutic agent must be available that can effectively control the growth of the androgen-independent human prostatic cancer cells.

Inability of present modalities to eliminate androgen-independent prostatic cancer cells

Unfortunately, there are no standard chemotherapeutic agents previously tested which effectively control the growth of human androgen-independent prostatic cancer cells (Raghaven, 1988). This inability has led to a search for new approaches to control androgen-independent prostatic cancer cells. The growth of any cancer cell is determined by the relationship between its rate of proliferation and death. Only when the rate of cell death is greater than cell proliferation is the cancer cell eliminated. A successful treatment for androgen-independent cancer cells can be obtained by either lowering the rate of proliferation and/or by raising the rate of cell death to a point where this exceeds the rate of cell proliferation.

There are a variety of antiproliferative chemotherapeutic agents which are cytostatic and/or cytotoxic to sensitive target cells. Unfortunately, these agents usually lead to death of cancer cells only during the subsequent cell proliferation (Shackney et al., 1978). Cancer cells not proliferating at the time of, or soon enough after, exposure are resistant to such cytotoxic agents since the cell has sufficient time to repair the damage induced (Shackney et al., 1978). Unfortunately, the majority (i.e. over 90%) of prostatic cancer cells within an individual patient are not actively proliferating (Helpap et al., 1974; Meyers et al., 1982; Nemoto et al., 1990) and are thus resistant to standard cytotoxic chemotherapy (Raghaven, 1988).

New approaches to therapy for androgen-independent prostatic cancer cells

What is needed is some type of cytotoxic therapy which induces the death of androgen-independent prostatic cancer cells not requiring cell proliferation. Is it possible to induce the death of cells without requiring them to attempt to divide? The answer to this question is yes. Recent studies have demonstrated that both androgen-dependent normal prostatic glandular cells and androgen-dependent prostatic cancer cells can be induced to undergo cell death following androgen ablation and this death process does not require the cells to be in the proliferative cell cycle (Isaacs, 1984a; English et al., 1989; Kyprianou et al., 1990). The death induced by androgen ablation in these non-proliferating androgen-dependent cells occurs as an energy-dependent process collectively referred to as 'programmed cell death' in which the cells actively commit 'suicide' (Kyprianou & Isaacs, 1988; Kyprianou et al., 1990). Associated with this programmed cell death pathway is the enhanced expression of a series of genes (Montpetit et al., 1986; Kyprianou & Isaacs, 1989a) and the fragmentation of the genomic DNA into nucleosomal oligomers (Kyprianou & Isaacs, 1988; Kyprianou et al., 1990). This fragmentation of genomic DNA is the irreversible commitment step in the death of the cell and is the result of the activation of Ca^{2+}, Mg^{2+}-dependent endonuclease present within the cell nucleus (Kyprianou et al., 1988; English et al., 1989). This activation is the result of a sustained elevation of intracellular free Ca^{2+} (Ca_i) induced following androgen ablation (Kyprianou et al., 1988; Martikainen & Isaacs, 1990). Following DNA fragmentation, the cells themselves fragment into membrane bound 'apoptotic' bodies which are phagocytized by neighbouring cells (Kerr & Searle, 1973; English et al., 1989).

Additional studies have demonstrated that androgen ablation does not induce this programmed death process in androgen-independent prostatic cancer cells due to a defect in the initiation step. Even with the defect, however, androgen-independent prostatic cancer cells retain the distal portion of this programmed cell death pathway (Kyprianou & Isaacs, 1989b). The inability of androgen ablation to induce programmed death of androgen-independent prostatic cancer cells appears to be due to the fact that such androgen ablation does not result in a sustained elevation in the intracellular free Ca^{2+} (Ca_i) cells. This conclusion is based upon the observation that androgen-independent prostatic cancer cells can be induced to undergo programmed death if an elevation of Ca_i of as small as only 3–6-fold above baseline induced by a calcium ionophore is sustained for over 12 h (Martikainen et al., 1991). Temporal analysis demonstrated that the death of these cells did not require cell proliferation and involves Ca^{2+}-induced fragmentation of genomic DNA into nucleosomal size pieces as the commitment step in this process. These results demonstrate that even non-proliferating androgen-independent prostatic cancer cells can be induced to undergo programmed cell death, if a modest elevation in the Ca_i is sustained for a sufficient time. These observations suggest that a new approach to the treatment of androgen-independent prostatic cancer cells should focus upon chemotherapeutic means to induce a sustained increase in the Ca_i in these cells. Approaches of this type in other cancers are discussed in Chapter 2.

An additional new approach to the better therapeutic management of androgen-independent prostatic cancer cells may lie in growth factor antagonists. There is an emerging body of experimental evidence implicating non-androgen growth factors (i.e. basic fibroblast growth factor (bFGF), epidermal growth factor (EGF), transforming growth factor-β_1 (TGF-β_1), platelet-derived growth factor (PDGF), and insulin-like growth

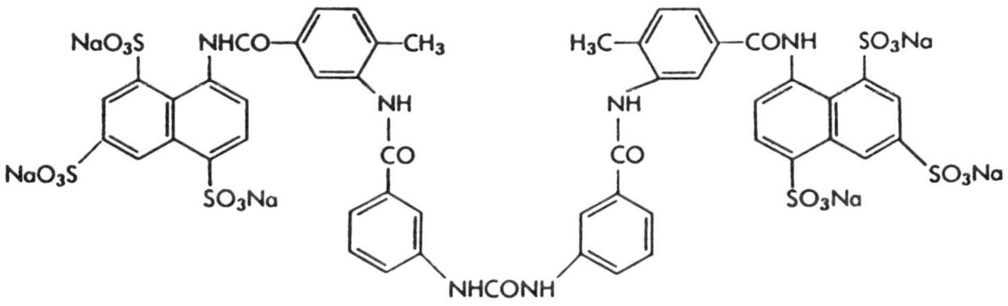

Fig. 13.6. Structure of suramin.

factor-I (IGF-I)) as important regulators of both normal and neoplastic prostatic cell growth (Isaacs *et al.*, 1991). Basic FGF has been shown to be a potent mitogen and autocrine motility factor in prostatic carcinoma *in vitro* (Isaacs *et al.*, 1991). Nonomura *et al* (1988) demonstrated that androgen-resistent cancer cells derived from an androgen-responsive mouse mammary cancer (Shionogi carcinoma 115), can be stimulated to grow by growth factors secreted by androgen-dependent cancer cells in a paracrine fashion. These growth factors have high heparin-binding affinity and appear to be FGF-like polypeptides.

Suramin (Fig. 13.6) is a polysulphonated naphthylurea (i.e. sym-*bis*(*m*-aminobenzoyl-*m*-amino-*p*-methylbenzoyl-1-naphthylamino-4,6,8,trisulphonate)carbamide) previously used in the therapy of trypanosomiasis and onchocerciasis. Suramin binds strongly to bFGF as well as PDGF, TGF-β_1 and EGF. This binding to growth factors inhibits the ability of the growth factors to bind to their receptors. Pienta *et al.* (1991) reported that suramin inhibits cell motility via its interaction with bFGF in *in vitro* models of prostatic cancer. La Rocca *et al.* (1991) reported that suramin inhibited the growth stimulatory effect of T and bFGF in human prostatic cancer cell lines *in vitro*. Protamine sulphate, a strongly basic low mol. wt protein, has many similar properties to suramin and is a more specific antagonist for bFGF and PDGF (Huang *et al.*, 1984; Neufeld & Gospodarowicz, 1987). Morton *et al.* (1990) treated androgen-independent rat prostatic adenocarcinomas with either suramin or protamine sulphate. Both treatment groups were able to inhibit but not completely suppress the *in vivo* growth of androgen-independent rat prostatic cancer. In recent phase II clinical trials, patients with hormone refractory metastatic prostatic cancer have been treated with suramin with objective tumour regression noted in some patients (Myers, 1989; Stein *et al.*, 1989). Toxicity with suramin can be quite severe and life threatening. The major toxicity is due to adrenal suppression, and dose-dependent coagulopathy and neuropathy. Recent studies have demonstrated that suramin's tumouricidal effects on human androgen-independent prostatic cancer cells *in vitro* can be synergized by combinations with other more standard chemotherapeutic agents (e.g. TNF, Adriamycin, etc.) thus allowing lower concentations of suramin to be effective (Freuhaf *et al.*, 1990). Such a combination approach could allow the dosage of suramin to be lowered to reduce host toxicity while producing effective antitumour response *in vivo*.

Conclusion

Presently, there are a large variety of pharmacological approaches which can effectively manage the androgen-dependent prostatic cancer cells within individual patients. These androgen-dependent cancer cells, however, are usually not the only type of cancer cell present within the patient. Androgen-independent cancer cells eventually develop which are resistant to androgen ablation therapy, regardless of the pharmacological approach used. Unfortunately, there is no pharmacological approach which has proven effective in management of the androgen-independent prostatic cancer cell present within the heterogeneous tumour of an individual with metastatic prostatic cancer. In order to make major progress in the management of metastatic prostatic cancer, much more attention needs to be focused upon developing effective non-androgen ablation pharmacological approaches to eliminate the androgen-independent prostatic cancer cell. While this development may not be easy or occur quickly, it is critical to start this search now. The area of 'programmed' cell death and growth factor antagonist therapy appear to be fertile areas to begin such a search.

References

Agardh, C.D., Nilsson-Ehle, P., Lundgren, R. & Gustafson, A. (1984). The influence of treatment with estrogens and estramustine phosphate on platelet aggregation and plasma lipoproteins in non-disseminated prostatic carcinoma. *Journal of Urology* **132**, 1021–1024.

Anderson, K.M. & Liao, S. (1968). Selective retention of dihydrotestosterone by prostatic nuclei. *Nature* **219**, 27–29.

Aro, J. (1991). Cardiovascular and all-cause mortality in prostatic cancer patients treated with estrogens or orchiectomy as compared to the standard population. *The Prostate* **18**, 131–137.

Beland, G., Elhilali, M., Fradet, Y., Laroche, B., Ramsey, E.W., Trachtenberg, J., Venner, P.M. & Tewari, H.D. (1990). A controlled trial of castration with and without nilutamide in metastatic prostatic carcinoma. *Cancer* **66**, 1074–1079.

Blackard, C.E. (1975). The Veterans Administration Cooperative Urological Research Group Studies of carcinoma of the prostate: a review. *Cancer Chemotherapy Report* **59**, 225–227.

Boring, C.C., Squires, T.S. & Tong, T. (1992). Cancer statistics, 1991. *Ca-A Cancer Journal for Clinicians* **42**, 19–38.

Brendler, C.B., Isaacs, J.T., Follansbee, A.L. & Walsh, P.C. (1984). The use of multiple variables to predict response to endocrine therapy in carcinoma of the prostate: a preliminary report. *Journal of Urology* **131**, 694–700.

Brooks, J.R., Berman, C., Primka, R.L., Reynolds, G.F. & Rasmusson G.H. (1986).

5α-reductase inhibitory and anti-androgenic activities of some 4-azasteroids in the rat. *Steroids* **47**, 1–19.

Bruchovsky, N. & Wilson, J.D. (1968). The conversion of testosterone to 5α-androstan-17β-ol-3-one by rat prostate *in vivo* and *in vitro*. *Journal of Biological Chemistry* **243**, 2012–2021.

Bruynseels, J., DeCoster, R., VanRooy, P., Wouters, W., Raeymaekers, A., Freyne, E., Sanz, G., Vanden Bussche, G. & Janssen, P.A.J. (1990). R75 251, a new inhibitor of steroid biosynthesis. *The Prostate* **16**, 345–357.

Byar, D.P. & Corle, D.K. (1988). Hormone therapy for prostate cancer: results of the Veterans Administration Cooperative Urological Research Group Studies. *National Cancer Institute Monographs* **7**, 165–170.

Carter, H.B. & Coffey, D.S. (1988). Prostate cancer: the magnitude of the problem in the United States. In Coffey, D.S., Resnick, M.I., Dorr, F.A. & Karr, J.P. (eds) *A Multidisciplinary Analysis of Controversies in the Management of Prostate Cancer*, pp. 1–7. Plenum Press, New York.

Catalona, W.J. & Scott, W.W. (1979). Carcinoma of the prostate. In Harrison, J.H., Gittes, R.F., Perlmutter, A.D., Stamey, T.A. & Walsh, P.C. (eds) *Campbell's Urology*, pp. 1085–1124. WB Saunders, Philadelphia.

Coffey, D.S. (1986). The biochemistry and physiology of the prostate and seminal vesicles. In Walsh, P.C., Gittes, R.F., Perlmutter, A.D. & Stamey, T.A. *Campbell's Urology*, 5th Edn, pp. 233–274. WB Saunders, Philadelphia.

Crawford, E.D., Eisenberger, M.A., McLeod, D.G., Spaulding, J.T., Benson, R., Dorr, F.A., Blemenstein, B.A., Davis, M.A. & Goodman, P.J (1989). A controlled trial of leuprolide with and without flutamide in prostatic carcinoma. *New England Journal of Medicine* **321**, 419–422.

Denis, L.J. (1991). Controversies in the management of localised and metastatic prostatic cancer. *European Journal of Cancer* **27**, 333–341.

Devesa, S.S. & Silverman, D.T. (1978). Cancer incidence and morbidity trends in the United States: 1935–1974. *Journal of the National Cancer Institute* **60**, 545–571.

Eisenberger, M.A., O'Dwyer, P.J. & Friedman, M.A. (1986). Gonadotropin hormone-releasing hormone analogues: a new therapeutic approach for prostatic cancer. *Journal of Clinical Oncology* **5**, 414–424.

Ellis, W.J. & Isaacs, J.T. (1985). Effectiveness of complete vs. partial androgen withdrawal therapy for the treatment of prostatic cancer as studied in the Dunning R-3327 system of rat prostatic carcinomas. *Cancer Research* **45**, 6041–6050.

English, H.F., Kyprianou, N. & Isaacs, J.T. (1989). Relationship between DNA fragmentation and apoptosis in the programmed cell death in the rat prostate following castration. *The Prostate* **15**, 233–251.

Fruehauf, J.P., Myers, C.E. & Sinha, B.K. (1990). Synergistic activity of suramin with tumor necrosis factor alpha and doxorubin of human prostate cancer cell lines. *Journal of the National Cancer Institute* **82**, 1206–1209.

Geller, J., Albert, J. & Yen, S.S.C. (1978). Treatment of advanced cancer of prostate with megestrol acetate. *Urology* **12**, 537–541.

George, F.W., Johnson, L. & Wilson, J.D. (1989). The effect of a 5α-reductase inhibitor on androgen physiology in the immature male rat. *Endocrinology* **125**, 2434–2438.

Glashan, R.W. & Robinson, M.R.G. (1981). Cardiovascular complications in the treatment of prostatic cancer. *British Journal of Urology* **53**, 624–631.

Hedlund, P.O., Gustafsson, H. & Sögren, S. (1980). Cardiovascular complications to treatment of prostate cancer with estramustine phosphate (Estracyt[R]) or conventional estrogen. *Scandinavian Journal of Urology and Nephrology* **55** (Suppl.), 103–105.

Helpap, B., Steins, R. & Bruhl, P. (1974). Autoradiographic *in vitro* investigations on prostatic tissue with C-14 and H-3 thymidine double labeling method. *Beitrage Zur Pathologischen Anatomie und Allgemeinen Pathologie* **151**, 65–72.

Holt, D.A., Levy, M.A. Oh, H.J., Erb, J.M., Heaslip, J.I., Brandt, M., Lan-Hargest, H.Y. & Metcalf, B.W. (1990). Inhibition of steroid 5α-reductase by unsaturated 3-carboxysteroids. *Journal of Medical Chemistry* **33**, 943–950.

Huang, J.S., Nishimura, J., Huang, S.S. & Deuel, T.F. (1984). Protamine inhibits platelet derived growth factor receptor activity but not epidermal growth factor activity. *Journal of Cell Biochemistry* **26**, 205–220.

Huggins, C., Stevens, R.E. & Hodges, C.V. (1941). Studies of prostatic cancer: II. The effects of castration on advanced carcinoma of the prostate gland. *Archives of Surgery* **42**, 209–223.

Isaacs, J.T. (1982). Cellular factors in the development of resistance to hormonal therapy. In Bruchovsky, N. & Goldie, J. (eds) *Drug and Hormone Resistance in Neoplasia* Vol. 1, pp. 139–156. CRC Press, Boca Raton.

Isaacs, J.T. (1984a). Antagonistic effect of androgen on prostatic cell the rat ventral prostate after castration. *Endocrinology* **122**, 552–562.

Isaacs, J.T. (1984b). The timing of androgen ablation therapy and/or chemotherapy in the treatment of prostatic cancer. *The Prostate* **5**, 1–18.

Isaacs, J.T. (1989). Relationship between tumor size and curability of prostate cancer by combined chemohormonal therapy. *Cancer Research* **49**, 6290–6294.

Isaacs, J.T. & Coffey, D.S. (1981). Adaptation vs. selection as the mechanism responsible for the relapse of prostatic cancer to androgen ablation as studied in the Dunning R-3327 H adenocarcinoma. *Cancer Research* **41**, 5070–5075.

Isaacs, J.T., Morton, R.A., Martikainen, P. & Isaacs, W.B. (1991). Growth factors effecting normal and malignant prostatic cells. In Schomberg, D.W. (ed) *Growth Factors in Reproduction*, pp. 167–184, Springer-Verlag, New York.

Iversen, P., Suciu, S., Sylvester, R., Christensen, I. & Denis, L. (1990). Zoladex and Flutamide versus orchiectomy in the treatment of advanced prostatic cancer. *Cancer* **66**, 1067–1073.

Jacobi, G.H., Altwein, J.E., Kurth, K.H., Basting, R. & Hohenfellner, H. (1980). Treatment of advanced prostatic cancer with parenteral cyproterone acetate: a phase II randomized trial. *British Journal of Urology* **52**, 208–215.

Johnson, D.E., Babaion, R.J., Eschenbach, A., Wisknow, K.I. & Tenney, D. (1988). Ketoconazole therapy for hormonally refractive metastatic prostate cancer. *Urology* **31**, 132–134.

Kerr, F.Fr. & Searle, J. (1973). Deletion of cells by apoptosis during castration-induced involution of the rat prostate. *Virchowa Archiv B* **13**, 87–102.

Klein, H., Bressel, M., Kastendieck, H. & Voigt, K.D. (1988). Quantitative assessment of endrogenous testicular and adrenal sex steroids of steroid metabolizing enzymes in untreated human prostatic cancerous tissue. *Journal of Steroid Biochemistry* **30**, 119–130.

Knuth, U.A., Hano, R. & Nieschllag, E. (1984). Effect of flutamide or cyproterone acetate on pituitary and testicular hormones in normal men. *Journal of Clinical Endocrinology and Metabolism* **59**, 963–969.

Korkut, E., Bokser, L., Comaru-Schally, A.M., Groot, K. & Schally, A.V. (1991). Inhibition of growth of experimental prostate cancer with sustained delivery systems (microcapsules and microgranules) of the luteinizing hormone-releasing hormone antagonist SB-75. *Proceedings of the National Academy of Sciences USA* **88**, 844–848.

Kung, T.T., Mingo, G.G., Siegel, M.I. & Watnick, A.S. (1988). Effect of andrenalectomy, flutamide and leuprolide on the growth of the Dunning R-3327 prostatic carcinomas. *The Prostate* **12**, 357–364.

Kyprianou, N. & Isaacs, J.T. (1988). Activation of programmed cell death in the rat ventral prostate after castration. *Endocrinology* **122**, 552–562.

Kyprianou, N. & Isaacs, J.T. (1989a). Expression of transforming growth factor-β in the rat ventral prostate during castration-induced programmed cell death. *Molecular Endocrinology* **3**, 1515–1522.

Kyprianou, N. & Isaacs, J.T. (1989b). Thymine-less death in androgen-independent prostatic cancer cells. *Biochemistry Biophysics Research Communications* **165**, 73–81.

Kyprianou, N., English, H.F. & Isaacs, J.T. (1988). Activation of a Ca^{2+} Mg^{2+}-dependent endonuclease as an early event in castration-induced prostatic cell death. *The Prostate* **13**, 103–118.

Kyprianou, N., English, H.F. & Isaacs, J.T. (1990). Programmed cell death during regression of PC-82 human prostate cancer following androgen ablation. *Cancer Research* **50**, 3748–3753.

La Rocca, R.V., Danesi, R., Cooper, M.R., Jamis Dow, C.A., Ewing, M.W., Linehan, W.M. & Myers, C.E. (1991). Effect of suramin on human prostate cancer cells *in vitro*. *Journal of Urology* **145**, 393–397.

Lamb, J.C., English, H., Levandoski, P.L., Rhodes, G.R., Johnson, R.K. & Isaacs, J.T. (1992a). Prostatic involution in rats induced by a novel 5α-reductase inhibitor, SK&F 105657: role for testosterone in the androgenic response. *Endocrinology* **130**, 685–694.

Lamb, J.C., Levy, M.A., Johnson, R.K. & Isaacs, J.T. (1992b). Response of rat and human prostatic cancers to the novel 5α-reductase inhibitor, SK&F 105657. *The Prostate* **21**, 15–34.

Lepor, H., Ross, A. & Walsh, P.C. (1982). The influence of hormonal therapy on survival of men with advanced prostatic cancer. *Journal of Urology* **128**, 335–340.

Levy, M.A., Brandt, M., Holt, D.A. & Metcalf, B.W. (1989). Interaction between rat prostatic steroid 5α-reductase and 3-carboxy-17 β-substituted steroids: novel mechanism of enzyme inhibition. *Journal of Steroid Biochemistry* **34**, 572–575.

Mackler, M.A., Liberti, J.P., Smith, M.J.V., Koontz, W.W. & Prout, G.R. (1972). The effect of orchiectomy and various doses of stilbestrol on plasma testosterone levels in patients with carcinoma of the prostate. *Investigative Urology* **9**, 423–425.

Mahler, C., Denis, L. & DeCoster, R. (1987). The endocrine effect of ketoconazole in high doses (KHD). In Murphy, G., Khoury, S., Kuss, R. *et al.* (eds) *Prostate Cancer Part A. Research, Endocrine Treatment and Histopathology*, pp. 291–297. New York, Alan R. Liss.

Martikainen, P. & Isaacs, J.T. (1990). Role of calcium in the programmed cell death of rat ventral prostatic glandular cells. *The Prostate* **17**, 175–187.

Martikianen, P., Kyprianou, N., Tucker, R.W. & Isaacs, J.T. (1991). Programmed death of non-proliferating androgen independent prostatic cancer cells. *Cancer Research* **51**, 4693–4700.

Mettlin, G. (1983). Epidemiology of prostate cancer in different population groups. *Clinics in Oncology* **2**, 287–300.

Meyers, J.S., Sufrin, G. & Martin, S.A. (1982). Proliferation activation of benign human prostate, prostatic andenocarcinoma and seminal vesicle evaluated by thymidine labeling. *Journal of Urology* **128**, 1353–1356.

Montpetit, M.L., Lawless, K.R. & Tenniswood, M. (1986). Androgen repressed messages in the rat ventral prostate. *The Prostate* **8**, 25–36.

Morton, R.A., Isaacs, J.T. & Isaacs, W.B. (1990). Differential effects of growth factor antagonists on neoplastic and normal prostatic cells. *The Prostate* **17**, 327–336.

Murray, R. & Pitt, P. (1985). Treatment of advanced prostatic cancer, resistant to conventional therapy, with aminoglutethimide. *European Journal of Cancer and Clinical Oncology* **21**, 453–458.

Myers, C. (1989). Three centers start phase 2 trials with suramin; NCI responses hold up. *Clinical Cancer Letter* **12**, 5–6.

Nemoto, R., Hattori, K., Uchida, K., Shimazui, T., Nishijima, Y., Koiso, K. & Harada, M. (1990). S-phase fraction of human prostate adenocarcinoma studied with *in vivo* bromodeoxyuridine labeling. *Cancer* **66**, 509–514.

Neufeld, G. & Gospodarowicz, D. (1987). Protamine sulfate inhibits mitogenic activities of the extracellular matrix and fibroblast growth factor, but potentiates that of epidermal growth factor. *Journal of Cell Physiology* **132**, 287–294.

Nonomura, N., Nakamura, N., Uchida, N., Noguchi, S., Sato, B., Sonoda, T. & Matsumoto, K. (1988). Growth stimulatory effect of androgen-induced autocrine growth factor(s) secreted from shionogi carcinoma 115 cells on androgen unresponsive cancer cells in a paracrine mechanism. *Cancer Research* **48**, 4904–4908.

Pienta, K.J., Isaacs, W.B., Vindwich, D. & Coffey, D.S. (1991). The effects of basic fibroblast growth factor and suramin on cell motility and growth of rat prostatic cancer cells. *Journal of Urology* **145**, 199–202.

Pollard, M., Luckert, P.H. & Sporn, M.B. (1991). Prevention of primary prostate cancer in Lobund–Wistar rats by *N*-(4-hydroxyphenyl)rentinamide. *Cancer Research* **51**, 3610–3611.

Ponder, B.A.J., Shearer, R.J., Pocock, R.D., Miller, J., Easton, D., Chilvers, C.E.D., Dowsett, M. & Jeffcoate, S.L. (1984). Response to aminoglutethimide and cortisone acetate in advanced prostatic cancer. *British Journal of Cancer* **50**, 757–763.

Pont, A. (1987). Long-term experience with high-dose ketoconazole therapy in patients with stage D2 prostatic carcinoma. *Journal of Urology* **137**, 902–904.

Prout, G.R., Kliman, B., Daly, J.J., MacLaughlin, R.A., Griffin, P.P. & Young, H.H. (1976). Endocrine changes after diethylstilbestrol therapy. Effects on prostatic neoplasm and pituitary–gonadal axis. *Urology* **7**, 148.

Raghaven, D. (1988). Non-hormone chemotherapy for prostate cancer: principles of treatment and application to the testing of new drugs. *Seminars in Oncology* **15**, 371–389.

Redding, T.W. & Schally, A.V. (1985). Investigation of the combination of the agonist D-Trp-6-LH-RH and the antiandrogen flutamide in the treatment of Dunning R-3327H prostate cancer model. *The Prostate* **6**, 219–232.

Rössner, S., Hedlund, P.O., Jogerstrand, T. & Säwe, U. (1985). Treatment of prostatic cancer: effects on serum lipoproteins and the cardiovascular system. *Journal of Urology* **133**, 53–57.

Schroeder, F.H., Lock, T.M., Chadha, D.R., Debruyne, F.M., Karthaus, H.F., De-Jong, F.H., Klijn, J.G., Matroos, A.W. & de-Voogt, H.J. (1987). Metastatic cancer of the prostate managed with buserelin versus buserelin plus cytoterone acetate. *Journal of Urology* **137**, 912–918.

Schulze, H., Isaacs, J.T. & Coffey, D.S. (1987a). A critical review of the concept of total androgen ablation in the treatment of prostatic cancer. In Murphy, G.P., Khory, S., Kuss, R., Chatelain, C. & Denis, L. (eds) *Prostate Cancer Part A: Research, Endocrine Treatment and Histopathology. Progress in Clinical and Biological Research* 243A, pp. 1–19. Alan R. Liss, New York.

Schulze, H., Isaacs, J.T. & Senge, T. (1987b). Inability of complete androgen blockade to increase survival of patients with advanced prostate cancer as compared to standard hormonal therapy. *Journal of Urology* **137**, 909–911.

Scott, W.W., Menon, M. & Walsh, P.C. (1980). Hormonal therapy of prostatic cancer. *Cancer* **435**, 1929–1936.

Seidman, H., Mushinski, M.H., Gelb, S.K. & Silverberg, E. (1985). Probabilities of eventually developing or dying of cancer: United States CA. *Cancer Journal for Clinicians* **35**, 36–56.

Shackney, S.E., McCormack, G.W. & Cuchural, G.J. (1978). Growth rate patterns of solid tumors and their relationship to responsiveness to therapy. *Annals of Internal Medicine* **89**, 107–115.

Sinha, A.A., Blackhard, C.E. & Seal, U.S. (1977). A critical analysis of tumor morphology and hormone treatment in the untreated and estrogen treated responsive and refractory human prostatic carcinoma. *Cancer* **40**, 2835–2850.

Smith, J.A. (1987). New methods of endrocine management of prostatic cancer. *Journal of Urology* **137**, 1–9.

Smolev, J.K., Heston, W.D.W., Scott, W.S. & Coffey, D.S. (1977). An appropriate animal model for prostatic cancer. *Cancer Treatment Reports* **61**, 273–287.

Stein, C.A., Larocca, R.V., Thomas, R., McAtee, N. & Myers, C.E. (1989). Suramin: an anticancer drug with a unique mechanism of action. *Journal of Clinical Oncology* **7**, 499–506.

Sufrin, G. & Coffey, D.S. (1976). Flutamide: mechanisms of action of a new nonsteroidal antiandrogen. *Investments in Urology* **13**, 429–434.

Svensson, M., Varenhorst, E. & Kagedal, B. (1986). Initial administration of cyproterone acetate to prevent the rise of testosterone concentration during treatment with an LH-RH agonist in prostatic cancer. *Anticancer Research* **6**, 379–384.

Swerdloff, R.S. (1986). Physiology of male reproduction: hypothalamic–pituitary function. In Walsh, P.C., Gittes, R.F., Perlmutter, A.D. & Stamey, T.A. (eds) *Campbell's Urology*, 5th edn, pp. 186–200. WB Saunders, Philadelphia.

The Leuprolide Study Group (1984). Leuprolide versus diethylstilbestrol for metastatic prostatic cancer. *New England Journal of Medicine* **311**, 1281–1286.

Tolis, G., Menta, A., Kinch, R., Comaru, A.M. & Schally, A.V. (1980). Suppression of sex steroids by an LH-Rh analogue in man. *Clinical Research* **28**, 676–680.

Trachtenberg, J. (1984). Ketoconazole therapy in advanced prostatic carcinoma. *Journal of Urology* **132**, 61–63.

Trachtenberg, J., Halpern, N. & Pont, A. (1983). Ketoconazole: a novel and rapid treatment of advanced prostatic cancer. *Journal of Urology* **130**, 152–153.

Tyrrell, C.J., Altwein, J.E., Klippel, F., Varenhorst, E., Lunglmayr, G., Boccardo, F., Holdaway, I.M., Haefliger, J.M., Jordann, J.P. & Sotarauta, M. for the International Prostate Cancer Study Group (1991). A multicenter randomized trial comparing the luteinizing hormone-releasing hormone analogue goserelin acetate alone and with flutamide in the treatment of advanced prostate cancer. *Journal of Urology* **146**, 1321–1326.

Van Ginckel, R., DeCoster, R., Wouters, W., Vanherck, W., van der Veer, R., Goeminnc, N., Jagers, E., Van Cauteren, H., Wouters, L., Distelmans, W. & Janssen, P.A.J. (1990). Antitumoral effects of R75251 on the growth of transplantable R3327 prostatic adenocarcinoma in rats. *The Prostate* **16**, 313–323.

Van Wauwe, J.P., Coene, M.C., Goossens, J., Cools, W. & Monbaliu, J. (1990). Effects of cytochrome P-450 inhibitors in the *in vivo* metabolism of all-trans-retinoic acid in rats. *Journal of Pharmacology and Experimental Therapeutics* **252**, 365–369.

Vermeulen, A., Schelfhout, W. & Desy, W. (1982). Plasma androgen levels after subcapsular orchiectomy or estrogen treatment for prostatic carcinoma. *The Prostate* **3**, 115–121.

Walsh, P.C. & Jewett, H.J. (1980). Radical surgery for prostate cancer. *Cancer* **45**, 1906–1910.

Walsh, P.C. & Sitteri, P.K. (1975). Suppression of plasma androgens by spironolactone in castrated men with carcinoma of the prostate. *Journal Urology* **114**, 254–256.

Waxman, J., Man, A., Hendry, W.F., Whitefield, H.N. & Besser, G.M. (1985). Importance of early tumour exacerbation in patients treated with long acting analogues of gonadotropin releasing hormone for advanced prostatic cancer. *British Medical Journal* **291**, 1387–1388.

Worgul, T.J., Santen, R.J., Samojlik, E., Veldhuis, J.D., Lipton, A., Harvey, H.A., Drago, J.R. & Rohner, T.J. (1983). Clinical and biochemical effect of aminoglutethimide in the treatment of advanced prostatic carcinoma. *Journal of Urology* **129**, 51–55.

Chapter 14
Cytokines in haemopoiesis: their application in oncology

Nydia G. Testa and T. Michael Dexter

Introduction

Mature functional haemopoietic cells are the end product of an orderly process of proliferation, differentiation and maturation that starts with the haemopoietic stem cells, and takes place in the blood forming tissues located in the bone marrow in the adult. This process culminates in the production of about 4×10^{11} haemopoietic cells per day in a normal individual, just to replace senescent cells, and of even higher numbers when there is increased demand in changed physiological or pathological circumstances. Cell production is mainly regulated by specific haemo-poietic growth factors which are the main part of an integrated and complex cytokine network, still not completely elucidated, where pleio-tropic cytokines also contribute stimulatory or inhibitory influences that may also play a role. In this chapter we will summarize the known roles of these factors, their present applications for treatment in oncology, and the possible new therapeutic options that the near future may bring.

The hierarchical structure of the haemopoietic tissue

The stem cells, characterized by their capacity to self-renew to maintain their own population through life (and which ultimately are the origin of all the lymphohaemopoietic cells in the adult), generate progenitor cells that become committed to one or other of the lymphohaemopoietic lineages; those cells in turn generate lineage-restricted cells that proliferate and give rise to a progeny that eventually mature into specialized cells. Modulation of mature cell production occurs usually at the later stages of differentiation, where demands for increased numbers of cells can be met by inducing extra cell divisions, shortening of cell cycle times and expanding areas of active cell production in the bone marrow, without necessarily affecting the stem cells or even the primitive progenitor cells (reviewed by Testa *et al.*, 1985; Lord & Testa, 1989). However, therapy for malignancy or accidental exposure to irradiation, where indiscriminate and perhaps extensive kill of stem cells takes place, would necessitate marked expansion of the surviving primitive cells, involving both self-renewal to regenerate their own population and differentiation to repopulate the haemopoietic tissue. Thus, knowledge of the regulation of haemopoietic cell proliferation at all levels of cell development has become an urgent necessity, especially in view of the aggressive treatments in oncology, where often the bone marrow is the tissue showing limiting toxicity.

The haemopoietic growth factors

The detection of the myeloid growth factors was due to their mandatory role in promoting the proliferation of progenitor cells *in vitro* resulting in the formation of clonal colonies. Those progenitor cells were called colony-forming cells (CFC) and the factors called colony-stimulating factors (CSFs) (reviewed by Metcalf, 1988). It later became apparent that the CSFs have multiple roles: they not only stimulate the proliferation of the CFC and of their progeny, but also enhance their survival *in vitro* and induce or increase the functional activity of the mature cells. The CSFs are grouped as a functional family of molecules: all are glycoproteins in their natural stage (although with the exception of erythropoietin non-glycosylated recombinant molecules are also functional) which act by binding to specific receptors, are able to influence the rate of production of other cytokines, to modulate their own receptors and those for the other CSFs, and may in some cases share common signalling pathways (Metcalf, 1988; Dexter *et al.*, 1990; Nicola, 1990). However, lack of homology within the group suggests that they are not derived from a common ancestral gene. In spite of this, there is considerable overlap in their target cells as demonstrated by the functional detection of receptors for many CSFs (maybe for all of them) in cells from purified marrow populations highly enriched for primitive CFC (Heyworth *et al.*, 1988). The high level of redundancy that this finding indicates may be explained by the fine adjustment of both cell proliferation and differentiation needed in a system that originates several cell lineages (Table 14.1).

Table 14.1. Haemopoietic growth factors

Growth factor	Major types of cells produced *in vitro*
IL-3	Neutrophilic granulocytes, monocytes–macrophages, eosinophils, basophils and mast cells; erythrocytes (if Epo also present); megakaryocytes
GM-CSF	Granulocytes, monocytes–macrophages, eosinophils, megakaryocytes, erythrocytes (with Epo)
G-CSF	Neutrophilic granulocytes, monocytes–macrophages (at high concentrations)
M-CSF	Macrophages, neutrophilic granulocytes (at high concentrations)
IL-5	Eosinophils
Epo	Erythrocytes

Epo, erythropoietin; G-CSF, granulocyte colony-stimulating factor; GM-CSF, granulocyte–macrophage colony-stimulating factor; IL, interleukin; M-CSF, macrophage colony-stimulating factor.

Regulation of proliferation and differentiation

There is a hierarchy in the CSFs with regard to their target cells (Fig. 14.1). Multi-CSF (also known as interleukin-3, or IL-3) can stimulate multi-potential cells and committed progenitor cells, and is able to induce the production of cells of all the myeloid lineages (Table 14.1). Granulocyte-macrophage (GM) CSF stimulates the development of progenitor cells, but only a proportion of multipotential cells, and induces the production of cells in most of the myeloid lineages, but not basophilic cells. The more

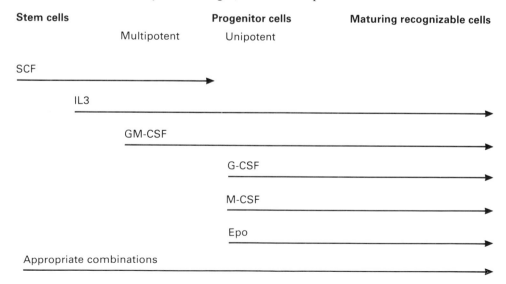

Fig. 14.1. Range of target cells for the haemopoietic growth factor.

lineage-specific factors, granulocyte (G) and macrophage (M) CSFs induce almost exclusively neutrophilic granulocytes or macrophages respectively (Metcalf, 1988). IL-5 induces only the formation of colonies of eosinophils (Sanderson, 1990). In highly purified populations of murine bone marrow cells enriched for primitive CFC, stimulation with IL-3 induces high numbers of colonies, but only a small proportion of the cells with the capacity to respond to IL-3 are able to respond to G- or M-CFC (Heyworth et al., 1988). Conversely, populations enriched for late CFC will respond preferentially to GM-CFC or to M-CFC (Cook et al., 1989; Baird et al., 1990). However, the pattern of response to combinations of growth factors is different. Synergistic or additive effects of growth factors have been described in several species including humans (McNiece et al., 1991). Primitive CFC which do not respond to M- or G-CSF when acting alone will proliferate if they are exposed to both factors, or to interleukin-1 (IL-1, not itself a CSF) plus M-CSF (Fig. 14.1). Potentiation between GM plus G-CSF can also be observed (Heyworth et al., 1988).

Another important point is that the balance of growth factors to which a cell is exposed will determine the lineage of differentiation. So, when factors are used in combination, not only the range of target cells is increased, but the cell lineages produced may be different. For example, the CFC which respond to IL-3 producing cells from several lineages, will produce only macrophages if stimulated with IL-1 plus M-CSF, or neutrophils and macrophages if stimulated with G plus M-CSF (Heyworth et al., 1988). This agrees with observations that the bone marrow is a highly structured tissue, with defined areas where different populations of stem and progenitor cells are found selectively, and where they may grow and differentiate preferentially in defined and different determinant microenvironments (Lord & Testa, 1989). These results also imply that the primitive haemopoietic cells may have receptors for many, if not all, of the growth factors from early stages of development, a concept relevant for the logical planning of clinical trials. These observations also indicate that the potential for differentiation is not a predetermined and intrinsic property of the primitive cells, but may be determined by the balance of factors present in the immediate cellular environment where not only the specific factors present but also their absolute and relative concentrations may be relevant (Testa & Dexter, 1990).

Effects on cell function

It is difficult to distinguish between the stimulation of proliferation and the induction of differentiation and function in maturing cells, as both processes occur concomitantly in the final cell divisions in the maturation sequence. However, it is now clear, from experiments done with cell lines (Heyworth et al., 1990; Metcalf, 1990) and with maturing cells (Gough &

Table 14.2. Effects of colony-stimulating factors on mature cells

Factor	Target cells	Effect
G-CSF	Neutrophils	↑ Antibody-dependent cell-mediated cytotoxicity ↑ Generation of superoxide anion ↑ Release of arachidonic acid in response to chemoattractants
GM-CSF	Neutrophils	↑ Priming of cells to activation by bacterial protein ↑ Antibody-dependent cell-mediated cytotoxicity ↑ Metabolic energy ↑ Phagocytosis (bacteria, parasites, yeast), inhibits migration ↑ Cell adhesiveness to endothelium ↑ Generation of superoxide ↑ Production of IL-1
	Monocytes	↑ Chemotaxis ↑ Release of prostaglandin E, plasminogen activator, interferons, tumour necrosis factor, M-CSF ↑ Cell adhesion

G-CSF, granulocyte colony-stimulating factor; GM-CSF, granulocyte–macrophage colony-stimulating factor; IL, interleukin; M-CSF, macrophage colony-stimulating factor.

Nicola, 1990), that several functions of the mature cells can be induced by growth factors (Table 14.2). Not all the CSFs are equally active in inducing cell function, with the more lineage-specific factors G- and M-CSF being most active in this respect. Also, the responses of a cell will not only depend on the particular factors to which it is exposed, but on their levels. For example, murine multipotential cell lines kept in high concentration of IL-3, self-reproduce but will not respond to G- or GM-CSF (Heyworth *et al.*, 1990), while low levels of IL-3 favour differentiation when acting together with G- or GM-CSF. Intermediate levels of IL-3 result in an equilibrium between self-renewal and differentiation. The mechanisms mediating these different effects are yet unknown. It is therefore reasonable to expect that sequential administration of IL-3, followed by GM- or G-CSF will potentiate the effect of the latter if IL-3 generates more target cells on which the other factors may act.

The cytokine network

A variety of cytokines, many of which were initially characterized by their actions on non-myeloid cells are known to stimulate directly or indirectly the development of several populations of haemopoietic cells (Table 14.3). One of the first characterized was IL-1, which as described above, may potentiate the effect of haemopoietic growth factors on primitive haemo-

Table 14.3. Main cytokines affecting the regulation of haemopoiesis

Cytokines	Target cells	Main effects in haemopoiesis
Stimulatory		
Il-1	Primitive multipotential cells	Potentiates effect of growth factors on colony formation
	Macrophages, endothelial cells	Increases cytokine production
IL-2	T cells	Cytokine production
IL-4	B, T mast cells, monocytes	Increases production of cytokines
	Progenitor cells	Potentiates the effect of growth factors on colony formation
IL-6	B, T cells, primitive multipotential cells	Potentiates the effect of growth factors on colony formation. Role in megakaryocyte development
Inhibitory		
TGF-β	Primitive multipotential cells, committed progenitors, maturing cells	Inhibits cycling of primitive and committed progenitors, down-modulates growth factor receptors
MIP-1α	Primitive multipotential cells Committed progenitors	Inhibits cycling May potentiate action of GM- and M-CSF

GM-CSF, granulocyte–macrophage colony-stimulating growth factor; IL, interleukin; M-CSF, macrophage colony-stimulating factor; MIP-1α, macrophage inflammatory protein-1α; TGF-β, transforming growth factor-beta.

poietic cells (Stanley *et al.*, 1986; Heyworth *et al.*, 1988; Iscove & Yan, 1990). Other cytokines, like IL-2 and IL-4 may act through activation of T or B cells which are then able to produce other cytokines and to initiate or modify cascade effects (Metcalf, 1988). IL-4 also has some effect potentiating colony formation induced by G-CSF and growth from committed erythroid progenitors when acting together with erythropoietin (Epo). However, it can also inhibit myeloid growth (Rennik *et al.*, 1987). IL-6 is a potent stimulus for the proliferation of primitive multipotential cells when acting together with IL-3 (Ikebuchi *et al.*, 1987) and also has a marked effect on megakaryocyte development (Quesenberry *et al.*, 1991).

The cytokines described previously have stimulatory effects on haemopoiesis. However, stable control of proliferating systems may require negative regulators to minimize cyclical variations in cell production. Although inhibitory factors (and in particular *specific* tissue inhibitors) are less well defined than the stimulators, several have been described, including prostaglandins, lactoferrins, interferons and tumour necrosis factor (Broxmeyer *et al.*, 1991). Two cytokines that share the capacity to prevent primitive multipotential cells into entering the cell cycle are transforming growth factor β (TGF-β) (Cheifetz *et al.*, 1987) and macrophage inflammatory protein-1α (MIP-1α). The former is a pleiotropic cytokine that inhibits the proliferation of multipotential haematopoietic progenitor cells both *in vitro* and *in vivo* (Migdalska *et al.*, 1991; Ruscetti *et al.*, 1991). This action is not cytotoxic, and is reversible, thus fulfilling the definition of a negative regulator. It is not, however, tissue specific: for example, inhibitory effects on cells of the intestinal epithelium are also seen (Migdalska *et al.*, 1991).

MIPs have been characterized as inflammation-mediators (Datavelis *et al.*, 1988). One molecule in this group, MIP-1α was identified by Graham *et al.* (1990) as the molecule originally described as a stem cell inhibitory factor (Lord *et al.*, 1976; Lord, 1988). Early experiments with partially purified preparations show that, although MIP-1α inhibited potential stem cells from entering into the S phase of the cell cycle, it did not affect the cycling status of committed progenitor cells (Tejero *et al.*, 1984). Indeed, it may enhance the proliferation of these progenitors when acting together with GM-CSF (Broxmeyer *et al.*, 1989). Although MIP-1α and TGF-β exert a similar effect on primitive murine haemopoietic cells, they do not appear to act through the same mechanism (Hampson *et al.*, 1989; Ruscetti *et al.*, 1991). The effect of MIP-1α can be detected after 4 h *in vitro* or *in vivo* treatment (B.I. Lord, personal communication) while TGF-β needs a considerably longer time: 5 days of *in vivo* treatment are required in mice before maximum numbers of quiescent cells are found (Migdalska *et al.*, 1991). These observations suggest that MIP-1α may exert its effects directly on primitive haemopoietic cells, a concept supported by the observation that highly purified populations of multipotential haemopoietic cells react to MIP-1α within the same time scale (B.I. Lord, personal communication). In contrast, the long time required by TGF-β may suggest indirect effects on the primitive cells (Migdalska *et al.*, 1991). The effects of TGF-β on haemopoiesis are multiple and complex: although it inhibits proliferation of primitive cells, it stimulates the development of progenitor cells responding to GM-CSF in both human and murine systems (Keller *et al.*, 1988; Hampson *et al.*, 1989; Ruscetti *et al.*, 1991), but has little or no effect on growth induced by G- or M-CSF.

Clinical applications of growth factors

Many haemopoietic growth factors are available in purified recombinant form, suitable for clinical use. Most are undergoing clinical trials at present, and two, Epo and G-CSF, have already been licenced for clinical use.

Effects on cell proliferation

The first clear indication for therapy was the use of erythropoietin to correct the anaemia of renal disease (mainly due to decreased production of Epo). This was proposed many years before the recombinant molecule became available for clinical use. At present, hundreds of patients have been treated with outstanding success, and Epo is now a clear indication for anaemic patients with renal pathology. Its prospective clinical use in oncology is related to correction of the anaemia due to cytotoxic treatment, and the possibility that platelet production may be increased by Epo administration, the latter based in experimental observations that Epo may increase the numbers of platelets in mice.

The obvious indication for the clinical use of the myeloid growth factors is to hasten haematopoietic recovery following chemotherapy, in order to minimize the period of cytopenia and thus reduce the risk of serious infection or haemorrhage and minimize the anaemia. The first aim, reducing the period of cytopenia, has now been achieved by the use of G- or GM-CSF, which produce respectively a selective rise of neutrophil production, or increases in neutrophils, monocytes and eosinophils (Bronchud et al., 1987; Gabrilove et al., 1988; Morstyn et al., 1988). These results make possible the intensification of chemotherapy, allowing the administration of increased drug dose or the completion of protocols in shorter periods of time (Bronchud et al., 1988). Another clinical situation in which acute regeneration of the haemopoietic tissue is accelerated is after allogeneic bone marrow transplantation, or after autologous bone marrow transplantation following intense chemotherapy (Brandt et al., 1988). Use of growth factors in these circumstances may shift the limiting toxicity from marrow tissue to endothelia.

Effects on differentiation and mature cell function

The induction of function in mature cells is one of the actions of the myeloid growth factors. In fact, the incidence of serious sepsis induced by chemotherapy may be markedly reduced when administration of growth factors follow such treatments (Bronchud et al., 1987). In myelodysplasia, long-term treatment with G-CSF resulted not only in higher neutrophil counts but also in decreased risk of bacterial infection (Negrin et al., 1990). However, this effect has not been observed in some trials.

The use of growth factors in myeloproliferative diseases such as myelodysplasia and acute myeloblastic leukaemia (AML), however, is not without risks. The imbalance between proliferation and differentiation

Table 14.4. *In vitro* responses of acute myeloblastic leukaemia (AML) cells to growth factors

Responses	Induced mainly by
Of the leukaemic colony-forming cells	
Colony formation	IL-3, GM-CSF, G-CSF, GM plus G-CSF
Improved survival	GM-CSF
Increased self-renewal	GM-CSF
Of the heterogeneous leukaemic cell population	
Stimulation of DNA synthesis	IL-3, GM-CSF, Epo (in erythroleukaemia)
Enhanced cell survival	IL-3, GM-CSF (M-CSF, Epo rarely)
Induction of differentiation	G-CSF, M-CSF

Epo, erythropoietin; G-CSF, granulocyte colony-stimulating factor; GM-CSF, granulocyte colony-stimulating factor; IL-3, interleukin-3; M-CSF, macrophage colony-stimulating factor.

characeristic of AML may be influenced by growth factors in a variety of ways (Table 14.4). However, the fact that, although clonal, the leukaemic cell population is heterogeneous, is reflected in the variety of growth patterns *in vitro*. A variable proportion of cells may proliferate to form colonies, and amongst those colony cells, a variable proportion may show self-reproduction capacity by forming new colonies upon replating, probably reflecting a hierarchy of cells at different stages of maturation (reviewed by Lowenberg *et al.*, 1990). Thus growth factors may stimulate the leukaemic process if cell proliferation is not accompanied by differentiation and maturation. In contrast, treatment with factors better able to induce differentiation, the more lineage-specific factors G- and M-CSF, may tilt the balance between proliferation and differentiation towards a possible control of the malignant process. However, as both myelodysplastic (preleukaemic) and leukaemic cells remain dependent on growth factors (Metcalf, 1988; Lowenberg *et al.*, 1990), the possibility of improving the leucocyte function remains a doubtful indication, except perhaps during life-threatening infections or in high-risk patients treated for relapse (Buchner *et al.*, 1990). However, other therapeutic approaches are possible: leukaemic cells recruited synchronously into cell division by the action of growth factors may then be the target of cell cycle-active therapy. If, at the same time, normal stem cells are protected by the use of MIP-1α or TGF-β, the goal of selective kill of leukaemic cells may be achieved. Observations that leukaemic cell lines are less sensitive than their normal equivalents to the action of these inhibitors (B.I. Lord, unpublished data; Keller *et al.*, 1988) support this concept.

   Prospective use of growth factors in AML is also complicated by the fact that in a proportion of patients, there is autocrine production of growth factors by leukaemic cells (reviewed by Metcalf, 1989; Lowenberg *et al.*, 1990; Testa & Dexter, 1990). More than one factor may be produced, and this complicates attempts at a logical approach to the use of factors in therapy, in view not only of the variability of the response of leukaemic cells (Table 14.4), but also of the effects of combinations of factors on cell development.

The stem cell population

It is unlikely that administration of the myeloid growth factors would exert a detectable influence on the stem cell population when correction of low numbers, for example in aplastic anaemia, is desired. Unfortunately, the mode of regulation of this population is less well known than that of the more mature progenitors (Fig. 14.1). Cytokines like IL-1 and IL-6 stimulate the growth of very primitive (stem?) cells *in vitro* when acting together with IL-3 (Ikebuchi *et al.*, 1987; Iscove & Yan, 1990). These factors promote their development, but whether they are also involved in stimulation of self-renewal is more difficult to ascertain. Polyclonal expansion of a severely depleted stem cell pool resulting from intense chemotherapy for malignancy may be desirable and may minimize the chance of development of secondary AML (a not inconsiderable risk after, for example, treatment for lymphoma). Long-lasting effects of chemotherapy on primitive haemopoietic cells are well recognized, and may be a target for therapy in the future (Testa & Gale, 1989).

A newly described factor, stem cell factor (SCF) has recently been identified and is available in recombinant form (reviewed by Witte, 1990). SCF is the ligand for the receptor encoded by the c-*kit* proto-oncogene, and is itself encoded in the S1 locus in mice. Mutations in this locus result in anaemia, but also in defects in primordial germ cells and melanocytes, indicating that SCF has a role to play in stem cell development not only in haemopoiesis, but also in other systems. *In vitro*, it synergizes with IL-1, IL-3, IL-6 and IL-7 (and also has some colony-stimulating activity on its own) to promote the development of haemopoietic lineages (McNiece *et al.*, 1991). Adminstered *in vivo* to mice it causes a modest increase in the numbers of neutrophils in blood, an effect potentiated by G-CSF. The numbers of multipotential cells in the spleen, and those migrating to the blood are also markedly increased, especially when SCF plus G-CSF are used (Molineux *et al.*, 1991). This migration of primitive cells into the blood stream has relevance in oncology, as these cells can be harvested for use in autologous transplantation.

Autologous transplants using peripheral blood stem cells

Transplantation of stem cells collected from peripheral blood is an attractive alternative to autologous bone marrow transplantation to rescue the haemopoietic tissue after ablative chemotherapy (reviewed by Henon *et al.*, 1991). However, engraftment may be unstable due to the lower capacity for marrow repopulation of the cells harvested from blood compared to those from the bone marrow (Micklem *et al.*, 1975). Nevertheless, the administration to mice of growth factors (G-CSF, GM-CSF, SCF, IL-3) alone or in combination, results not only in higher numbers of progenitor and stem cells in the blood, which may have an enhanced capacity (as a population) to reconsititute haemopoiesis in the long term (Molineux *et al.*, 1990). This may also be the case in humans, as we have observed an enhanced capacity to reconstitute haemopoiesis when peripheral blood cells collected after G-CSF administration (following treatment for lymphoma) are seeded *in vitro* on irradiated bone marrow stroma (Demuynck *et al.*, 1992). Available data show that the reinfusion of harvested blood cells in addition to bone marrow in autologous transplant results in accelerated regeneration (Gianni *et al.*, 1989). Although this accelerated recovery is likely to be due to the large number of committed progenitor cells found in the blood of patients treated with G- or GM-CSF, the mobilization of repopulating cells is likely to ensure the long-term grafting of reinfused circulating cells.

Evaluation of clinical data

The neutropenia following most chemotherapeutic regimes in oncology, and the concomitant risks of serious infections can now be ameliorated by the use of G- or GM-CSF (Table 14.5). Treatment results in shorter times with critically low numbers of neutrophils in blood and accelerated rate of recovery. The same is seen after bone marrow transplantation. Correction of anaemia, that may be serious after some treatments, is also achieved with Epo. However, stimulation of platelet production has not been achieved consistently, although modest responses have been observed in some cases after GM-CSF or IL-3. Trials adding Epo to combinations of factors, (IL-3 plus GM-CSF, IL-3 plus G) or IL-3 may give better results. Positive results will be of great clinical importance as the need for platelet transfusions is often the most serious critical manifestation of marrow toxicity in patients whose marrow recovery is assisted by growth factors. Phase I trials with IL-6 have started recently.

One bonus resulting from the administration of myeloid growth factors is the migration of stem and progenitor cells into the blood stream. Collection of peripheral blood cells for autologous transplant following chemotherapy is at present being performed in several centres. This offers practical advantages (like no need of general anaesthesia, or possibility of harvesting in patients who had received pelvic irradiation) when compared to a marrow harvest, and may in addition offer a cell population less

Table 14.5. Growth factors used in oncology

Aim	Factors
Present	
To accelerate regeneration of leucocytes following chemotherapy or bone marrow transplantation	G-CSF, GM-CSF
To allow dose intensification	G-CSF
To prevent or treat infection	G-CSF, GM-CSF, M-CSF
To treat anaemia	Epo
To promote migration of primitive cells into the blood (to harvest for autologous transplant)	G-CSF, GM-CSF
To improve cell production and cell function in myelodysplasia	G-CSF, GM-CSF, IL-3
Planned, or in early stages	
To stimulate thrombopoiesis	IL-6, combinations with IL-3, GM-CSF, Epo
To recruit AML cells synchronously into cell cycle	G-CSF, GM-CSF, IL-3
Possible	
To induce differentiation in AML	G-CSF, M-CSF
To normalize stem cell numbers	SCE, IL-6, IL-1

AML, acute myeloblastic leukaemia; Epo, erythropoietin; G-CSF, granulocyte colony-stimulating factor; GM-CSF, granulocyte–macrophage colony-stimulating factor; IL, interleukin; M-CSF, macrophage colony-stimulating factor; SCF, stem cell factor.

contaminated with malignant cells when there is metastatic disease. Our theoretical calculations indicate that in certain patients, about 500 ml of blood may contain enough primitive cells for a successful autologous transplant and thus the use of relatively small volumes of blood also minimizes the risk of contamination with malignant cells (Demuynck *et al.*, 1992). These studies also demonstrate that the cells harvested from blood after chemotherapy and G-CSF are, on a cell for cell basis, at least as good as bone marrow cells in repopulating irradiated bone marrow stroma *in vitro* (and presumably *in vivo*). The results also imply that the risk of late bone marrow failure after autologous transplantation may be much smaller than that reported in the literature after autologous transplants of circulating cells obtained without previous administration of growth factors.

The use of combinations of growth factors is also being investigated.

Table 14.6. Possible problems after administration of colony-stimulating factors (CSFs)

General
  Toxic granulation, vacuolization of granulocytes (G-CSF)
  ↑ Uric acid (G-CSF)
  Lower mobility of granulocytes (GM-CSF) (may be desirable in local infection)
  Hypertension (Epo)
  Leak capillary syndrome (GM-CSF)
  Bone pain (GM-CSF, G-CSF)

Dependent on the type of malignancy
  Presence of receptors in cells from a proportion of solid tumours
  (G-CSF, GM-CSF)
  Increase in blasts in myelodysplasia (IL-3, GM-CSF, G-CSF)
  Stimulation of leukaemic cells (IL-3, GM-CSF, G-CSF; Epo in erythroleukaemia)

Epo, erythropoietin; G-CSF, granulocyte colony–stimulating factor; GM-CSF, granulocyte–macrophage colony-stimulating factor; IL-3, interleukin-3.

This will allow a reduction in the dose of each factor, the tailoring of treatment protocols to specific needs and a better approximation to the way these factors act *in vivo*. It is important to point out, however, that while present data establish beyond doubt the usefulness of growth factors for treatment in oncology by allowing both better and faster recovery from treatment and dose-intensification, no data are yet available indicating longer remissions or higher numbers of patients cured.

Possible problems after administration of growth factors

The undesirable side effects of growth factors have in general been minor and tolerable (Table 14.6), the most serious being capillary leak syndrome observed after GM-CSF (which depended mainly on the i.v. route of administration, and which can be avoided by appropriate protocols), hypertension in the early Epo trials (also controllable by lowering the dose and adapting the schedules) and bone pain that may on occasion be serious.

The possible problems that the myeloid growth factors may cause in accelerating myelodysplasia or AML have already been mentioned. The factors to use if induction of differentiation is contemplated are probably G- or M-CSF or Epo in erythroleukaemia (reviewed in Testa & Dexter, 1990). However, the most logical use of growth factors in leukaemia at present appear to be for recruiting cells into cell cycle before using cycle-active agents.

Another potential problem concerns the finding of receptors for IL-3, GM- or G-CSF in various non-haemopoietic malignant cell lines including non-small cell lung carcinoma, osteosarcoma and carcinoma of the breast (reviewed by Hanauske, 1990). However, the majority of malignant cell lines do not apparently express receptors and it is not clear whether expression of receptors may lead to a proliferative response to growth factors. On the occasions in which such a response has been observed, the concentration of growth factors required to elicit such a response has usually been very high. Less data are available on receptors from samples of primary tumours, but in about 25–35% of a sample of 42 various solid tumours examined, tumour-colony growth *in vitro* was stimulated by GM-, G-CSF or IL-3 (Jaraschewitz *et al.*, 1990). We have detected receptors for G-CSF in two out of 12 breast carcinomas (J. Hampson, unpublished data). There are not, however, reports of tumour growth stimulation in the clinical trials; also, anecdotal evidence of stabilization or even partial regression (that might be attributable to macrophage activation) in phase I trials of GM-CSF have been recorded (Steward *et al.*, 1991). However, determination of receptors in tumour samples may be sensible in a minority of patients, especially since no data are yet available on the effects of combination of cytokines on primary tumour cells.

Future developments

The availability of relatively large amounts of recombinant material allows the planning of the structure/function analysis of growth factors, in studies which may have different aims. The identification of regions of the molecules which bind to the receptor is a first step for the design of analogues which may be administered orally, or of antagonists that may block the receptors. The development of antibodies (some are already available) may allow epitope mapping, and detection of the sequences responsible for the variety of actions exerted by each factor. Some data using mutagenesis for the analysis of the residues that are necessary for biological activity of murine GM-CSF are already available (Gough *et al.*, 1987), although it is not known whether the loss of biological activity is due to conformational changes in the three-dimensional structure of the molecule which interferes with its capacity to bind to its receptor. Work with synthetic proteins (Clark-Lewis *et al.*, 1988) and with constructs of human–murine hybrid factors (Kaushansky *et al.*, 1989) is also aimed at characterizing the sequences determining the interaction of GM-CSF with its receptor. It is also possible that, as has been shown for IL-1, natural receptor antagonists binding to specific growth factor receptors and blocking the response to them may be found (Ju *et al.*, 1991). In the case of IL-1 using site-specific mutagenesis the receptor antagonist was converted into a partial agonist, which showed some, but not all of the effects of IL-1 in different biological assays (Ju *et al.*, 1991). It is tempting to speculate that this is a possible way of manipulating the different effects of growth factors, selecting for example differentiation over proliferation, or vice versa.

New molecules may act at the level of receptor binding needing different proportions of receptor occupancy, or by influencing signal transduction proteins, or modifying subsequent events. Another possible area of manipulation is by recognizing receptor domains capable of interactions leading to receptor self-association, or binding to other proteins. For example, the G-CSF receptor has been implicated in some adhesion or recognition events occurring at the cell surface, in addition to the binding of G-CSF (Larson *et al.*, 1991), a suggestion of particular importance in view of the binding of growth factors to matrix proteins.

Differential splicing of the receptor may result in tissue-specific expression, an area yet largely unexplored which may have important implications in development. High levels of M-CSF are found in the placenta (Pollard *et al.*, 1987) and expression of the M-CSF receptor is found in choriocarcinoma cell lines (Rettenmier *et al.*, 1986), and in endometrial carcinomas (Kacinski *et al.*, 1990).

The experimental approaches summarized here will increase our fundamental knowledge of the haemopoietic system, but may also have some more immediate clinical implications. The finding of receptors for haemopoietic growth factors in non-haemopoietic cells makes more studies on malignant cells advisable. In some malignancies like endometrial carcinoma, measurement of circulating levels of growth factors produced by the tumour may aid diagnosis or management, especially if they act in an autocrine or paracrine fashion. If molecules with partial agonistic effects become available, it is tempting to envisage their use to suppress unwanted effects, especially of the pleiotropic molecules such as IL-1 or TGF, while conserving the desired therapeutic actions.

The more immediate future will bring trials with combinations of cytokines to manipulate selectively haemopoietic lineages and to add possible antitumour effects. Selective protection of normal cells by inhibitors (preferably tissue-specific) is also envisaged. Indeed, it is likely that the importance of inhibitors will become more apparent as our knowledge increases.

Finally, it is a matter of satisfaction to the numerous workers involved with molecules whose effects could be described some years ago as *in vitro* artefacts, to see their clinical applications within one generation.

References

Baird, M.C., Hendry, J.H. & Testa, N.G. (1990). Radiosensitivity increases with differentiation states of murine haemopoietic progenitor cells selected using enriched marrow subpopulations and recombinant growth factors. *Radiation Research* **123**, 292–298.

Brandt, S.J., Peters, W.P., Altnater, S.K., Kurtzberger, J., Borowitz, M.J., Jones, R.B., Shpall, E.J., Bast, R.C., Colleen, J.G. & Oette, D.H. (1988). Effect of recombinant human granulocyte-macrophage colony-stimulating factors on hematopoietic reconstitution after high-dose chemotherapy and autologous bone marrow transplation. *New England Journal of Medicine* **318**, 869–876.

Bronchud, M.H., Potter, M.R., Morgenstern, G., Blasco, M.J., Scarffe, J.H., Thatcher, N., Crowther, D., Souza, L.M., Alton, N.K., Testa, N.G. & Dexter, T.M. (1988). *In vitro* and *in vivo* analysis of the effects of recombinant human granulocyte colony-stimulating factors in patients. *British Journal of Cancer* **58**, 64–69.

Bronchud, M.H., Scharffe, J.H., Thatcher, N., Crowther, D., Souza, L.M., Alton, N.K., Testa, N.G. & Dexter, T.M. (1987). Phase I/II study of recombinant human granulocyte colony-stimulating factors in patients receiving intensive chemotherapy for small cell lung cancer. *British Journal of Cancer* **56**, 809–813.

Broxmeyer, H.E., Najman, A. & Dainiak, N. (1991). Summary of meeting on negative regulators of hematopoiesis. *Experimental Haematology* **19**, 149–152.

Broxmeyer, H.E., Sherry, B., Lu, L., Cooper, S., Carow, C., Wolpe, C.D. & Cerami, A. (1989). Myelopoietic enhancing effects of murine macrophage inflammatory proteins 1 and 2 on colony formation *in vitro* by murine and human bone marrow granulocyte/macrophage progenitor cells. *Journal of Experimental Medicine* **170**, 1583–1594.

Buchner, T., Hiddemann, W., Koenigsmann, H., Zuhlsdorf, M., Worman, B., Bockman, A., Agnion-Freine, E., Innig, G., Maschmeyer, G., Ludwig, W.D., Sauerland, C.M. & Schultz, G. (1990). Effect of chemotherapy followed by GM-CSF for acute leukaemias at higher age or after relapse. In Freund M., Liuk, H. & Welte, K. *Cytokines in Hemopoiesis, Oncology and AIDS*, pp. 387–401. Springer-Verlag, Berlin.

Cheifetz, S., Weatherbee, J.A., Tsang, M.L.S., Anderson, J.K., Mole, J.E., Lucas, R. & Massagué, J. (1987). The transforming growth factor-beta system, a complex pattern of cross-reactive ligands and receptors. *Cell* **48**, 409–415.

Clark-Lewis, I., Lopez, A.F., To, L.B., Vadas, M.A., Schrader, J.W., Hood, L.E. & Kent, S.B.H. (1988). Structure–function studies of human granulocyte-macrophage colony-stimulating factor. *Journal of Immunology* **141**, 881–889.

Cook, N., Dexter, T.M., Lord, B.I., Cragoe, E.J. & Whetton, A.D. (1989). Identification of a common signal associated with cellular proliferation stimulated by 4 haemopoietic growth factors in a highly enriched population of granulocyte-macrophage colony-forming cells. *European Journal of the Molecular Biology Organisation* **8**, 2967–2974.

Datavelis, G., Tekamp-Olson, P., Wolpe, S.D., Hermsen, K., Luedbe, C., Gallegos, C., Coit, D., Merryweather, J. & Cerami, A. (1988). Cloning and characterisation of a cDNA for murine macrophage inflammatory (MIP): a novel monokine with inflammatory and chemokinetic properties. *Journal of Experimental Medicine* **167**, 1939–1944.

Demuynck, H., Pettengell, R., de Campos, E., Dexter, T.M. & Testa, N.G. (1992). The capacity of peripheral blood stem cells mobilised with chemotherapy plus G CSF to repopulate irradiated marrow stroma *in vitro* is similar to that of bone marrow. *European Journal of Cancer*, **28**, 381–386.

Dexter, T.M., Garland, J. & Testa, N.G. (eds) (1990). *Colony Stimulating Factors: Molecular and Cellular Biology*. Marcel Dekker, New York.

Gabrilove, J.L., Jakubowski, A., Scher, H., Stenberg, C., Wong, G., Grous, J., Yagosa, A., Fain, K., Moore, M.A.S., Clarkson, B., Oettgen, H.F., Alton, K., Welte, K. & Souza, L. (1988). Effect of granulocyte colony-stimulating factor on neutropenia and associated morbidity due to chemotherapy for transitional-cell carcinoma of the urothelium. *New England Journal of Medicine* **318**, 1414–1422.

Gianni, A.M., Sierra, S., Bregni, M., Tarella, C., Stern, A.C., Pilem, A. & Bonadona, G. (1989). Granulocyte-macrophage colony stimulating factor to harvest circulating hemopoietic stem cells for autotransplantation. *Lancet* **i**, 580–585.

Gough, N.M. & Nicola, N. (1990). Granulocyte-macrophage colony stimulating factor. In Dexter, T.M., Garland, J.M. & Testa N.G. (eds) *Colony Stimulating Factors: Molecular and Cellular Biology*, pp. 231–256. Marcel Dekker, New York.

Gough, N.M., Grail, D., Gearing, D.P. & Metcalf, D. (1987). Mutagenesis of murine granulocyte/macrophage colony stimulating factor reveals critical residues near the N terminus. *European Journal of Biochemistry* **169**, 353–358.

Graham, G.J., Wright, E.G., Hewick, R., Wolpe, S.D., Wilkie, N.M., Donaldson, D., Lorimore, S. & Pragnell, I.B. (1990). Identification and characterisation of an inhibitor of haemopoiesis stem cell proliferation. *Nature* **344**, 442–444.

Hampson, J., Ponting, I.L.O., Cook, N., Vodinelich, L., Redmonds, S., Roberts, A.B. & Dexter, T.M. (1989). The effect of TGFβ on haemopoietic cells. *Growth Factors* **1**, 193–202.

Hanauske, A.R. (1990). Target cell specificity of hematopoietic growth factors. In Freund, M., Liuk, H. & Welte, K. *Cytokines in Hemopoiesis, Oncology and AIDS*, pp. 162–171. Springer-Verlag, Berlin.

Henon, P.R., Butturini, A. & Gale, R.P. (1991). Blood-derived haematopoietic cell transplants: blood to blood? *Lancet* **337**, 961–963.

Heyworth, C.M., Dexter, T.M., Kan, O. & Whetton, A.D. (1990). The role of hemopoietic growth factors in self-renewal and differentiation of IL-3 dependent multipotential stem cells. *Growth Factors* **2**, 197–211.

Heyworth, C.M., Ponting, I.L.O. & Dexter, T.M. (1988). The response of haemopoietic cells to growth factors: developmental implications of synergistic interactions. *Journal of Cell Science* **91**, 239–247.

Ikebuchi, K., Wong, G.G., Clark, S.C., Ihle, J.N. Hirai, Y. & Ogawa, M. (1987). Interleukin 6 enhancement of interleukin 3-dependent proliferation of multipotential haemopoietic progenitors. *Proceedings of the National Academy of Sciences USA* **84**, 9035–9039.

Iscove, N.N. & Yan, X.Q. (1990). Precursors (pre-CFC-multi) of multilineage hemopoietic colony forming cells quantitated *in vitro*. *Journal of Immunology* **145**, 190–195.

Jaraschewitz, M., Trijssenaar, J., Freund, M., Neukam, D., Krumwieh, D., Meyer, H.J., Poliwoda, H. & Hanauske, A.R. (1990). Effects of recombinant cytokines on clonogenic cells from primary human tumors. In Freund, M., Liuk, H. & Welte, K. *Cytokines in Hemopoiesis, Oncology and AIDS*, pp. 189–195. Springer-Verlag, Berlin.

Ju, G., Labriola-Tompkins, E., Campen, C.A., Benjamin, W.R., Karas, J., Plocinski, J., Biondis, D., Kaffka, K.L., Kilian, P.L., Eisenberg, S.P. & Evans, R.J. (1991). Conversion of the interleukin 1 receptor agonist into an agonist by site-specific mutagenesis. *Proceedings of the National Academy of Sciences USA* **88**, 2658–2662.

Kacinski, B.M., Setsuko, K., Chambers, M.D., Stanley, E.R., Carter, D., Tseng, P., Scata, K.A., Chang, D.H.Y., Pirro, M.H., Nguyen, J.T., Ariza, A., Rohrschneider, L.R. & Rothwell, V.M. (1990). The cytokine CSF1 (M-CSF) expressed by endometrial carcinomas *in vivo* and *in vitro* may also be a circulating tumour marker of neoplastic disease activity in endometrial carcinoma patients. *International Journal of Radiation Oncology, Biology and Physics* **19**, 619–626.

Kaushansky, K., Shoemaker, S.G., Alfaro, S. & Brown, C. (1989). Hematopoietic activity of granulocyte-macrophase colony-stimulating factor is dependent upon two distinct regions of the molecule. Functional analysis based upon the activities of interspecies hybrid growth factors. *Proceedings of the National Academy of Sciences USA* **86**, 1213–1217.

Keller, J.R., Sing, G.K., Ellingsworth, L.R. & Ruscetti, F.W. (1988). Transforming growth factor beta: possible roles in the regulation of normal and leukemic hematopoietic cell growth. *Journal of Cellular Biochemistry* **39**, 175–184.

Larson, A., Davis, T., Curtis, B.M., Gimpel, S., Sims, J.E., Cosman, D., Park, L., Sorensen, E., March, C.J. & Smith, C.A. (1991). Expression cloning of a human granulocyte colony stimulating factor receptor: a structural mosaic of hematopoietin receptor, immunoglobulin and fibronectin domains. *Journal of Experimental Medicine* **172**, 1559–1570.

Lord, B.I. (1988). Feedback regulators in normal and tumour tissues. In Lord, B.I. & Dexter, T.M. (eds) *Stem Cells*, pp. 231–242. *Journal of Cell Science* (Suppl. 10).

Lord, B.I. & Testa, N.G. (1989). The hemopoietic system: structure and regulation. In Testa, N.G. & Gale, R.P. (eds) *Haematopoiesis: Long-term Effects of Chemotherapy and Radiation*, pp. 1–26. Marcel Dekker, New York.

Lord, B.I., Mori, K.J., Wright, E.G. & Lajtha, L.G. (1976). An inhibitor of stem cell proliferation in normal bone marrow. *British Journal of Haematology* **34**, 441–445.

Lowenberg, B., Delwel, R. & Tuow, I. (1990). Hematopoietic growth factors and progenitor cells in human acute leukemia. In Dexter, T.M., Garland, J. & Testa, N.G. (eds) *Colony Stimulating Factors: Molecular and Cellular Biology*, pp. 277–296. Marcel Dekker, New York.

McNiece, I.K., Langley, K.E. & Zsebo, K.M. (1991). Recombinant human stem cell factor synergises with GM-CSF, G-CSF, IL-3 and Epo to stimulate human progenitor cells of the myeloid and erythroid lineages. *Experimental Haematology* **19**, 226–231.

Metcalf, D. (1988). *The Molecular Control of Blood Cells*. Harvard University Press, Cambridge, Massachusetts.

Metcalf, D. (1989). The roles of stem cell renewal and autocrine growth factor production in the biology of myeloid lineages. *Cancer Research* **49**, 2305–2311.

Metcalf, D. (1990) Colony stimulating factors: past and future. In Freund, M., Liuk, H. & Welte, K. (eds) *Cytokines in Hemopoiesis, Oncology and AIDS*, pp. 3–7. Springer-Verlag, Berlin.

Micklem, H.S., Anderson, N. & Ross, E. (1975). Limited potential of circulating hemopoietic stem cells. *Nature* **256**, 41–43.

Migdalska, A., Molineux, G., Demuynck, H., Evans, G.S., Ruscetti, F. & Dexter, T.M. (1991). Growth inhibitory effects of transforming growth factor-β1 *in vivo*. *Growth Factors* **4**, 239–245.

Molineux, G. Migdalska, A., Szmitkowski, M., Zsebo, K. & Dexter, T.M. (1991). The effects upon haemopoiesis of recombinant stem cell factor (ligand for c-*kit*) administered *in vivo* to mice either alone or in combination with G-CSF. *Blood* **78**, 961–966.

Molineux, G., Pojda, Z., Hampson, I., Lord, B.I. & Dexter, T.M. (1990). Transplantation potential of peripheral blood stem cells induced by granulocyte colony stimulating factor. *Blood* **76**, 860–866.

Morstyn, G., Souza, L.M., Keech, J., Sheridan, W., Campbell, L., Alton, N.K., Green, M., Metcalf, D. & Fox, R. (1988). Effect of granulocyte colony-stimulating factor on neutropenia induced by cytotoxic chemotherapy. *Lancet* **i**, 667–672.

Negrin, R.S., Haeuber, D.H., Nagler, A., Kobayashi, Y., Sklar, J., Donlon, T., Vincent, M. & Greenberg, P.L. (1990). Maintenance treatment of patients with myelodysplastic syndromes using recombinant granulocyte colony-stimulating factor. *Blood* **76**, 36–43.

Nicola, N.A. (1990). Granulocyte colony stimulating factor. In Dexter, T.M., Garland J. & Testa, N.G. (eds) *Colony Stimulating Factors: Molecular and Cellular Biology*, pp. 77–109. Marcel Dekker, New York.

Pollard, J.W., Bartocci, A., Arceci, R., Orlovsky, A., Ladner, M.B. & Stanley, E.R. (1987). Apparent role of the macrophage growth factor CSF1 in placental development. *Nature* **330**, 484–486.

Quesenberry, P.J., McGrath, H.E., Williams, M.E., Robinson, B.E., Deacon, D.H., Clark, S., Urdal, D. & McNiece, I.K. (1991) Multifactor stimulation of megakaryocytopoiesis: effects of interleukin 6. *Experimental Hematology* **19**, 35–41.

Rennick, D., Jang, G., Muller-Sieberg, C., Smith, C., Arai, N., Takabe, Y. & Gemmel, L. (1987). IL-4 (B-cell stimulatory factor 1) can enhance or antagonise the factor-dependent growth of hemopoietic progenitor cells. *Proceedings of the National Academy of Sciences USA* **84**, 6889–6893.

Rettenmier, C.W., Sacca, R., Turmman, W.L., Roussel, M.F., Holt, J.T., Nienhuis, A.W., Stanley, E.R. & Sherr, C.J. (1986). Expression of the human C-FMS protooncogene product (colony stimulating factor 1-receptor) on peripheral blood mononuclear cells and choriocarcinoma cell lines. *Journal of Clinical Investigation* **77**, 1740–1746.

Ruscetti, F.W., Dubois, C., Falk, L.A., Jacobsen, S.E., Sing, G., Longo, D.L., Wiltrout, R.H. & Keller, J.R. (1991). *In vivo* and *in vitro* effects of TGF-β1 on normal and neoplastic haemopoiesis. In Bock, G.R. & Marsh, J. (eds) *Clinical Applications of TGF-β*, pp. 212–227. John Wiley, Chichester.

Sanderson, C.J. (1990). Eosinophil differentiation factor (Interleukin 5). In Dexter, T.M., Garland, J.M. & Testa, N.G. (eds) *Colony Stimulating Factors: Molecular and Cellular Biology*, pp. 231–256. Marcel Dekker, New York.

Stanley, E.R., Bartolin, A., Patinkin, D., Rosendaal, M. & Bradley, T.R. (1986). Regulation of very primitive multipotential haemopoietic cells by haemopoietin-1. *Cell* **45**, 667–674.

Steward, W.P., Bronchud, M.H., Scarffe, J.H., Howell, A., Thatcher, N., Dirix, L.Y., Testa, N.G., Dexter, T.M. & Crowther, D. (1991). Hemopoietic colony stimulating factors in patients receiving radiotherapy. In Peters, W.P. (ed.) *Hematopoietic Growth Factors*. Futura Press, New York.

Tejero, C., Testa, N.G. & Lord, B.I. (1984). The cellular specificity of haemopoietic stem cell proliferation regulators. *British Journal of Cancer* **50**, 335–341.

Testa, N.G. & Dexter, T.M. (1990). Haemopoietic growth factors and haematological malignancies. *Clinical Endocrinology and Metabolism* **4**, 177–189.

Testa, N.G. & Gale, R.P. (eds) (1989). *Hematopoiesis: Long-term Effects of Chemotherapy and Radiation*. Marcel Dekker, New York.

Testa, N.G., Hendry, J. & Molineux, G. (1985). Long-term bone marrow damage in experimental systems and in patients after radiation or chemotherapy. *Anticancer Research* **5**, 101–110.

Witte, O.N. (1990) Steel locus defines new multipotent growth factor. *Cell* **63**, 5–6.

Index